# Endovascular and Hybrid Management of the Thoracic Aorta

# Endovascular and Hybrid Management of the Thoracic Aorta

## A Case-based Approach

by

### Edward B. Diethrich, MD
Arizona Heart Institute & Hospital
Phoenix, AZ, USA

### Venkatesh G. Ramaiah, MD
Arizona Heart Institute
Phoenix, AZ, USA

### Jacques Kpodonu, MD
Bluhm Cardiovascular Institute
Division of Cardiac Surgery
Northwestern Memorial Hospital
Chicago, IL, USA

### Julio A. Rodriguez-Lopez, MD
Arizona Heart Institute
Phoenix, AZ, USA

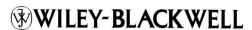

WILEY-BLACKWELL

A John Wiley & Sons, Ltd., Publication

This edition first published 2008, © 2008 by Blackwell Publishing Ltd

Blackwell Publishing was acquired by John Wiley & Sons in February 2007. Blackwell's publishing program has been merged with Wiley's global Scientific, Technical and Medical business to form Wiley-Blackwell.

*Registered office:* John Wiley & Sons Ltd, The Atrium, Southern Gate, Chichester, West Sussex, PO19 8SQ, UK

*Editorial offices:* 9600 Garsington Road, Oxford, OX4 2DQ, UK
　　　　　　　　The Atrium, Southern Gate, Chichester, West Sussex, PO19 8SQ, UK
　　　　　　　　111 River Street, Hoboken, NJ 07030-5774, USA

For details of our global editorial offices, for customer services and for information about how to apply for permission to reuse the copyright material in this book please see our website at www.wiley.com/wiley-blackwell

**Library of Congress Cataloguing-in-Publication Data**

Endovascular and hybrid management of the thoracic aorta / by Edward B. Diethrich . . . [et al.].
　　　p.　;　cm.
　　Includes bibliographical references and index.
　　ISBN 978-1-4051-7535-7 (alk. paper)
　　1. Aorta–Surgery.　2. Thoracic arteries–Surgery.　3. Endarterectomy.　I. Diethrich,
　　Edward B., 1935–
　　[DNLM: 1. Aorta, Thoracic–surgery–Case Reports.　2. Aortic Diseases–surgery–Case Reports.
　　3. Vascular Surgical Procedures–methods–Case Reports.　WG 410 E557 2008]
　　RD598.65.E53 2008
　　617.4′13–dc22　　　　　　　　　　　　　　　　　　　　　　　　　　　　2008010765

ISBN: 9781405175357

A catalogue record for this book is available from the British Library.

Set in 9.5/12pt Minion by Aptara Inc., New Delhi, India
Printed in Singapore by COS Printers Pte Ltd

1　2008

# Contents

# Preface

When the Arizona Heart Institute's endovascular program was initiated well over two decades ago, no one could have envisioned its current acceptance by all disciplines given its checkered beginning, with skepticism and resistance to move from traditional therapies. Today, radiologists, vascular surgeons, vascular medicine specialists, cardiologists, and more recently cardiovascular surgeons have all recognized the enormous benefits of the endovascular approach to cardiovascular disease. Interventional technology has been proven to shorten hospitalization, reduce morbidity and mortality, speed recovery, and hasten return to normal life. Clinical investigations have shown these procedures to be favorable over open surgical techniques in most situations.

Despite these findings and the worldwide movement toward less invasive techniques, our training and educational programs have lagged behind the technology explosion. The core curricula in our current training residencies and fellowships in the majority of cases were not designed to easily accommodate the rapid evolution in endovascular technology. Hence, the need to revamp and expand our educational process to assure that current and future endovascular interventionalists will have adequate fundamental knowledge and skill sets.

Didactic lectures, simulations, hands-on training, and observation of the experts are all essential in this training paradigm. Importantly, learning by case example has been a hallmark in cardiovascular surgery training for decades. To assure an optimum result, the pathophysiology and anatomy of the disease process must be appreciated. Modern diagnostic tools, particularly new imaging modalities, must be understood and applied appropriately. Interventionalists today must have not only an acquaintance with the growing variety of endovascular techniques, but also a working knowledge of their efficacy. In an effort to address these needs, we have called upon our vast endovascular experience to assemble this textbook of thoracic endovascular interventions. It is important to note that most cases in this textbook were performed under an investigational protocol with Institutional Board Review oversight. We earnestly believe that informed patients who adhere to a follow-up protocol will generate the much-needed data that can help us address the pressing questions in this blossoming field.

We recognize that certain limitations exist currently regarding thoracic endografting techniques and their application to thoracic aortic pathologies. There is every indication, however, that most thoracic aortic pathologies will be treated with these less invasive procedures in the future, and so this textbook should prove useful as this segment of the field expands. Our particular institution has been fortunate enough to be at the forefront of this technological revolution.

With this in mind, the textbook has been organized to begin with the currently accepted procedures and progress to those techniques for which proof of principle exists. It then proceeds to evolving areas of treatment in which further understanding and investigation are needed. The final chapters address the challenges of the ascending aortic arch, with recommendations for future endovascular technology. There is no substitute for learning from experience. It is our hope that endovascular management of the thoracic aorta with its case study approach will provide a useful tool for practitioners as they plan and execute treatment of patients with these thoracic aortic pathologies.

Edward B. Diethrich, MD
Venkatesh G. Ramaiah, MD
Jacques Kpodonu, MD
Julio A. Rodriguez-Lopez, MD

# Foreword

How do you teach new procedures involving brand-new, still evolving technologies to a diverse group of physicians? Dr Ted Diethrich and colleagues from the Arizona Heart Institute have successfully addressed this daunting problem in their comprehensive new textbook. Endovascular and hybrid management of thoracic aortic diseases have been rapidly advancing and these practitioners are clearly at the leading edge of this revolution. The authors use an interesting "case based" approach of approximately 50 cases that are very well illustrated with appropriate references. They range from relatively common problems, such as thoracic aortic aneurysms and chronic Type B aortic dissections, to more rare and challenging problems such as ascending aortic pseudoaneurysms. The authors make use of their outstanding background and clinical experience with the surgical treatment of aortic pathology add in new advanced imaging techniques such as 64-slice CT imaging and intravascular ultrasound, and show how endovascular and hybrid approaches can be applied to a variety of pathological conditions. The text itself is very well written and well illustrated and for those learning about this new field or those already with some experience, this is an important reference.

The publication is timely because of the rapid advancement and expansion of these approaches outside of traditional academic medical centers to a variety of clinical practices. The text should be of great interest to cardiovascular surgeons, cardiologists, vascular medicine specialists, and interventional radiologists. Dr Diethrich and his colleagues have done a tremendous service dedicating the time and effort into amassing this clinical experience and disseminating it through the medical community at this early phase using this new technology.

Patrick M. McCarthy, MD
Heller-Sacks Professor of Surgery
Chief of Cardiothoracic Surgery and Co-director
Bluhm Cardiovascular Institute
at Northwestern Memorial Hospital
Chicago, IL

# Foreword

The authors have presented a comprehensive, state-of-the-art review of the current status of thoracic aortic endografting. The format of the book is based on case reviews including indications for the procedure, concise discussions of therapeutical alternatives, and methods used during the procedure. The book covers the entire spectrum of thoracic pathologies and therapeutic options from fully endovascular repairs to the hybrid inventions combining endovascular approaches and conventional vascular surgical techniques. The text has excellent illustrations demonstrating not only the pathology being addressed, but appropriately selected procedural and post-intervention studies that illustrate not only the techniques and outcomes but also appropriate imaging modalities and imaging quality that is required for optimal outcomes.

The text contains approximately 50 case discussions. The text begins with a review of the approved Gore TAG device and the Food and Drug Administration–approved indications. This device is used in the majority of patients treated in the case studies. Other devices are described as they were used as part of ongoing clinical trials that were not completed at the time of the publication. The Gore TAG chapter outlines the approved indications and follow-up data regarding the outcomes that are available. The subsequent chapters each deal with a major thoracic pathology or with techniques that can be used to extend the utility of thoracic endoluminal devices, such as extending the proximal and distal landing zones and describing utility of hybrid techniques. There is also sections dealing with complications and addressing associated additional pathologies including ascending aortic and transverse thoracic arch pathologies. The text fully addresses all the approved current indications, developing therapies, and future indications for application of thoracic endografts.

The text is written with a style and excellence that characterizes the Arizona Heart Institute. It contains well-illustrated cases and discussions as well as easily assimilated and exceptionally well-illustrated teaching modules. The comprehensive nature of the pathologies and endovascular techniques displayed can only be exhibited in this manner by the team at Arizona Heart Institute lead by Dr Ted Diethrich.

The development of thoracic endograft technologies promises to be a major advance in medical therapy significantly reducing patient morbidity and mortality in the critical spectrum of pathologies, including aneurysm, dissections, and traumatic lesions. The publication is an exceptionally well-written and timely endeavor and provides an easily assimilated, comprehensive view of the subject for all who are interested in this rapidly developing field.

Rodney A. White, MD
Chief of Vascular Surgery
Harbor-UCLA Medical Center
Torrance, California

# Acknowledgments

The authors would like to recognize the following people whose contributions to this project made this book possible: Dr John A. Sutherland, Director of Imaging Services, Arizona Heart Institute; and James P. Williams, Research Coordinator, Arizona Heart Institute.

# Current status of thoracic endografting

## Gore TAG thoracic endoprosthesis

The Gore Excluder thoracic endoprosthesis (W.L. Gore & Associates, Flagstaff, AZ) was the first thoracic endograft to enter clinical trials in the United States in 1998 with a feasibility trial. This was followed by the pivotal study in 1999. The Gore TAG excluder device gained Food and Drug Administration (FDA) approval in March 2005 for the commercial use for the treatment of thoracic aortic aneurysms (Figure 1).

## Device design

The TAG endoprosthesis is a symmetrical expanded polytetrafluoroethylene (ePTFE) tube reinforced with ePTFE/FEP (fluorinated ethylene propylene) film and an external nickel–titanium (nitinol) self-expanding stent along the entire surface of the graft (Figure 2). The stent is attached to the graft with ePTFE/FEP bonding tape. A circumferential PTFE sealing cuff is located on the external surface of the endograft at the base of each flared, scalloped end. Flares are designed to help with conforming to tortuous anatomy. Each cuff is circumferentially attached on one edge with FEP, thus allowing the other end to remain free to enhance sealing of the endoprosthesis to the aortic wall and help eliminate endoleaks.

The original TAG device graft material was constructed from two ePTFE layers with two longitudinal wires for support during deployment. The modified TAG device is constructed from three ePTFE layers. The additional layer, similar to that incorporated into the excluder bifurcated endoprosthesis, is sandwiched between the two original layers and provides support that was formerly provided by the deployment wires. At the base of the flares are two radiopaque gold bands, which serve as a guide during implantation and in follow-up. The devices are available in 26–40 mm diameters that accommodate aortic diameters between 23 and 37 mm and require 20-F (20-French) through 24-F introducer sheaths, depending on the device size. Recently a 45-mm-diameter device has been introduced under investigational device protocol.

Deployment of the TAG device is unique. A sleeve made of ePTFE/FEP film is used to constrain the endograft. A deployment knob is located at the control end of the delivery catheter and has a deployment line that runs the entire length of the catheter connecting it to the sleeve. Turning and pulling the deployment knob removes the deployment line from the endograft, thereby deploying it. The device is deployed rapidly from the middle of the endograft toward both ends of the prosthesis. The device is then secured in position with a specially designed trilobed balloon, which allows continuous blood flow during inflation.

## Feasibility study

The first trial to be conducted in the United States was the feasibility study to establish preliminary device safety data. This study was performed at two sites in the United States and enrolled a total of 28 patients between 1998 and 1999. The 30-day mortality rate was 3.6% ($n = 1$). At 1 year, the mortality rate was 21% without any paraplegia or stroke. Renal failure and myocardial infarction were noted in 1 patient each (3.6%). Through a 5-year follow-up period, two additional adverse events were reported between 2 and 5 years. All-cause mortality at 5 years was 25%. Endoleaks were noted at

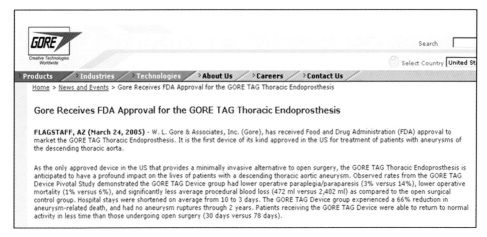

**Figure 1**  Federal drug administration approves use of thoracic endoluminal graft for treatment of thoracic aneurysms.

any time in 21% of the patients, and aneurysm sac growth was noted in 18%. Stent fractures were noted in 32%. There was one conversion and there were two reinterventions over time to place additional devices. No aneurysm ruptures, device migration, extrusion, erosion, lumen obstruction, or branch vessel occlusions were reported.

Once device safety was demonstrated with the feasibility study, the pivotal phase II trial was undertaken.

## Pivotal (phase II) trial

### Objectives and hypotheses

The objectives were to determine the safety and efficacy of the TAG endoprosthesis for the treatment of descending thoracic aneurysm as compared with open surgical repair controls. The primary safety hypothesis was that the percentage of subjects with one or more major adverse events (MAEs) through 1 year after treatment would be lower in the TAG group as compared with the surgical control group. The primary efficacy hypothesis was that freedom from any major device-related events through 1 year

of follow-up for the TAG device group would be better than 80%. A predefined point estimate of 80% for the endovascular group was considered to be a reasonable efficacy outcome, because the device was expected to show a considerable improvement in safety profile. The efficacy for the surgical procedure was assumed to be 100%. The secondary hypotheses were that the procedural blood loss, intensive care unit (ICU) and hospital stay, and convalescence to normal activities would be lower in the TAG device group as compared with the surgical control group. The primary efficacy end point of this pivotal study was the percentage of subjects who were free from major device-related events through 1 year of follow-up for the TAG device group.

### Study design

This study was a prospective, nonrandomized, controlled multicenter trial. The study enrolled 140 study patients and 94 control subjects between September 1999 and May 2001 through 17 clinical sites in the United States. The control group consisted of 44 patients acquired prospectively during the study and 50 historical patients acquired by

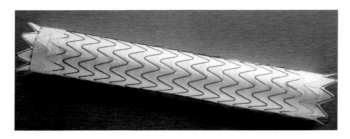

**Figure 2**  Gore TAG thoracic endoprosthesis.

**Table 1** Inclusion criteria.

| Criterion | Gore TAG |
| --- | --- |
| Age (yr) | >21 |
| Women | Must be infertile |
| Open surgical candidate | Yes |
| Neck length | Minimal 2 cm proximal and distal |
| Aneurysm | Fusiform descending thoracic aorta at least twice the size of normal thoracic aorta; saccular |
| Penetrating ulcer | No |
| Proximal landing zone location | 20 mm distal to left common carotid artery |
| Distal landing zone location | 20 mm proximal to celiac axis |
| Landing zone diameter (mm) | 23–37 |

selecting the most recent surgical patients in reverse chronological order. Inclusion and exclusion criteria are detailed in Tables 1 and 2.

## Follow-up

All patients are to be followed for 5 years. Computed tomography (CT) scans, plain radiographs, and

**Table 2** Exclusion criteria.

| Criterion | Gore TAG |
| --- | --- |
| Creatinine (mg/dL) | >2.0 |
| Unstable rupture | Yes |
| Mycotic aneurysm | Yes |
| Connective tissue disease | Yes |
| Significant landing zone thrombus | Yes |
| Previous descending aortic surgery or endovascular repair of descending thoracic aneurysm or abdominal aortic aneurysm | N/A |
| Aortic dissection | Yes |
| Coagulopathy | Yes |
| Myocardial infarction/cerebrovascular accident | <6 wk |
| Major operation within 30 days | Yes |
| Participation in another investigational study | <1 yr |

N/A, not applicable.

physical examinations were obtained at 1-month, 6-month, and 12-month intervals and yearly thereafter. A 3-month visit with a CT scan was conducted for patients with early endoleaks. A core laboratory reviewed all imaging studies. Clinical data were reported by individual centers and monitored by sponsor representatives. Major adverse effects were adjudicated by the Clinical Events Committee and defined as clinical events that required therapy or that resulted in an unintended increase in the level of care, prolonged hospitalization, permanent adversity, or death [5]. Minor adverse events were those that did not require any therapy or those with no consequences.

## Results of the pivotal study

### Clinical materials

The TAG group and the surgical group were very similar in all major demographic and clinical variables (Table 3). The average age of the patients was 71 years in the TAG group and 68 years in the control group. Men accounted for 58% of the patients in the TAG group and 51% in the control group.

Baseline aortic morphology was also well matched between the groups, except for the smaller diameter of the proximal and distal necks in the TAG device group, which was expected because of the requirements for sealing. Baseline comorbidities were also quite similar between the TAG device group and the control group (Table 4). Although coronary artery disease seemed to be more prevalent among the TAG group, this difference was not significant. Symptomatic aneurysms, however, were significantly more prevalent in the control group than in the TAG group. The risk classifications performed on the basis of the standard American

**Table 3** Patient demographics.

| Variable | TAG group | Surgical control |
| --- | --- | --- |
| Male (%) | 57 | 51 |
| Age (yr) | 71 | 68 |
| Ethnicity (%) | | |
| White | 87 | 86 |
| Black | 8 | 10 |
| Other | 5 | 4 |
| Height (cm) | 170 | 170 |
| Weight (kg) | 76 | 78 |

**Table 4** Comparison of early complications between TAG and open surgical controls in the Gore pivotal study.

| Variable | TAG device (%) | Surgical control (%) | p value |
|---|---|---|---|
| Coronary artery disease | 49 | 36 | .06 |
| Cardiac arrhythmia | 24 | 31 | .23 |
| Stroke | 10 | 10 | >.95 |
| PVOD | 16 | 11 | .33 |
| Prior vascular intervention | 45 | 55 | .14 |
| Symptomatic aneurysm | 21 | 38 | <.01 |
| Other concomitant aneurysms | 28 | 28 | >.95 |
| COPD | 40 | 38 | .89 |
| Smoking | 84 | 82 | .86 |
| Renal dialysis | 1 | 0 | .52 |
| Hepatic dysfunction | 2 | 1 | .65 |
| Paraplegia | 1 | 0 | >.95 |
| Cancer | 19 | 13 | .21 |

PVOD, peripheral vascular occlusive disease; COPD, chronic obstructive pulmonary disease.

Society of Anesthesiologists classification and the Society of Vascular Surgery risk score showed no significant difference in either classification.

## Operative data

Of 142 patients recruited (140 in the pivotal trial and 2 extended access), 139 (98%) underwent successful implantation of the TAG device. The three failures were all due to poor iliac access. A conduit was placed to facilitate access in 21 patients (15%). More than one device was used in 77 patients (55%): 61 patients (44%) received two devices, 11 patients (8%) received three devices, and 5 patients (4%) received four devices.

Prophylactic left carotid/subclavian bypass grafting was performed in 28 patients in preparation for planned left subclavian artery coverage with the device. Unplanned subclavian artery and visceral artery coverage occurred in one patient each. The latter underwent an open abdominal explantation of the device and redeployment of a new device without sequelae.

## Early adverse events

### Mortality

Operative mortality, defined as death within 30 days of the procedure or on the same hospital admission, occurred in 3 patients (2.1%) after TAG implantation (Table 5). One death was due to a postoperative

stroke and another to a cardiac event that occurred on postoperative day 11. The third death occurred after 7 months of a protracted hospital course as a result of anoxic brain injury after a respiratory arrest. The patient died of septic complications from an aortoesophageal fistula. Six deaths (6.4%) occurred in the surgical control group.

## Spinal cord ischemia

Spinal drainage was not routinely used in either group. In the TAG group, spinal cord ischemia (SCI) was noted in 4 patients. One was noted immediately after the procedure, and the deficit persisted despite all supportive measures. Three were delayed in onset, and all these regained motor function (one complete and two partial) and were ambulatory at last follow-up. It should be noted that multiple pieces of TAG endografts were used in 3 of 4 patients and that 2 of 4 patients had had previous infrarenal aortic aneurysm repair. The incidence of SCI did not differ between those with and without

**Table 5** Operative complications.

| Variable | TAG | Open surgical |
|---|---|---|
| Death | 2.1% | 11.7% |
| Paraplegia/paraparesis | 3 | 14 |
| Stroke | 4 | 4 |

prior abdominal aortic aneurysm repair (4.7% vs 2%, respectively). The incidence of SCI in the control group was significantly higher (13.8%). Of 13 patients, 8 had paraplegia, of whom 6 died. One case of paraplegia resolved completely.

### Cerebrovascular accidents

Perioperative stroke was noted in 5 patients (3.5%). One was fatal. Three were right-sided. Four of the five strokes occurred in patients who had proximal aneurysms requiring extension of the TAG to the left carotid and coverage of the subclavian artery; all four underwent carotid/subclavian bypass. Of the 28 patients with proximal aneurysms who had planned subclavian artery coverage, 4 (14%) had a stroke, compared with 1 (1%) of 114 with disease distal to the subclavian artery ($p < .001$). The overall incidence of cerebrovascular accident (4.3%) was similar in the two groups.

### Endoleaks

Early endoleaks were seen in 5 patients. One patient had a proximal type I endoleak and was treated with endovascular revision and additional grafts. The remaining endoleaks were thought to be type II.

### Other MAEs

The other most common MAEs were bleeding, cardiopulmonary events, and intraoperative vascular injury. Both bleeding and pulmonary events were significantly reduced in the TAG group compared with the surgical control group, due to a high percentage of procedural bleeding and respiratory failure in the latter.

The incidence of vascular injuries was 14% in the TAG group, which was significantly higher than in the control group (4%). This was related to the introduction of large introducer sheaths through the iliac system.

### Hospital length of stay

The average ICU stay was significantly shorter in the TAG group compared with the control group (2.6 ± 14.6 days vs 5.2 ± 7.2 days; $p < .001$), as was the total length of stay (7.4 ± 17.7 days vs 14.4 ± 12.8 days; $p < .001$).

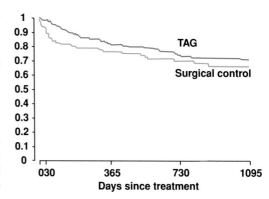

**Figure 3** Comparison of Kaplan-Meier estimates for all-cause mortality through the 3-year follow-up between the Gore TAG and surgical control groups.

### Late outcome

*Late survival*

All-cause mortality through 3 years did not differ in the two groups (Figure 3). The causes of death were commensurate with associated comorbidities in this elderly population. No ruptures have been reported.

With respect to aneurysm-related mortality, defined as death before hospital discharge, death within 30 days of the primary procedure or within 30 days of any secondary procedure to treat the original aneurysm, or death due to aneurysm rupture, there was one late death in the TAG group. This patient had an aneurysm growth in the setting of graft infection at 2 months. The patient underwent an open conversion and was found to have an aortoesophageal fistula, which was treated by graft excision and an extra-anatomic bypass, only to experience a respiratory arrest on postoperative day 13 with resultant anoxic brain injury. The patient died 3 days later. In the open surgical group, three additional deaths occurred during the first 6 months of follow-up. Freedom from aneurysm-related mortality through 3 years was 97% for the TAG device group and 90% for the open surgical controls ($p = .024$). No mortalities were noted in either group after the first year (Figure 4).

*Major adverse events*

The Kaplan-Meier estimates of the probability of freedom from MAEs were significantly higher with TAG treatment (58%) than with open surgical

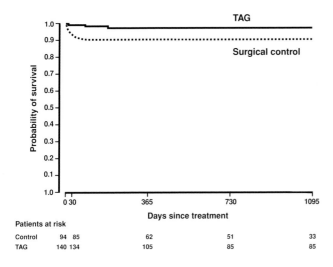

Patients at risk

| | | | | |
|---|---|---|---|---|
| Control | 94  85 | 62 | 51 | 33 |
| TAG | 140 134 | 105 | 85 | 85 |

**Figure 4** Comparison of Kaplan-Meier estimates for aneurysm-related mortality through 3-year follow-up between the Gore TAG and surgical control groups.

controls: 48% versus 20% at 3 years, respectively (Figure 5). In fact, 70% of all MAEs occurred within 30 days of the original procedure. A similar observation was made in the feasibility study, in which 63% of all events over 5 years were noticed in the first 30 days.

### Device-related events

During a 3-year follow-up, 5 patients underwent endovascular revisions and 1 patient underwent surgical conversion. Three of the revisions occurred after 24 months of follow-up. Device migrations, three proximal and four components, were noted without clinical compromise at the 2-year follow-up. Sac shrinkage of greater than 5 mm was observed in 38% (24/64) and sac expansion in 17% (11/64) of patients. Three of the 11 patients with sac enlargement had endoleaks at some point during follow-up. Twenty fractures were noted in 19 patients: 18 in the longitudinal spine and 2 in the apical nitinol support rings. Clinical sequelae developed in only 1 patient, who developed a type III endoleak that was treated with an endograft. No ruptures were noted at a follow-up extending to 2 years. No device-related deaths were noted through 3 years.

## Confirmatory study

### Objectives and hypotheses

The confirmatory study was launched to demonstrate that deployment and early results with the modified device are comparable to those with the original device. The safety and efficacy hypotheses were the same as in the pivotal trial except for using a 30-day end point. This earlier safety end point was chosen as an appropriate measure on the basis of the results of the pivotal study, in which most MAEs occurred within the 30-day period. Almost all major device-related events were also identified in the first 30 days during the pivotal trial. Although 30-day study end points were used, all patients are to be followed up to 5 years. Inclusion and exclusion criteria were identical to those used in the pivotal study.

### Study design

The confirmatory study was a prospective, nonrandomized trial with all test subjects treated with the modified TAG device. The study was performed at 11 sites, all but one of which had participated in the pivotal trial. Fifty-one patients were enrolled in this study, and their results were compared with the same 94 control subjects used in the pivotal study.

### Results of the confirmatory study

#### Clinical materials

Baseline demographics and aortic morphology were quite similar in the TAG device group and the surgical control group. Comorbidities were also well matched. In this comparison, the symptomatic aneurysm difference did not reach statistical

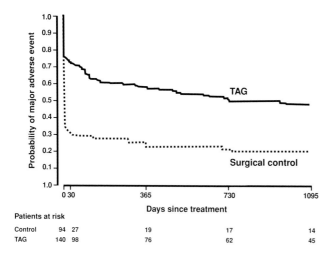

Figure 5 Comparison of Kaplan-Meier estimates for freedom from MAEs through the 3-year follow-up between the Gore TAG and surgical control groups.

significance. However, there was a higher prevalence of cancer or a history of cancer in the TAG device group compared with the surgical control group. Risk classification according to the American Society of Anesthesiologists was very well matched between the TAG and the surgical control groups. The Society of Vascular Surgery risk score was slightly higher in the TAG device group, and this was significant.

### Early MAEs

At 30 days, the incidence of MAEs was 12% in the TAG group and 70% in the controls, a highly significant difference corresponding to an 83% risk reduction for those treated with the TAG device. No early deaths were noted in the TAG group. The rate of vascular complications was not significantly different in this cohort compared with the surgical controls.

Kaplan-Meier estimates of the probability of freedom from MAEs through 30 days showed a significant advantage for the TAG device group compared with the surgical control group ($p < .001$).

### Device-related events

No major device-related events were reported through the 30-day follow-up in the test subjects compared with six (4%) reported for the pivotal study test subjects.

Hospital length of stay was shorter with the TAG device compared with the control group (3 days vs 10 days, respectively). The time to return to normal activities was shortened in the TAG group to 15 days versus 78 days for the control group.

Results from the Gore TAG trials [1, 2] have shown that the safety of endovascular repair of thoracic aortic aneurysm is superior to open surgical repair at short-term and mid-term results, with operative mortality and morbidity and SCI lower than those observed for open surgical repair. Patients treated with the endovascular approach had a lower length of hospital stay, lower length of ICU stay, lower blood transfusions, rapid recovery rates, lower aneurysm-related deaths, and fewer device-related complications.

The incidence of SCI though lower than with open surgical repair is still a major source of morbidity and mortality. Potential risk factors include extensive coverage of the descending thoracic aorta, open abdominal aneurysm repair with extensive coverage of descending thoracic aorta [3–5], and possibly coverage of the left subclavian artery with extensive coverage of the descending thoracic aorta.

Vascular complications were more frequent in the endovascular group compared to the open surgical group. Small access vessels especially in females who comprised 50% of the thoracic aneurysm group are at risk of potential rupture when large sheaths are inserted. Conduits should be readily used as prophylactic procedure when small, tortuous, and calcified vessels are anticipated.

The risk of endoleak requires lifelong surveillance of patients with regular chest roentgenogram to detect device-related complications like migration or stent fracture and CT scans to follow endoleaks, aneurysm sac regression, or expansion.

In conclusion, the Gore TAG US trial has shown the efficacy of the Gore TAG excluder device for the treatment of thoracic aortic aneurysm. The application of this technology to other aortic pathologies is still under investigative trial protocols. Long-term data are required to establish better outcomes in the management of patients with thoracic aortic aneurysms. The evolution of more flexible end grafts, smaller delivery sheaths, and branched endografts would expand the application of this technology to patients with varied thoracic aortic pathologies.

# References

1 Makaroun MS, Dillavou ED, Kes ST *et al*. Endovascular treatment of thoracic aortic aneurysms: results of the phase II multicenter trial of the Gore TAG thoracic endoprosthesis. *J Vasc Surg* 2005; **41**: 1–9.

2 Gore TAG Thoracic Endoprosthesis Annual Clinical Update, September 2006.

3 Greenberg R, Resch T, Nyman U *et al*. Endovascular repair of descending thoracic aortic aneurysm: an early experience with intermediate-term follow-up. *J Vasc Surg* 2000; **31**: 147–156.

4 Moon MR, Mitchell RS, Dake MD, Zarins CK, Fann JL, Miller DG. Simultaneous abdominal aortic replacement and thoracic stint graft placement for multilevel aortic disease. *J Vasc Surg* 1997; **25**: 332–340.

5 Gravereaux EC, Faries PL, Burks JA *et al*. Risk of spinal cord ischemia after endograft repair of thoracic aortic aneurysms. *J Vasc Surg* 2001; **31**: 997–1003.

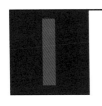

# SECTION I
# Thoracic aortic aneurysms

## CASE 1

# Endovascular repair of descending thoracic aortic aneurysms using the Gore TAG stent graft

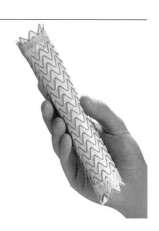

## Introduction

A descending thoracic aneurysm (DTA) is defined as a localized or diffuse dilation of an artery with a diameter at least 50% greater than an adjacent normal size artery. Thoracic aortic aneurysms are estimated to affect 10 per 100,000 elderly adults with 30–40% of those occurring in the descending portion of the thoracic aorta. The consensus size for intervention is generally 5.5 cm in the ascending aorta and somewhere in the range of 6.0–7.0 cm in the descending aorta. The most common risk factors include smoking, hypertension, atherosclerosis, bicuspid or unicuspid aortic valves, and genetic disorders. Potential symptoms from DTAs include back pain localized between the scapulae and midback and epigastric pain located at the level of the diaphragmatic hiatus. DTAs and thoracoabdominal aneurysms may compress the trachea or bronchus, cause stridor, wheezing, or dysphagia through compression of the esophagus. Erosion into surrounding structures may result in hemoptysis, hematemesis, or gastrointestinal bleeding. Erosion into the spine may cause back pain or instability. Spinal cord compression or thrombosis of spinal arteries may result in neurologic symptoms of paraparesis or paraplegia. DTAs may thrombose or embolize clot and atheromatous debris distally to visceral, renal, or lower extremities. The most common complications of thoracic aortic aneurysms are acute rupture or dissection. Some patients present with tender or painful nonruptured aneurysms. Although debate continues, these patients are thought to be at increased risk for rupture and should undergo surgical repair on an emergent basis. Endovascular stent grafting is fast becoming the accepted treatment modality for managing DTAs [1, 2] and has been approved for the US market since March 2005 (Figure 1).

## Case scenario

A 71-year-old lady was diagnosed with a DTA of 4.4 cm × 5.2 cm approximately 18 months before intervention. She was now symptomatic with a complaint of chest pain that would radiate to the back. Her medical history was significant for hypertension, emphysema requiring nocturnal oxygen supplementation and a 120-pack year smoking history. Her medications included a couple of antihypertensive medications and inhalers for her emphysema. The remainder of her history and physical examination were essentially normal. A CT scan of the chest conducted within 3 months of intervention demonstrated a DTA of 6.0 × 5.3 cm (Figure 2a and 2b). Due to the expansion of the aneurysm and her prohibitive medical history, she was referred for endovascular repair.

## Recommendation

Due to the patient's requirement for home oxygen and other severe comorbidities, she was felt to be a prohibitive risk for open surgery. Measurements

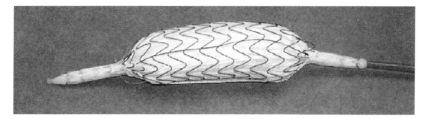

**Figure 1** Illustration of a partially deployed Gore-TAG device.

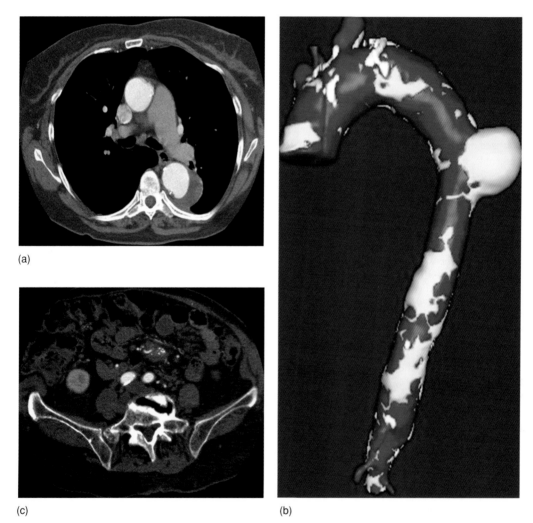

(a)

(c)

(b)

**Figure 2** (a) A CT scan of the chest with IV contrast demonstrating a DTA with mural thrombus measuring 6.0 cm × 5.3 cm in diameter. (b) A 3-D reconstruction showing the patient's anatomy and dimensions of the proximal and distal landing zones. (c) An axial CT image demonstrating adequate-sized iliac arteries with mild calcification in the posterior wall of right iliac artery.

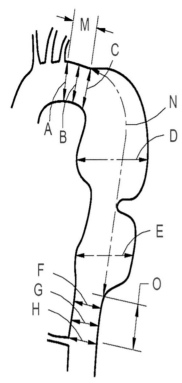

**Figure 3** A preoperative worksheet to evaluate the candidacy for stent-graft placement. A, proximal implantation site, 30 mm; B, 1 cm proximal to implantation site; C, 2 cm from implantation site, 32 mm; D, aneurysm diameter, 60 mm; E, secondary aneurysm N/A; F, 2 cm distal to implantation site; G, 1 cm from distal implantation site, 29 mm; H, distal implantation site, 28 mm; N, distal neck, distance from aneurysm to celiac axis, 3 cm; O, total treatment length 9 cm.

obtained from the diagnostic CT scans of the chest, abdomen, and pelvis indicated that the patient met the criteria for endoluminal stent grafting using the preoperative work sheet (Figure 3). A Gore TAG endoluminal graft (W.L. Gore & Associates, Flagstaff, AZ) 34 mm × 15 cm would provide a 10–15% oversizing in the landing zones (Table 1) and would be adequate in length to exclude the aneurysm. A CT scan of the pelvis helped assess the size, tortuosity, and amount of calcification of the iliac vessels. The iliac arteries were 10 mm in diameter and free of significant disease or tortuousity (Figure 2c) and were adequately sized for deployment of an endograft (Table 2).

**Table 1** Gore TAG sizing chart.

| Device diameter (mm) | Vessel diameter (mm) | Oversizing (%) |
| --- | --- | --- |
| 26 | 23–24 | 8–14 |
| 28 | 24–26 | 8–17 |
| 31 | 26–29 | 7–19 |
| 34 | 29–32 | 9–16 |
| 37 | 32–34 | 9–16 |
| 40 | 34–37 | 9–18 |

## Procedure

Under general anesthesia, open retrograde cannulation of the right common femoral artery was performed with an 18-G needle and a 0.035-in. soft-tip angled glide wire (Medi-tech/Boston Scientific, Natick, MA) was passed into the distal thoracic aorta and exchanged to a 9-F (French) sheath under fluoroscopic visualization. Percutaneous access of the left common femoral artery was similarly performed with a 5-F sheath. Five thousand units of heparin were given to keep the activated clotted time greater than 200 seconds. A 5-F pigtail catheter was advanced through the left groin sheath into the thoracic aorta. The fluoroscopic C-arm was positioned in a left anterior oblique angle, and an oblique thoracic arch aortogram was performed to visualize the arch vessels and the descending thoracic aortic aneurysm (Figure 4). Intravascular ultrasound (IVUS) is routinely performed in our institution using an IVUS 8.2-F probe (Volcano Therapeutics, Inc., Rancho Cordova, CA). The IVUS probe was advanced through the right groin sheath to confirm the size of the aneurysm, presence or absence of thrombus, proximal neck diameter and length, and distal neck diameter and length. The 34 mm × 15 cm

**Table 2** Recommended iliac diameter for the introduction of Gore delivery sheaths.

| Size (F) | ID (mm) | OD (mm) |
| --- | --- | --- |
| 20 | 6.7 | 7.6 |
| 22 | 7.3 | 8.3 |
| 24 | 8.1 | 9.1 |

ID, inner diameter; OD, outer diameter.

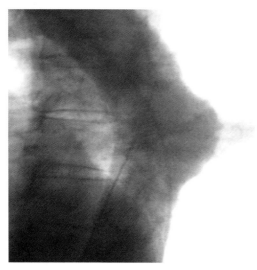

**Figure 4** An aortogram demonstrating a descending thoracic aortic aneurysm with adequate proximal and distal neck length.

TAG stent graft was chosen (Figure 5). The IVUS catheter was exchanged for an extra-stiff 260-cm double curve Lunderquist wire (Cook Inc., Bloomington, IN). The right 9-F sheath was exchanged for a 22-F Gore sheath and a 34 mm × 15 cm TAG stent-graft device was advanced through the Gore sheath (Figure 6). Prior to deployment, the proximal and distal landing zones were identified and marked on angiographic road map. At the time of deployment

of the endoluminal graft, a systolic blood pressure of 90 mm Hg is achieved to decrease the "windsock" effect in the thoracic aorta. We have not felt the need for adenosine-induced asystole. A Gore trilobe balloon (Figure 7) was used to perform post-deployment balloon angioplasty to both the proximal and distal segments of the graft for good fixation. A completion angiogram demonstrated exclusion of the aneurysm with no endoleak (Figure 8). All wires and sheaths were removed from the right common femoral artery with the incision closed in a transverse fashion. A 6-F angioseal vascular closure device (St. Judes Medical, Inc., St. Paul, MN) was deployed to the left common femoral artery. At the end, the patient had bilateral peripheral pulses was extubated prior to leaving the OR and transferred to the recovery room. She was discharged on post-operative day (POD) 2 in satisfactory condition. A CT scan of the chest performed on POD 1 showed exclusion of the 6-cm aneurysm with no evidence of an endoleak (Figure 8a and 8b).

## Discharge CT scan

## Discussion

The management of DTAs has traditionally been by open surgical repair. Open surgical repair requires performing a left thoracotomy, aortic cross clamping, possible left heart bypass, and some degree of

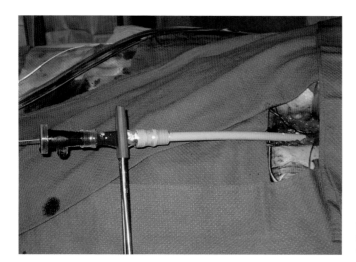

**Figure 5** A 22-F Gore delivery sheath introduced through the femoral artery for deployment of endoluminal graft.

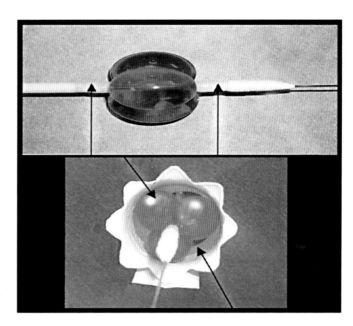

**Figure 6** Gore trilobed balloon used for profiling the Gore TAG stent graft.

hypothermia that can increase the morbidity and mortality of the procedure. Thoracic endoluminal grafting has recently gained wide acceptance as a treatment modality for managing various aortic pathologies including DTAs [2–4]. From September

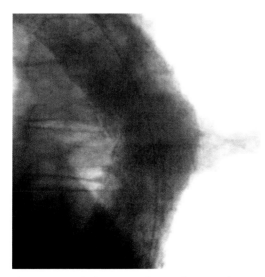

**Figure 7** A postdeployment angiogram demonstrating exclusion of the thoracic aneurysm.

1999 through May 2001, 140 patients with DTAs were evaluated and enrolled at 17 sites across the United States. An open surgical control arm consisting of 94 patients was identified by enrolling both historical controls and concurrent subjects. Results of this US multicenter comparative trial (TAG 99-01) [5] showed a perioperative mortality in the endograft arm of 2.1% ($n = 3$) versus 11.7% ($n = 11$, $p < .001$) in the open surgery cohort. A 30-day analysis revealed a statistically significant lower incidence of the following complications in the endovascular cohort versus surgical cohort: spinal cord ischemia (3% vs 14%), respiratory failure (4% vs 20%), and renal insufficiency (1% vs 13%). The endovascular group had a higher incidence of peripheral vascular complications (14% vs 4%). The mean intensive care and hospital stay were shorter in the endovascular cohort group. Accepted, commercial indications for a thoracic endoluminal graft include DTAs deemed to warrant surgical repair, fusiform aneurysm greater than two times diameter of normal adjacent aorta, and saccular aneurysms. A minimum of 2-cm nonaneurysmal segment in both the proximal and distal landing areas are needed for successful deployment of a thoracic endoluminal graft. Angles less than 60°

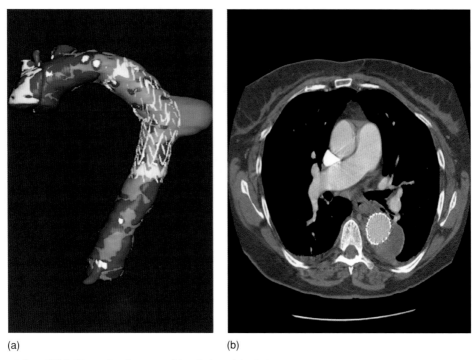

(a)                                         (b)

**Figure 8** (a and b) A CT scan showing successful exclusion of the DTA.

between the aortic arch and the descending thoracic aorta may require additional length of nonaneurysmal segment, and coverage of the left subclavian artery may be required. Late complications associated with endografting include aortic wall perforation from the proximal bare spring configuration of earlier devices, device collapse from oversizing the endograft greater than 20% of the thoracic aortic neck diameter metal fracture, fabric erosion, and suture breakage associated with circumferential, radial, and tensional stresses from repetitive aortic pulsations [6]. Two-year follow-up data from the TAG 01 US multicenter trial showed a 6% endoleak rate detected at 1 year and 9% endoleak at 2 years postprocedure. During that time, three reinterventions in the endograft cohort were done with none in the open surgical cohort [7]. Five-year follow-up data show freedom from device-related complications to be very low with no aneurysm-related deaths, conversions, or ruptures for the control subjects enrolled in the pivotal and confirmatory studies (TAG 99-01 and TAG 03-03) [8]. Recommendations for endograft surveillance include a 4-view chest X-ray to assess for device migration or stent fracture and a CT scan of the chest at periodic intervals (1 mo, 6 mo, 1 yr, and annually thereafter).

## References

1 Ramaiah V, Rodriguez-Lopez JA, Diethrich EB. Endografting of the thoracic aorta: a single center experience with technical considerations. *J Card Surg* 2003; **18**: 444–453.

2 Dake MD, Miller DC, Semba CP, Mitchell RS, Walker PJ, Liddell RP. Transluminal placement of endovascular stent grafts for the treatment of descending thoracic aneurysms. *N Eng J Med* 1994; **331**: 1729–1734.

3 Greenberg R, Resch T, Nyman U, Lindh M *et al.* Endovascular repair of descending thoracic aortic aneurysm: an early experience with intermediate-term follow-up. *J Vasc Surg* 2000; **31**: 147–156.

4 Wheatley GH, III, Gurbuz AT, Rodriguez-Lopez JA *et al.* Midterm outcome in 158 consecutive Gore TAG thoracic endoprostheses: single center experience. *Ann Thorac Surg* 2006; **81**(5): 1570–1577; discussion 1577.

5 Makaroun MS, Dillavou ED, Kes ST *et al.* Endovascular treatment of thoracic aortic aneurysms: results of the phase II multicenter trial of the Gore TAG thoracic endoprosthesis. *J Vasc Surg* 2005; **41**: 1–9.

6 Kasirajan K, Milner R, Chaikof E. Late complications of thoracic endografts. *J Vasc Surg* 2006; **43**: 94A–99A.

7 Bavaria JE, Appoo JJ, Makaroun MS, Verter J, Zi-Fan Yu, Scott Mitchell RS. Endovascular stent grafting versus open surgical repair of descending thoracic aortic aneurysms in low-risk patients: a multicenter comparative trial. *J Thorac Cardiovasc Surg* 2007; **133**: 369–377.

8 Gore TAG Thoracic Endoprosthesis Annual Clinical Update, September 2006.

## CASE 2

# Endovascular management of thoracic aortic aneurysm using a Cook Zenith TX2 endograft

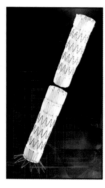
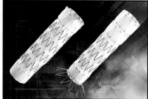

## Introduction

With the introduction of the first commercially available endograft, two additional endoprosthesis are in the process of being evaluated for Food and Drug Administration approval. The Cook TX2 stent graft is designed as a two-piece system that incorporates hooks and barbs, distal fixation, and a proximal controlled deployment. Thoracic stent-graft treatment of thoracic aortic pathologies, including thoracic aortic aneurysms, has been associated with migration of both proximal and distal fixation points [1], erosion of uncovered proximal portion through the aortic arch [2], component separation with modular devices [2, 3]. These problems have been described with most of the thoracic endoprosthesis implanted for thoracic aortic pathologies [3–5]. The ideal thoracic stent graft currently does not exist but would need to be flexible enough to accommodate the tortuosity of the arch, incorporate a fixation system that is secure both proximally

and distally, seal within both straight and tortuous segments, be readily deliverable and have favorable effects on the excluded region of the aorta. Additionally, delivery of the device would optimally not require the induction of hypotension or bradycardia even in the setting of extreme tortuousity. The Cook TX1 and TX2 device has been designed to attempt to solve some of these issues but currently at this time is not approved as a commercial device in the United States.

## Device description

The Zenith endograft is a one-piece (TX1) or two-piece (TX2) modular endovascular graft (Figure 1). The device composition is of Dacron (DuPont, Wilmington, DE) fabric sewn to self-expanding stainless steel Z-stents with braided polyester and monofilament polypropylene sutures. The graft is fully stented with an intention to provide columnar stability and expansile force. It consists of a

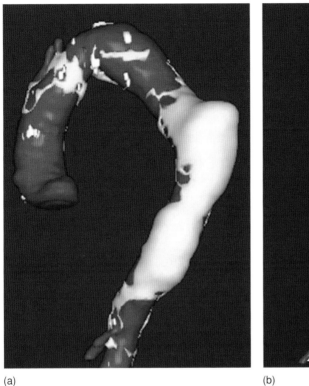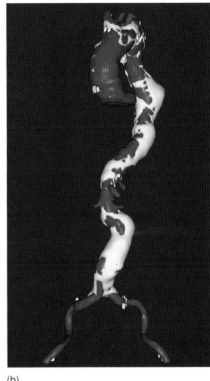

(a)                                                         (b)

**Figure 1** Reconstructed CT scan of the chest demonstrating a thoracic aortic aneurysm measuring 6.0 cm in diameter with adequately sized iliac vessels with minimal tortuosity and calcium.

proximal (TX2P) and a distal (TX2D) component, with a minimal overlap of two stents between them. The proximal part of the TX2P is covered and contains a series of 5-mm-long, staggered, caudally oriented barbs to prevent distal migration. Proximally, the distal TX2 component has a two-stent overlap zone in which the stents are sutured to the internal surface of the fabric. Distally, there is an uncovered Gianturco Z-stent with cranially oriented barbs to help prevent proximal migration. Four gold radiopaque markers are stationed near the edge of the graft material to enhance visualization of graft ends. The graft diameters range from 28 to 42 mm, and the graft profile ranges from 20 to 22-F (French). The proximal components can either be tapered or nontapered. The device is deployed by manually retracting the outer sheath of the delivery system while holding the stent graft in position. Additional ancillary endovascular components (proximal and distal main body extensions) are available. The TX2 ancillary components are cylindrical components constructed from the same polyester fabric and materials. At the distal and proximal graft margins, the Z-stents are attached to the inner surface. Elsewhere, the Z-stents are sutured on the external surface.

## Case scenario

An 80-year-old man presented with a 40-pack-year smoking history and past medical history of open abdominal aortic aneurysm repair, coronary artery disease with recent coronary artery bypass graft surgery, chronic obstructive lung disease with steroid and oxygen dependency, hypertension, and left ventricular dysfunction. He was found to have a thoracic aortic aneurysm of the mid and descending thoracic aorta on a chest X-ray performed for evaluation of a lung nodule. A CT scan of the chest performed demonstrated a 6.0-cm thoracic aortic aneurysm with mural thrombus (Figure 1). Due to the extensive comorbidities he was felt to be a

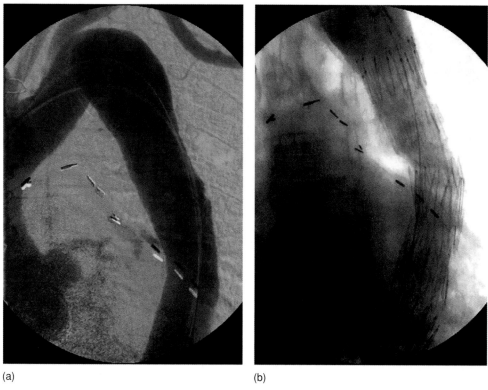

(a)                                                                         (b)

**Figure 2** (a and b) A pre- and post-endoluminal graft thoracic aortogram demonstrating an angulated and tortuous arch and exclusion of the aneurysm.

high-risk candidate for open surgical repair and enrolled in the multicenter TX2 trial.

## Endovascular procedure

The right common femoral artery was exposed through a small oblique incision and cannulated with a 9-F sheath. Percutaneous access of the left common femoral artery was performed and a 5-F sheath was introduced. Oblique thoracic aortogram was performed through the left groin sheath via a 5-F pigtail angiographic catheter to delineate the arch and the descending thoracic aorta aneurysm (Figure 2a). Intravascular ultrasound (IVUS) was performed using an 8.2-F probe (Volcano Therapeutics, Inc., Rancho Cordova, CA) through the right groin sheath to confirm the size of aneurysm, presence or absence of thrombus, proximal neck diameter and length; distal neck diameter and length. The proximal neck and distal neck diameter were measured at 30 mm. Based on the measurements,

a 36-mm Cook Zenith TX2 thoracic endoluminal graft was chosen for exclusion of the thoracic aortic aneurysm. An extra-stiff Lunderquist wire (Cook Inc., Bloomington, IN) was exchanged through the IVUS catheter. The right 9-F sheath was exchanged for a Cook Zenith TX2 device (Cook Inc., Bloomington, IN) measuring 36 mm × 152 mm and deployed 2-cm distal to the left subclavian artery with at least a 3-cm proximal neck. A second Cook Zenith device 36 mm × 136 mm was deployed distally with adequate overlap between grafts to a level just above the celiac trunk. A completion angiogram demonstrated satisfactory exclusion of the thoracic aortic aneurysm with no endoleak (Figure 2b). All wires and sheaths were removed. The right common femoral artery was closed in a transverse fashion with restoration of flow. A vascular closure device was deployed to the left common femoral artery. The patient had bilateral palpable pulses at the end of the procedure was extubated and transferred to recovery room. A postoperative CT scan

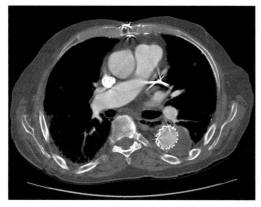

(a)

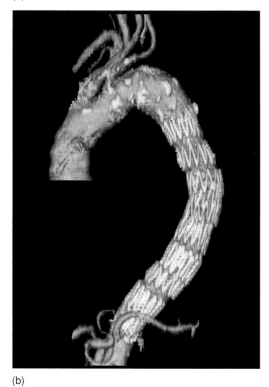

(b)

**Figure 3** (a and b) Postoperative CT scan of the chest demonstrating satisfactory exclusion of aneurysm.

demonstrated adequate exclusion of thoracic aortic aneurysm with no endoleak (Figure 3a).

## Discussion

Endovascular repair of descending thoracic aneurysms is a progression of technology first introduced for the management of infrarenal abdominal aneurysms in 1991 [6, 7]. It was first used to treat a thoracic aortic aneurysm by Dake *et al.* [8]. The Gore TAG thoracic stent was approved for use in the United States in March 2005 for the treatment of thoracic aortic aneurysms based on favorable data from the phase II multicenter trial [9]. The application of thoracic stent-graft technology to various aortic pathologies including aneurysms, acute dissections, chronic dissections, penetrating aortic ulcers, and aortobronchial fistulae are less defined than infrarenal aneurysms. With the decreased blood loss, hospital stay, paraplegia rates, and morbidity and mortality, endovascular repair can be viewed as a favorable alternative to open surgical repair. Complications unique to endovascular repair include endoleaks, device migration, and increased secondary intervention rates.

The most recent version of the Cook Zenith TX2 device for the treatment of thoracic aortic aneurysms and penetrating aortic ulcers underwent a United States phase II multicenter trial. It is commercially available in Europe, Australia, and Canada.

Greenberg *et al.* [10] studied 100 patients (42% women) under a single-site device exemption protocol to assess the technical success and outcomes of patients with thoracic aortic pathology at high risk for conventional therapy using the Cook Zenith TX1 and TX2 thoracic stent graft between 2001 and 2004. The study population consisted of patients at high risk for conventional surgical therapy presenting with chronic aortic dissections, thoracic aneurysms, aortobronchial or aortoesophageal fistulae. Follow-up studies included radiographic evaluation before discharge and at 1, 6, 12, and 24 months. Most patients (55%) included in the study had undergone prior aortic aneurysm repair. The pathology treated included 81 aneurysms, 15 aortic dissections (with aneurysms), 2 patients with fistulous connections (1 aortobronchial and 1 aortoesophageal), 1 subclavian artery aneurysm, and 1 aortic rupture. Mean aneurysm size was 62 mm and patients had a 14-month mean follow-up. Hybrid interventions were necessary to create adequate implantation sites in 29% patients, including 14 elephant trunk/arch reconstructions, 18 carotid–subclavian bypasses, and 4 visceral vessel bypasses. Iliac conduits were required in 19 patients. Overall mortality in this cohort group was 17%, and aneurysm-related mortality was 14% at 1 year. Sac regression (>5 mm maximum diameter decrease) was observed in 52 and 56% at 12 and 24 months. Growth was noted in 1 patient (1.6%) at 12 months. Endoleaks were detected in 8 patients (8.5%) at 30 days and 3 patients (6%) at 12 months. Secondary interventions were required in 15 patients. Migration (>10 mm) of the proximal or distal stent was noted in 3 patients (6%) (2 proximal and 1 distal), none of which required treatment or resulted in an adverse event. These authors concluded that acceptable intermediate-term outcomes have been achieved in the treatment of high-risk patients in the setting of both favorable and challenging anatomic situations with these devices.

## The STARZ trial

The STARZ-TX2 trial (Study of Thoracic Aortic Aneurysm Repair with the Zenith TX2 TAA Endovascular Graft) is a North American multicenter, nonrandomized, prospective clinical trial. It is seeking to enroll 270 patients at 35 sites in the United States and Canada. It includes a control group consisting of patients with concurrent and recent historical open surgical procedures. Subject selection is based on the inclusion and exclusion criteria listed in Tables 1 and 2. Control subjects are those who do not meet the anatomic inclusion criteria for the endovascular treatment group but otherwise fit the study criteria.

The primary safety hypothesis is that the subjects treated with the Zenith device will have 30-day survival rates equivalent to those of the surgical control group. The secondary hypothesis under investigation is that patients treated with the TX2 stent graft will have equivalent or fewer complications compared with the surgical arm up to 30 days after the procedure. Other outcome measures include 12-month survival, aneurysm-related survival, incidence of rupture and conversion, aneurysm size reduction, rates of major adverse effects, device-related events, and secondary intervention rates.

The screening process includes a thorough history and physical, an ankle/brachial index, and a preoperative Short Form-36 quality-of-life questionnaire, as well as a preoperative angiography

**Table 1** Inclusion criteria.

| Criterion | Cook TX2 |
|---|---|
| Age (yr) | >18 |
| Women | Negative pregnancy test 7 days before treatment |
| Open-surgical candidate | Yes |
| Neck length | Minimal 3-cm proximal and distal |
| Aneurysm | Fusiform DTA at least twice the size of normal thoracic aorta |
| Penetrating ulcer | |
| Proximal landing zone location | 30 mm distal to left CCA |
| Distal landing zone location | 20 mm proximal to celiac axis |
| Landing zone diameter (mm) | 24–38 |

CCA, common carotid artery; DTA, descending thoracic aortic aneurysm.

or a contrast-enhanced CT scan. Follow-up physical examination, Short Form-36 quality of life, ankle/brachial index, chest radiograph, and a CT scan of the chest are obtained before discharge at 1, 6, and 12 months after implantation with annual

**Table 2** Exclusion criteria.

| Criterion | Cook TX2 |
|---|---|
| Creatinine (mg/dL) | N/A |
| Unstable rupture | Yes |
| Mycotic aneurysm | Yes |
| Connective tissue disease | Yes |
| Significant landing zone thrombus | Yes |
| Previous descending aortic surgery or endovascular repair of DTA or AAA | Yes |
| Aortic dissection | Yes |
| Coagulopathy | Yes |
| MI/CVA | <3 mo |
| Major operation within 30 days | Yes |
| Participation in another investigational study | <30 days |

DTA, descending thoracic aortic aneurysm; AAA, abdominal aortic aneurysm; MI, myocardial infarction; CVA, cerebrovascular accident; N/A, not applicable.

follow-up thereafter up to 5 years. The study started enrolling patients in March 2004 and has completed its enrollment targets at this time. Results of this multicenter trial are currently not available to make any meaningful conclusion. It is hoped that within the next few months, the Federal Drug Administration will grant approval of the Cook Zenith TX1 and TX2 device approval for use in the United States to treat thoracic aortic aneurysm.

## References

1 Greenberg R, Resch T, Nyman U *et al.* Endovascular repair of descending thoracic aortic aneurysms (an early experience with intermediate-term follow-up). *J Vasc Surg* 2000; **31**(1): 147–156.

2 Malina M, Brunkwall J, Ivancev K *et al.* Late aortic arch perforation by graft-anchoring stent (complication of endovascular thoracic aneurysm exclusion). *J Endovasc Surg* 1998; **5**(3): 274–277.

3 Criado FJ, Clarke NS, Barnaton M. Stent-graft repair in the aortic arch and descending thoracic aorta (a 4-year experience). *J Vasc Surg* 2002; **36**: 1121–1128.

4 White RA, Donayre CE, Walot L, Kopchok G, Woody J. Endovascular exclusion of descending thoracic aortic aneurysms and chronic dissections (initial clinical results with the AneuRx device). *J Vasc Surg* 2001; **33**: 927–934.

5 Dake MD, Miller DC, Mitchell RS. The first generation of endovascular stent grafts for patients with descending thoracic aortic aneurysms. *J Thorac Cardiovasc Surg* 1998; **116**: 689–704.

6 Parodi J, Palmaz J, Barone H. Transfemoral intraluminal graft implantation for abdominal aortic aneurysms. *Ann Vasc Surg* 1991; **5**: 491–499.

7 Volodos NL, Karpovich IP, Troyan VI *et al.* Clinical experience of the use of self-fixing synthetic prostheses for remote endoprosthetics of the thoracic and abdominal aorta and iliac arteries through the femoral artery and as intraoperative endoprosthesis for aortic reconstruction. *Vasa Suppl* 1991; **33**: 93–95.

8 Dake MD, Miller DC, Semba CP, Mitchell RS, Walker PJ, Liddell RP. Transluminal placement of endovascular stent-grafts for the treatment of descending thoracic aortic aneurysms. *N Engl J Med* 1994; **331**: 1729–1734.

9 Makaroun MS, Dillavou ED, Kee ST *et al.* Endovascular treatment of thoracic aortic aneurysms (results of the phase II multi-center trial of the GORE TAG thoracic endoprosthesis) [abstract]. *J Vasc Surg* 2005; **41**: 1–9.

10 Greenberg RK, O'Neill S, Walker E *et al.* Endovascular repair of thoracic aortic lesions with the Zenith TX1 and TX2 thoracic grafts (intermediate-term results). *J Vasc Surg* 2005; **41**: 589–596.

# Endovascular management of a thoracic aortic aneurysm using a Medtronic Talent thoracic graft (VALOR trial)

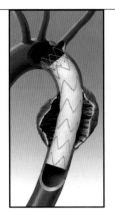
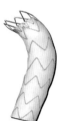

## Introduction

Endovascular management of thoracic aortic aneurysms has been shown to result in lower morbidity and mortality than open surgical repair [1, 2] and has become established as a first-line treatment for pathological conditions affecting the distal arch and the descending thoracic aorta. The Gore TAG stent graft (W.L. Gore & Associates, Flagstaff, AZ) is the only available commercially Food and Drug Administration approved graft for the treatment of thoracic aortic aneurysms.

The Talent thoracic stent-graft system (Medtronic, Santa Rosa, CA) is a self-expanding endoprosthesis consisting of circumferential nitinol stent springs arranged as a tube and covered on its exterior with a Dacron graft. It recently was involved in a multicenter trial in the United States. The tube is customized with respect to width, length, and the configuration of each end (as a bare spring or a covered web for optimal conformance with the aorta) and is compressed in a 22–25 F (French) polytetrafluoroethylene sheath. The nitinol rings are interconnected by a longitudinal wire to ensure stabilization and separation of all the rings and to prevent twisting.

## Case scenario

A 44-year-old woman with past medical history significant for hypertension and diabetes mellitus presented to an outside facility with severe chest and lower back pain. Her cardiac work-up was negative for ischemic heart disease. Her physical examination was significant for moderately elevated blood pressure with equal bilateral femoral pulses. A CT scan of the chest and abdomen demonstrated a type B dissecting thoracic aneurysm measuring 9 cm with a dissecting flap distal to the left subclavian artery to the celiac axis. She was felt to be at high risk for an open surgical repair and considered a candidate for endoluminal graft therapy. An angiogram and an intravascular ultrasound (IVUS) were scheduled to determine the pathophysiology of the dissection in relation to the aneurysm and to determine proximal and distal landing zones.

## Intravascular ultrasound and angiogram

Patient was taken to the operating room; after local sedation, percutaneous access of the right common femoral artery was performed with the introduction of a 9-F sheath under fluoroscopic guidance. A 5-F pigtail catheter (Cordis Corporation, a Johnson & Johnson company, Miami, FL) was advanced into the thoracic arch. The fluoroscopic C-arm was angled in a left anterior oblique view and an oblique thoracic aortogram was performed which demonstrated a large thoracic aortic dissecting aneurysm distal to the left subclavaian artery with an adequate

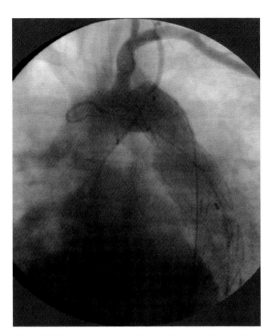

**Figure 1** Thoracic aortogram demonstrating a descending thoracic aortic aneurysm measuring 9.0 cm in its maximum diameter.

proximal and distal landing zones (Figure 1). The ascending aorta was normal and the innominate, left common carotid and the left subclavian arteries appeared within normal limits. Two dissecting thoracic aortic aneurysms were identified distal to the left subclavian artery. The angiographic pigtail catheter was exchanged for an IVUS 8.2-F probe (Volcano Therapeutics, Inc., Rancho Cordova, CA) and advanced into the thoracic aorta to determine the length of thoracic aorta to be covered as well as the proximal and distal neck length and diameter. The thoracic dissecting aneurysm originated about 3.5-cm distal to the left subclavian artery. The bigger aneurysm measured 9 cm with mural thrombus present in the aneurysm sac with the smaller aneurysm measured at 4.5 cm. A proximal neck diameter of 29 mm × 29 mm was measured and a distal neck diameter of 23 mm × 20 mm about 6 cm proximal to the celiac axis. The total length of thoracic aorta to be excluded was measured at 30 cm. The right common iliac artery was measured at 9 mm and was mildly calcified. The measurements obtained were used for the selection of an appropriately sized endoluminal graft.

## Surgical planning

1 *Proximal neck diameter D1.* Based on the proximal neck diameter, a Talent (Medtronic, Santa Rosa, CA) endoluminal graft 34 mm × 15 cm was chosen. The presence of 3.5 cm neck length was adequate for a proximal landing zone without the need to cover the left subclavian artery. The lack of a tortuous thoracic aortic arch and descending thoracic aorta would allow the device to track smoothly along the thoracic aortic curve with good apposition of the endograft to the aortic wall (Figure 2a and 2b).

2 *Distal neck diameter D3.* Due to the difference in the proximal and distal neck diameters, two different-sized devices would need to be used with deployment of the larger 34 mm × 28 mm × 15 cm device proximally and telescoping the second 32 mm × 28 mm × 15 cm device into the more proximal device.

3 *Tortuous, calcified iliac artery.* An iliac artery of 9.0 mm would tolerate the passage of a 25-F sheath which is needed to deploy the largest 44-mm-diameter Talent thoracic endograft. The presence of tortuous vessels may make tracking of the device sheath more difficult than usual and any difficulty encountered should prompt urgent conversion to a retroperitoneal conduit with a 10-mm limb for delivery of endoluminal graft to the thoracic aorta (Figure 3).

## Endovascular procedure

Open retrograde cannulation of the right common femoral artery was performed with an 18-G needle and a 0.035-in. soft-tip angled glide wire (Medi-tech/Boston Scientific, Natick, MA) was passed into the distal thoracic aorta and exchanged to a 9-F sheath under fluoroscopic visualization. Percutaneous access of the left common femoral artery was similarly performed and a 5-F sheath introduced. Five thousand units of heparin were given to keep the activated clotted time greater than 200 seconds. A 5-F pigtail catheter was advanced through the left groin sheath into the thoracic aorta. The fluoroscopic C-arm was positioned in a left anterior oblique angle and an oblique thoracic arch aortogram was performed to visualize the orifices of the arch vessels and the descending thoracic aortic

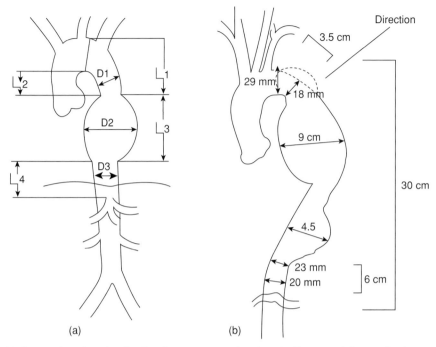

**Figure 2** (a) Planning sheet for Talent (Medtronic, Santa Rosa, CA) endograft. (b) An actual diagram for the patient treated with a Talent endograft.

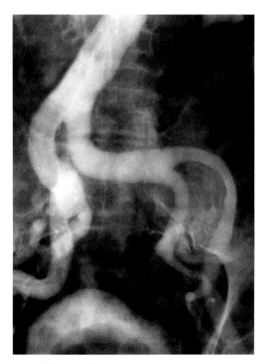

**Figure 3** Tortuous iliac vessels.

dissecting aneurysm. IVUS performed previously using an IVUS 8.2-F probe (Volcano Therapeutics, Inc., Rancho Cordova, CA) confirmed the location of the type B dissection to be 3.5-cm distal to the left subclavian artery with a 29-mm proximal and a 23-mm distal neck diameter with 30 cm of thoracic aorta to be covered to exclude the two aneurysms measured at 9.0 and 4.5 cm. An extra-stiff 260-cm Lunderquist wire (Cook Inc., Bloomington, IN) was advanced into the thoracic aorta with the help of a guiding catheter. The right 9-F sheath was exchanged for a 34 mm × 28 mm × 150 cm Talent device which was advanced into the thoracic aorta and deployed distal to the left subclavian artery as demarcated on an earlier road map angiogram. A second device 32 mm × 28 mm × 150 mm Talent stent-graft device was deployed 2-cm proximal to the celiac trunk by telescoping the device with 3 cm of overlap between devices. Balloon angioplasty with a 40-mm balloon of the proximal, distal segments, and area of overlap of the grafts was performed for aortic wall fixation. A completion angiogram demonstrated exclusion of the aneurysm

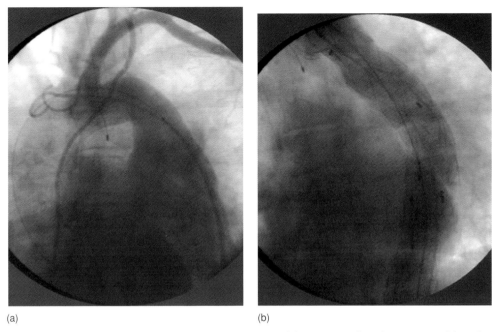

(a)                                               (b)

**Figure 4** (a and b) Completion angiogram demonstrating exclusion of thoracic aortic dissecting aneurysm with a Talent endograft.

with no endoleak (Figure 4a and 4b). All wires and sheaths were removed from the right common femoral artery and closed in a transverse fashion with restoration of flow. Patient was discharged on postoperative day (POD) 2 in satisfactory condition. A CT scan of the chest performed on POD 1 showed exclusion of the 9-cm aneurysm with no identifiable endoleak (Fig 5a and 5b).

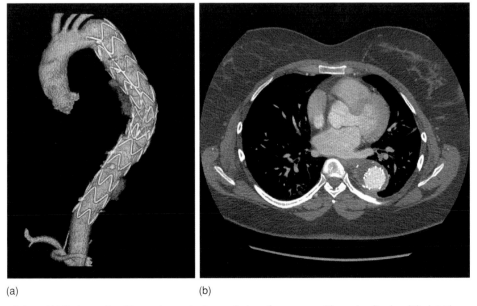

(a)                                               (b)

**Figure 5** (a and b) Postoperative CT scan demonstrating exclusion of aneurysm with no visualized endoleak and satisfactory position of endoluminal graft.

## Discussion

The Talent device allows for the treatment of larger necks with its 44-mm-diameter graft. The delivery sheaths range from 20 to 25 F and do require large access vessels for introduction.

## The VALOR trial (vascular Talent thoracic stent-graft system for the treatment of thoracic aortic aneurysms)

The VALOR trial is a prospective, multicenter study with three arms conducted at 35 sites in the United States. Enrollment for the study concluded in June 2005 with 394 patients with final VALOR trial results made available in late 2007 and expected Federal Drug Administration (FDA) approval in the early part of 2008.

The primary objective of the study is to determine the safety and efficacy of the Talent device in the treatment of descending thoracic aortic aneurysm (DTA) in subjects who are otherwise eligible for standard open repair. The safety end point compares the all-cause mortality of DTA repair with the Talent endograft against the literature control for open surgical repair within 1 year of follow-up. The efficacy end point measures the proportion of subjects with successful aneurysm treatment at the 12-month follow-up. The secondary safety and efficacy end points evaluate the technical success rate, the percentage of subjects with major adverse effects, device-related events, and aneurysm rupture rates at 30 days and at 12 months. Additional data analysis will include blood loss, blood product transfusion, operative time, ICU stay, and overall length of hospital stay. The VALOR trial reached its enrollment target in June 2005, and no results are yet available.

Subject screening required a minimum of a contrast-enhanced spiral CT scan of the chest, abdomen, and pelvis with optional 3-D reconstruction or contrast-enhanced magnetic resonance arteriography. History and physical, chest radiograph, and CT or magnetic resonance arteriography of the chest were obtained at 1, 6, and 12 months and yearly thereafter.

The test group ($n = 144$) consisted of patients who were diagnosed with DTA and were considered candidates for open surgical repair with low- to moderate-risk Society for Vascular Surgery/International Society for Cardiovascular Surgery criteria. The test group inclusion/exclusion criteria are listed in Tables 1 and 2. No surgical

**Table 1** Inclusion criteria.

| Criterion | Medtronic Talent |
|---|---|
| Age (yr) | >18 |
| Women | Negative pregnancy test 7 days before treatment |
| Open surgical candidate | Yes |
| Neck length | Minimal 2 cm proximal and distal |
| Aneurysm | Fusiform DTA at least twice the size of normal thoracic aorta; saccular |
| Penetrating ulcer | Yes |
| Proximal landing zone location | 20 mm distal to left CCA |
| Distal landing zone location | 20 mm proximal to celiac axis |
| Landing zone diameter | 18–42 mm |

CCA, common carotid artery; DTA, descending thoracic aortic aneurysm.

**Table 2** Exclusion criteria.

| Criterion | Medtronic Talent |
|---|---|
| Creatinine (mg/dL) | N/A |
| Unstable rupture | N/A |
| Mycotic aneurysm | Yes |
| Connective tissue disease | Yes |
| Significant landing zone thrombus | Yes |
| Previous descending aortic surgery or endovascular repair of DTA or AAA | Yes |
| Aortic dissection | Yes |
| Coagulopathy | Yes |
| MI/CVA | <3 mo |
| Major operation within 30 days | Yes |
| Participation in another investigational study | <30 days |

DTA, descending thoracic aortic aneurysm; AAA, abdominal aortic aneurysm; MI, myocardial infarction; CVA, cerebrovascular accident; N/A, not applicable.

control arm was included, and the comparative open control arm would be derived from the established literature. In addition to the test group, two additional observational treatment group registries were conducted concurrently. The registry group ($n = 150$) enrolled subjects who were open surgical candidates with complicated type B thoracic aortic dissections, aneurysmal degeneration from dissection, pseudoaneurysms, and chronic, stable traumatic injuries. The last arm was a high-risk group ($n = 100$). Patient eligibility included patients considered at high risk for open surgery, nonsurgical candidates not associated with Society for Vascular Surgery scoring, and subjects with traumatic thoracic aortic injuries. Only the data from the test arm will be used in device safety and efficacy analysis. The information from the registries will be descriptive in nature and may serve as the basis for future phase III clinical investigations. The VALOR trial lacks a concurrently enrolled open surgical control arm and therefore differs from the Gore TAG trial. Depending on the results of the high-risk registry group in the VALOR trial, a wider application of thoracic endoluminal grafts for the treatment of various aortic pathologies may occur to be more in line with worldwide usage. No device-specific results are available at this time.

The first reported case of thoracic endografting for the treatment of a thoracic aortic aneurysm with a customized graft was reported by Dake et al. [3].

## Clinical experience

At the Arizona Heart Institute, we have treated over 500 patients [4, 5] with various aortic pathologies using various customized and commercial endoluminal grafts between October 2000 and March 2007. The Talent (Medtronic) thoracic endoluminal graft was used to treat 34 patients within that time period under an investigational device exemption protocol. Thoracic aortic pathologies treated included thoracic aortic aneurysms in 19 patients (55.9%), type B dissections in 10 patients (29.4%), contained rupture in 2 patients (5.9%), transaction in 1 patient (2.9%), and endoluminal graft repair in 2 patients (5.9%). Delivery of sheath was achieved through femoral access in 28 patients (82.4%) and iliofemoral conduit in 6 patients (17.6%). The 30-

day operative mortality was 8.8% (3 patients). There was 1 conversion to open surgical repair. There were 2 patients who developed a type I endoleak at 30 days follow-up. Complications included paraplegia in 2 patients, stroke in 1 patient, impaired renal function in 6 patients, and pulmonary related in 3 patients.

Our results with the use of the Talent (Medtronic) stent graft in a high-risk population of patients to treat various thoracic aortic pathologies including thoracic aortic aneurysms and type B dissection seem favorable. The recently completed VALOR trial, using the Talent thoracic aortic device, will provide useful information concerning the role of endoluminal stent graft in the management of both high-risk and low-risk patients with DTAs. Similarly, results of the recently completed investigation of stent grafts in patients with type B aortic dissection (INSTEAD) trial [6] in Europe and the recently completed high-risk arm of the VALOR trial in the United States should further clarify the role of aortic stent grafting in the treatment of acute descending thoracic aortic dissections.

## References

1 Makaroun MS, Dillavou ED, Kes ST *et al.* Endovascular treatment of thoracic aortic aneurysms: results of the phase II multicenter trial of the Gore TAG thoracic endoprosthesis. *J Vasc Surg* 2005; **41**: 1–9.

2 Bavaria JE, Appoo JJ, Makaroun MS, Verter J, Zi-Fan Yu, Scott Mitchell RS. Endovascular stent grafting versus open surgical repair of descending thoracic aortic aneurysms in low-risk patients: a multicenter comparative trial. *J Thorac Cardiovasc Surg* 2007; **133**: 369–377.

3 Dake MD, Miller DC, Semba CP, Mitchell RS, Walker PJ, Liddell RP. Transluminal placement of endovascular stent grafts for the treatment of descending thoracic aneurysms. *N Eng J Med* 1994; **331**: 1729–1734.

4 Wheatley GH, III, Gurbuz AT, Rodriguez-Lopez JA *et al.* Midterm outcome in 158 consecutive Gore TAG thoracic endoprostheses: single center experience. *Ann Thorac Surg* 2006; **81**(5): 1570–1577; discussion 1577.

5 Ramaiah V, Rodriguez-Lopez JA, Diethrich EB. Endografting of the thoracic aorta: a single center experience with technical considerations. *Card Surg* 2003; **18**: 444–453.

6 Nienaber CA, Zanetti S, Barbeiri B *et al.* Investigation of stent grafts in patients with type B aortic dissection: design of the INSTEAD trial-A prospective, multicenter, European randomized trial. *Am Heart J* 2005; **149**: 595–599.

# Endovascular management of thoracic aortic aneurysms with coverage of the left subclavian artery

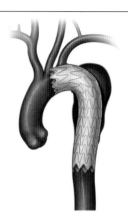

## Introduction

Endovascular management of thoracic aortic aneurysms is associated with a lower morbidity, mortality, shorter hospital and ICU stay, decreased blood loss, and a lower paraplegia rate when compared to open surgical repair [1–3]. The Gore TAG stent graft was recently approved for commercial use in the United States for the management of thoracic aortic aneurysms with other endografts, namely Talent (Medtronic) and Cook Zenith TX2 (Bloomington, IN) in the closing stages of their investigational trials. A significant proportion of patients with acute and chronic pathologies who are managed by an endovascular approach have aortic pathologies adjacent to or close to the left subclavian artery [4, 5]. Anatomical presentations like this may require the coverage of the left subclavian artery, with or without revascularization, to extend the proximal landing zone and allow endograft exclusion of these more proximal thoracic aortic lesions. Coverage of the left subclavian artery without extra anatomic revascularization has become increasingly more popular [6–14]. Contraindications to occlusion of the left subclavian artery without a preprocedural carotid subclavian bypass include an aberrant left vertebral artery, a dominant left vertebral artery blood supply to the basilar system, previous coronary artery bypass procedure with a patent left internal mammary artery, and a functioning arteriovenous fistula in the left upper extremity. For patients who develop significant left upper

extremity ischemia, revascularization can be performed in an expedient manner. For patients whose symptoms are less pronounced, expectant management is appropriate. Endovascular management of thoracic aortic pathologies with coverage of the left subclavian artery can be performed safely without any sequalae.

## Case scenario

An 84-year-old woman presented to her physician for chest discomfort. A chest X-ray demonstrated a wide mediastinum (Figure 1). She denied any history of trauma in the past. Her history and physical examination were also significant for non-insulin-dependent diabetes mellitus, hypertension, atrial fibrillation, and previous cholecystectomy. Computed tomography imaging detected the presence of a thoracic aortic aneurysm in close proximity to the left subclavian artery (Figure 2a and 2b and Figure 3b). She was further studied with an abdominal and pelvic CT scan to assess iliac vessel size, tortuosity, and calcification (Figure 4).

## Access vessel

### Surgical considerations required for endografting

1 To achieve a 2-cm proximal neck, the left subclavian artery would have to be covered. Contraindications to left subclavian coverage include a patent internal mammary to left anterior

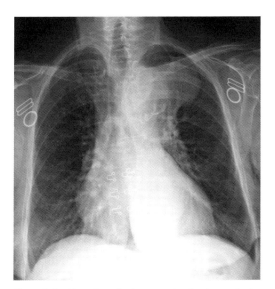

**Figure 1** A widened mediastinum as visualized on a chest X-ray.

descending artery bypass graft, dominant left vertebral artery. In those instances, a left carotid artery to left subclavian artery bypass graft is necessary prior to the deployment of an endoluminal graft.

2 Severe angulation of arch or a tortuous aorta may require the choice of an extra-stiff wire or the use of a right brachiofemoral wire for the graft to track up the arch.

3 Extreme angulation of the fluoroscopic C-arm toward a left anterior oblique view with angles up to 60° may need to be performed to align the fluoroscopic C-arm perpendicular to the arch for adequate visualization of the takeoffs of each branch vessel.

4 A retroperitoneal iliac conduit or an "endoconduit" may be necessary in tortuous, calcified small arteries to prevent iliac artery rupture during the process of advancing or withdrawing the delivery sheath.

## Surgical planning

1 Open cut down on right common femoral artery.
2 Retrograde percutaneous access on left common femoral artery.
3 Intravascular ultrasound (IVUS) to determine the diameters of the proximal neck, distal neck, common iliac vessels and the length of aorta to be covered.

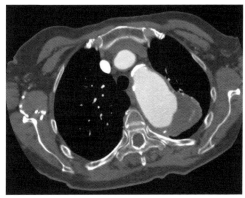

(a)

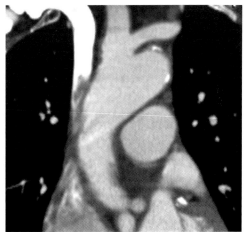

(b)

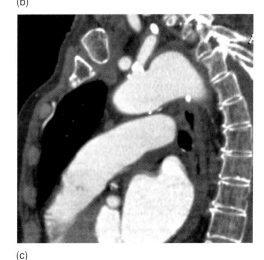

(c)

**Figure 2** (a) A 6.5-cm aneurysm shown on a CT scan of the chest. (b) An oblique view of the bovine arch. (c) An oblique view showing the approximate start of the aneurysm.

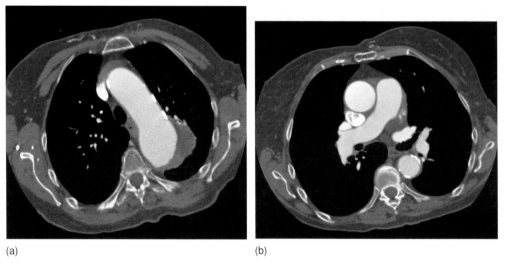

(a)                                                    (b)

**Figure 3** (a) A CT scan image showing the intended proximal landing zone for the graft. The diameter was 31–33 mm. (b) A CT scan image showing the intended distal landing zone for the graft. The diameter was 27–29 mm.

**4** Coverage of left subclavian artery (Do you need a left carotid to left subclavian bypass?)

## Endovascular technique

Under general anesthesia, open retrograde cannulation of the right common femoral artery was performed with an 18-G needle (Cook Inc., Bloomington, IN) and 0.035-in. soft-tip angled glide wire was passed in the aorta and exchanged to a 9-F (French)

sheath after 5000 units of heparin were given. Percutaneous access of the left common femoral artery was similarly performed and a 5-F sheath was introduced. A 5-F pigtail angiographic catheter was advanced through the left groin sheath into the thoracic aorta. An oblique thoracic arch aortogram was performed which demonstrated a thoracic aortic aneurysm just distal to the left subclavian artery (Figure 5). IVUS was performed using a Volcano

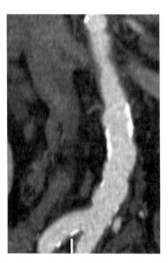

**Figure 4** An oblique, longitudinal view of a mildly tortuous iliac vessels with mild calcification.

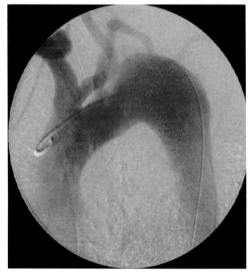

**Figure 5** An angiogram demonstrating a descending thoracic aneurysm in a bovine arch.

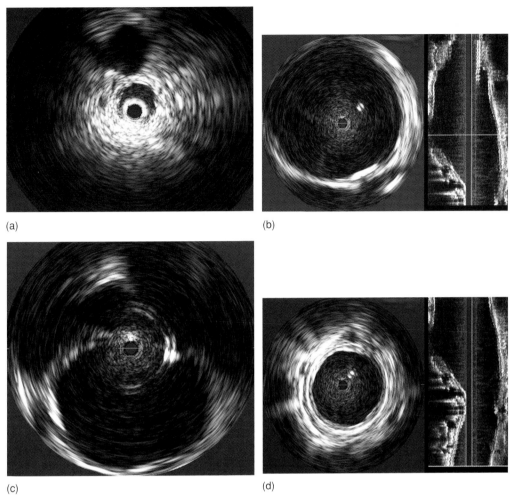

(a)

(b)

(c)

(d)

**Figure 6** (a) IVUS demonstrating a common iliac artery measuring 8.5 mm with no thrombus and mild calcification. (b) IVUS demonstrating thoracic aortic aneurysm. (c) IVUS demonstrating proximal neck of the thoracic aortic aneurysm. (d) IVUS demonstrating distal neck of thoracic aortic aneurysm with no demonstrable thrombus.

Therapeutics probe through the right groin sheath. The right common iliac artery was measured at 8.5 mm (Figure 6a). The descending thoracic aortic aneurysm was measured at 6.0 cm (Figure 6b). The aorta proximal to the aneurysm and just distal to the left carotid artery was 33 mm (Figure 6c). The distal was approximately 3 cm distal to the thoracic aortic aneurysm with a width of 29 mm (Figure 6d). The aortic arch was tight angled with a near horizontal configuration. The total length of aorta to be covered was measured at 15 cm. The IVUS probe was exchanged for a Lunderquist wire (Cook Inc.,

Bloomington, IN). To exclude the aneurysm, a total of two devices would be needed. The difference in the landing zone diameters indicated different graft sizes would need to be used with the smaller graft deployed first. The right 9-F sheath was exchanged for a 24-F sheath. An oblique thoracic aortogram was performed and a road map obtained with a guiding needle placed at both the proximal and distal landing zones. After ensuring the mean blood pressure was lower than 50 mm Hg, a 34 mm × 10 cm Gore TAG graft was advanced through the sheath and deployed successfully distal and through

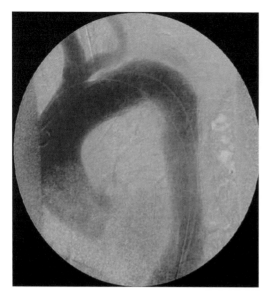

**Figure 7** A completion angiogram demonstrating exclusion of aneurysm with coverage of the left subclavian artery with a slight blush of contrast in the aneurysm sac consistent with an endoleak.

the aneurysm. A 37 mm × 15 cm Gore TAG stent graft was subsequently deployed within the 34-mm graft extending proximally to the point where the top portion of the graft landed in healthy, normal aortic tissue excluding the thoracic aortic aneurysm as well as covering of the left subclavian artery. The 24-F sheath was exchanged to a 14-F sheath and a 40-mm Coda balloon (Cook Inc., Bloomington, IN) was advanced into the endoluminal graft and balloon angioplasty was conducted at the distal, the interdevice junction, and at the proximal portions of the graft. A completion angiogram showed partial exclusion of the thoracic aortic aneurysm with a small type II endoleak (Figure 7). A decision was made to follow the type II endoleak clinically. Persistence of the type II endoleak with aneurysm sac expansion would require coiling of the left subclavian artery to resolve the endoleak. All wires and sheaths were removed; the right common femoral artery was closed in a transverse fashion with restoration of flow. A 6-F angioseal (St. Jude Medical, Inc., St. Paul, MN) vascular closure device was deployed to the left common femoral artery. Prior to leaving the operating room, the patient had bilateral palpable pulses in the legs and was extubated. A

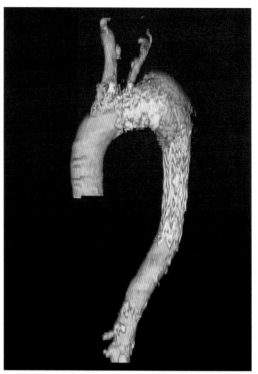

(a)

(b)

**Figure 8** (a and b) Postoperative CT scans demonstrating exclusion of aneurysm with an endoleak coming in a retrograde fashion from the left subclavian artery.

postoperative CT scan demonstrated successful exclusion of aortic pathology by the endoluminal graft and a small type II endoleak (Figure 8). The patient was discharged from the hospital with a follow-up examination consisting of a chest X-ray and contrast-enhanced CT scan around 1 month after the procedure.

## Discussion

With increasing experience with thoracic stent grafting for the treatment of thoracic aortic pathologies of the distal arch and proximal descending thoracic aorta coverage of the subclavian artery has been necessary to increase length of the proximal landing zone [15]. In the early experience with thoracic endografting, the left subclavian artery was routinely revascularized before endograft coverage owing to concerns about the potential for left upper extremity ischemia and vertebrobasilar insufficiency [16–20]. The Gore TAG phase 2 study treated 142 patients with an endoluminal graft with 28 patients (19.7%) requiring a prophylactic left subclavian carotid bypass procedure prior to coverage of the left subclavian artery to achieve an adequate proximal landing zone to exclude a thoracic aortic aneurysm. As more experience with thoracic endografting has occurred, prophylactic revascularization prior to coverage of the left subclavian artery has been found not to be necessary [6–14].

When symptoms occur after left subclavian artery coverage, they include neurologic signs consistent with vertebrobasilar insufficiency as well as left upper extremity hypoperfusion, such as claudication, rest pain, or ischemia. To identify patients with possible likelihood of complications, preprocedural carotid and vertebral duplex ultrasound imaging, digital subtraction angiography, CTA, or MRA to evaluate for the patency, size, and location of the contra lateral vertebral artery as well as to rule out an aortic arch origin of the left vertebral artery. The carotid arteries should also undergo concomitant evaluation to rule out stenosis. Cerebral angiography or MRA has a role in determining the presence of an intact circle of Willis to exclude a dominant left vertebral artery system and to ensure sufficient collateral blood flow.

At the Arizona Heart Institute, we have treated 304 patients with a thoracic stent graft over a 6-year period (2000–2006). The Talent (Medtronic) graft was implanted in 31 patients and the Gore TAG stent graft (W.L. Gore & Associates, Flagstaff,

AZ) in 276 patients. Coverage of the left subclavian artery was performed in 73 patients (24%) with 14 of those patients (19.2%) having a preoperative carotid subclavian bypass. Aortic pathology treated included type B dissection in 32 patients, thoracic aortic aneurysm in 24 patients, pseudoaneurysm in 7 patients, traumatic disruption in 2 patients, aortobronchial fistula in 2 patients, penetrating aortic ulcers in 2 patients, treatment of a proximal type I endoleak in 2 patients, and a contained rupture in 1 patient. There were 7 early deaths (9.6%). Of 59, 5 patients developed left arm claudication with 2 patients requiring a postoperative carotid subclavian bypass. Given that the vertebral artery supplies the superior portion of the anterior spinal artery, coverage of the left subclavian artery may disrupt an important collateral source of spinal perfusion in patients with prior abdominal aortic aneurysm repair as well as in those who will undergo extensive thoracic aortic coverage. In our series, there were no patients that developed a posterior circulation stroke or paraplegia. There were 11 patients (15.1%) who developed an endoleak with a type I endoleak in 6 patients and a type II endoleak in 5 patients. Coverage of the left subclavian artery accounted for 3/5 (60%) of the type II endoleaks. The type II endoleaks were successfully treated with coil embolization in 2 patients and ligation of the subclavian artery in the other patient. Our results clearly demonstrate the low incidence of arm complications and type II endoleaks with coverage of the left subclavian artery. A 5-year Kaplan-Meier survival curves comparing patients who had left subclavian artery coverage with those patients who did not have the subclavian coverage did not show any stastistical significance (Figure 9).

With the advancement of technology, it is likely that branched and scalloped endografts will offer another option for dealing with the left subclavian artery. Advanced techniques to fenestrate the endograft material and deploy stents into the great vessels are being pioneered in some institutions [21, 22]. There is currently no consensus regarding how best to handle cases with proximal thoracic aortic pathology. Most experts agree that preventing significant proximal endoleaks is critical for durable success of thoracic endografting in treating thoracic aortic pathologies. Preserving vertebral and

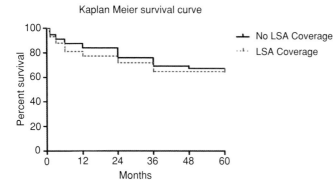

**Figure 9** Kaplan-Meier survival curve. LSA, left subclavian artery.

mammary circulation is critical especially in patients with a dominant left vertebral system and patients with a patent internal mammary bypass graft.

## References

1 Makaroun MS, Dillavou ED, Kes ST *et al.* Endovascular treatment of thoracic aortic aneurysms: results of the phase II multicenter trial of the Gore TAG thoracic endoprosthesis. *J Vasc Surg* 2005; **41**: 1–9.

2 Wheatley GH, III, Gurbuz AT, Rodriguez-Lopez JA *et al.* Midterm outcome in 158 consecutive Gore TAG thoracic endoprostheses: single center experience. *Ann Thorac Surg.* 2006; **81**(5): 1570–1577; discussion 1577.

3 Bavaria JE, Appoo JJ, Makaroun MS, Verter J, Zi-Fan Yu, Scott Mitchell RS. Endovascular stent grafting versus open surgical repair of descending thoracic aortic aneurysms in low-risk patients: a multicenter comparative trial. *J Thorac Cardiovasc Surg* 2007; **133**: 369–377.

4 DeSanctis RW, Dorgoghazi RM, Austen WG, Buckley MJ. Medical progress (aortic dissection). *N Engl J Med* 1987; **317**: 1060–1067.

5 Duhaylongsod FG, Glower DD, Wolfe WG. Acute traumatic aortic aneurysm: the Duke experience from 1970 to 1990. *J Vasc Surg* 1992; **15**: 331–343.

6 Gorich J, Asquan Y, Seifarth H *et al.* Initial experience with intentional stent-graft coverage of the subclavian artery during endovascular thoracic aortic repairs. *J Endovasc Ther* 2002; **9**: II39–II43.

7 Hausegger KA, Oberwalder P, Tiesenhausen K *et al.* Intentional left subclavian artery occlusion by thoracic aortic stent-grafts without surgical transposition. *J Endovasc Ther* 2001; **8**: 472–476.

8 Tiesenhausen K, Hausegger KA, Oberwalder P *et al.* Left subclavian artery management in endovascular repair of thoracic aortic aneurysms and aortic dissections. *J Card Surg* 2003; **18**: 429–435.

9 Dake MD. Endovascular stent-graft management of thoracic aortic diseases. *Eur J Radiol* 2001; **39**: 42–49.

10 Cambria RP, Brewster DC, Lauterbach SR *et al.* Evolving experience with thoracic aortic stent graft repair. *J Vasc Surg* 2002; **35**: 1129–1136.

11 Rehders TC, Petzsch M, Ince H *et al.* Intentional occlusion of the left subclavian artery during stent-graft implantation in the thoracic aorta: risk and relevance. *J Vasc Surg* 2004; **11**: 659–666.

12 Lambrechts D, Casselman F, Schroeyers P, DeGeest R, D'Haenens P, Degrieck I. Endovascular treatment of the descending thoracic aorta. *Eur J Vasc Endovasc Surg* 2003; **26**: 437–444.

13 Moore RD, Brandschwei F. Subclavian-to-carotid transposition and supracarotid endovascular stent graft placement for traumatic aortic disruption. *Ann Vasc Surg* 2001; **15**: 563–566.

14 Burks JA, Faries PL, Gravereaux EC, Hollier LH, Marin ML. Endovascular repair of thoracic aortic aneurysms (stent-graft fixation across the aortic arch vessels). *Ann Vasc Surg* 2002; **16**: 24–28.

15 Criado FJ, Barnatan MF, Rizk Y, Clark NS, Wang CF. Technical strategies to expand stent-graft applicability in the aortic arch and proximal descending thoracic aorta. *J Endovasc Ther* 2002; **9**: II32–II38.

16 Czerny M, Zimpfer D, Fleck T *et al.* Initial results after combined repair of aortic arch aneurysms by sequential transposition of the supra-aortic branches and consecutive endovascular stent-graft placement. *Ann Thorac Surg* 2004; **78**: 1256–1260.

17 Shigemura N, Kato M, Kuratani T, Funakoshi Y, Kaneko M. New operative method for acute type B dissection (left carotid artery-left subclavian artery bypass combined with endovascular stent-graft implantation). *J Thorac Cardiovasc Surg* 2000; **120**: 406–408.

18 Quinones-Baldrich WJ, Marelli D, Esmalian F. Distal aortic arch replacement for aneurysmal disease (the value of

preparatory carotid subclavian reconstruction). *Ann Vasc Surg* 2003; **17**: 148–151.

19 Heijmen RH, Deblier IG, Moll FL *et al.* Endovascular stent-grafting for descending thoracic aortic aneurysms. *Eur J Cardiothorac Surg* 2002; **21**: 5–9.

20 Grabenwoger M, Hutschala D, Ehrlich MP *et al.* Thoracic aortic aneurysms (treatment with endovascular self-expandable stent grafts). *Ann Thorac Surg* 2000; **69**: 441–445.

21 Saito N, Kimura T, Odashiro K *et al.* Feasibility of the In-oue single-branched stent-graft implantation for thoracic aortic aneurysm or dissection involving the left subclavian artery (short- to medium-term results in 17 patients). *J Vasc Surg* 2005; **41**: 206–212.

22 Inoue K, Hosokawa H, Iwase T *et al.* Aortic arch reconstruction by transluminally placed endovascular branched stent graft. *Circulation* 1999; **100**: II316–II321.

# Endovascular management of a thoracic aortic aneurysm with tortuous aorta and calcified iliac arteries using the brachiofemoral wire approach

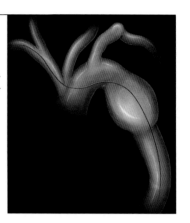

## Introduction

The presence of tortuous, calcified or small femoral, or iliac vessels along with a tortuous, elongated thoracic aorta and an angulated arch pose a technical challenge to deliver an endoluminal graft to the target site. Despite the availability of a flexible delivery sheath system, adjunct techniques are necessary to deal with extremely tortuous thoracic aortas or small, tortuous calcified iliac vessel. The use of a 260-cm brachiofemoral wire with tension applied at both ends of the wire may be a more useful technique than the use of a super-stiff wire in an angulated thoracic arch. Techniques for the small, tortuous, calcified iliac artery including balloon angioplasty and stenting, direct common iliac artery access, common carotid access, trial sheath insertion, retroperitoneal conduit, endoconduit, and direct surgical exposure of the thoracic or abdominal aorta should be part of the tool kit of every practicing endovascular specialist.

## Case scenario

A 75-year-old man with past medical history significant for hypertension, hyperlipidemia, coronary artery disease, chronic obstructive lung disease, and prostate cancer postradiation therapy had been followed regularly for a thoracic aortic aneurysm. A CT scan of the chest performed revealed a thoracic aortic aneurysm had increased in size from 4.0 to 7.0 cm in diameter (Figure 1). He also had a very tortuous aorta and calcified iliac arteries. He was felt to be at an increased risk of rupture and given his numerous comorbidities was felt not to be an open surgical candidate. The presence of a very tortuous thoracic aorta along with calcified iliac arteries increases the technical complexity of deployment of an endoluminal graft.

## Endovascular procedure

Bilateral radial arterial lines were placed and under general anesthesia open retrograde cannulation of the right common femoral artery was performed. Five thousand units of heparin were given.

Percutaneous access of the left common femoral artery was performed and a 9-F (French) sheath was introduced. Bilateral iliac angiograms were performed through each groin sheath. Diffuse stenosis and calcification of both common and external iliac

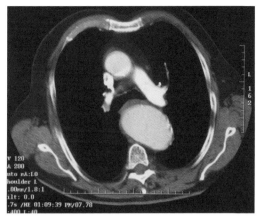

**Figure 1** A CT scan of the chest demonstrating a thoracic aortic aneurysm with a diameter of 7.0 cm.

arteries were identified with a significant pressure gradient compared to bilateral radial arterial lines (Figure 2). An OPTA Pro 10 mm × 40 mm balloon was used to balloon both areas of stenosis with a satisfactory angiographic result and resolution of pressure gradient (Figure 3a and 3b). Due to the severe tortuosity of the aorta, there was great difficulty passing the 5-F pigtail catheter to the thoracic aorta. An oblique thoracic aortogram demonstrated a thoracic aortic aneurysm juxtadistal to the left subclavian artery with a very tortuous angled arch (Figure 4). Intravascular ultrasound was performed

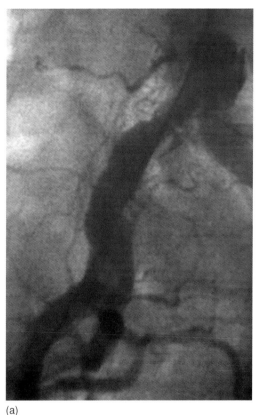

(a)

(b)

**Figure 3** (a and b) An angiogram of both iliac arteries postballoon angioplasty with resolution of stenosis.

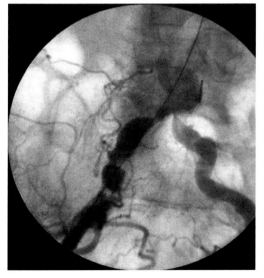

**Figure 2** Retrograde iliac angiogram demonstrating tortuous iliac arteries with areas of stenosis.

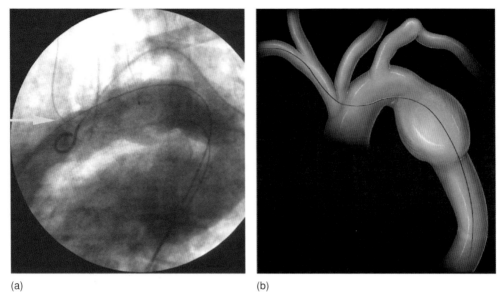

(a)                                                    (b)

**Figure 4** (a and b) Angiogram and illustration demonstrating an extremely angulated arch with a large thoracic aortic aneurysm and a brachiofemoral wire (yellow arrow) in place.

using an 8.2-F probe (Volcano Therapeutics, Inc., Rancho Cordova, CA) through the right groin sheath. A proximal neck diameter at the level of the left carotid artery measured 31 mm × 24 mm and a distal neck diameter at the level of the celiac trunk measured 27 mm × 24 mm. There was thrombus in the aneurysm sac but both proximal and distal landing zones were free of thrombus. Due to the extreme tortuousity of the thoracic arch aorta, it was evident that a thoracic endograft would not be able to negotiate the aortic arch curve and a brachiofemoral wire conduit was required to help navigate the tortuous aortic arch. A retrograde percutaneous right brachial approach was performed with a 6-F 35-cm sheath. Using a 5-F Bernstein catheter as a guiding catheter, a 260-cm-long, 0.035-in. soft-tip angled glide, wires was negotiated into the tortuous descending thoracic aorta under fluoroscopic guidance. The wire was subsequently secured through the right groin sheath with the help of a snare (Microvena). A glide catheter was exchanged over the 260-cm-long, 0.035-in. soft-tip angled glide wire and an exchange to a stiff Lunderquist wire (Cook Inc., Bloomington, IN) was performed. The 9-F sheath in the right groin was exchanged to a 22-F sheath which was advanced into the distal abdominal aorta. The fluoroscopic C-arm was angled in an extreme left anterior oblique angle and an oblique thoracic aortic angiogram was performed through the left groin sheath pigtail catheter and a road map obtained. By keeping a constant tension on the brachiofemoral wire conduit from the right brachial end and the right common femoral end a 34 mm × 20 cm Gore TAG device (W.L. Gore & Associates, Flagstaff, AZ) was advanced through the tortuous descending aorta into the arch and deployed distal to the left carotid artery covering partially the left subclavian artery. A 31 mm × 15 cm Gore TAG device was subsequently deployed distally just above the celiac trunk after an aortogram had been performed to demarcate the distal landing zone on road map. A third device, 34 mm × 15 cm Gore TAG device, was necessary to cover the area of overlap between the proximal and distal endografts. A completion angiogram demonstrated successful exclusion of the thoracic aortic aneurysm with no endoleak (Figure 5). The 22-F sheath was then exchanged to a 9-F sheath and bilateral iliac angiograms demonstrated no extravasation of contrast. Bilateral express 10 mm × 37 cm self-expandable stents were subsequently deployed at the area of previous balloon angioplasty. Completion angiogram demonstrated

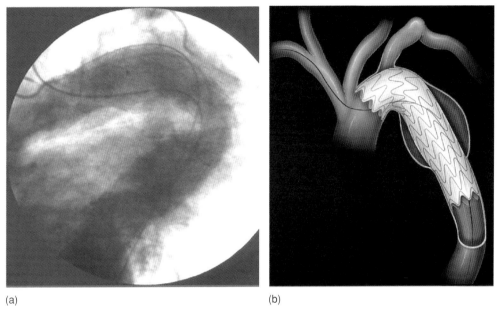

(a)            (b)

**Figure 5** (a) A completion angiogram demonstrating exclusion of thoracic aortic aneurysm with no demonstrable endoleak. (b) Illustration of endoluminal graft deployed using a brachiofemoral wire.

satisfactory angiographic pictures with brisk flow through the iliac vessels and no pressure gradient. Sheaths and wires were removed and the right common femoral artery was closed in a transverse fashion with restoration of flow. A 6-F angioseal closure device (St. Jude Medical, Inc., St. Paul, MN) was deployed to the left common femoral artery. Patient had bilateral palpable pulses at the end of the procedure. He was extubated and transferred to the recovery room. A postoperative CT scan (Figure 6) demonstrated no endoleak with exclusion of thoracic aortic aneurysm.

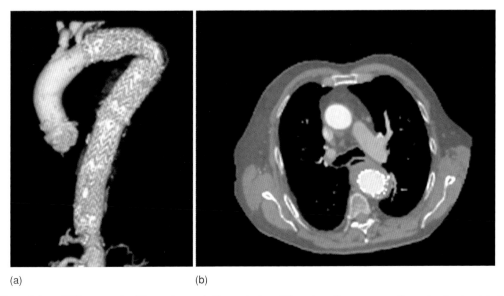

(a)            (b)

**Figure 6** (a and b) Postoperative CT scan demonstrating exclusion of thoracic aortic aneurysm with no visualized endoleak.

## Discussion

Despite improved surgical techniques, the operative mortality with open surgical repair of descending thoracic aortic aneurysms is between 4.8 and 20% [1, 2]. Many authors [3–6] have confirmed the decreased morbidity and mortality with thoracic stent grafts to treat thoracic aortic aneurysms. Results of the recent multicenter phase II trial [7–9] further confirmed that patients treated with a Gore TAG stent graft (W.L. Gore & Associates, Flagstaff, AZ) for the management of a thoracic aortic aneurysm had a decreased mortality 2.1% versus 11.7% ($p <$ .001) compared to open surgical repair. Conduits were required in 15% of the TAG group to provide access for sheath delivery. Intraoperative vascular complications occurred more commonly in the TAG group 14% versus 4% in the control open surgical group.

Problems relating to vascular access for stent grafts occur up to 28% of cases and are prevalent in patients with iliofemoral occlusive disease, small vessels size, iliofemoral tortuosity, and calcified vessels [10, 11]. Vascular access issues were responsible in close to half of the failures to qualify for a stent graft in one study [12]. Adequate preoperative imaging is paramount for planning access during endovascular repair of the thoracic aorta using a stent graft. Use of CT angiography provides satisfactory examination of iliofemoral lumen size; presence of vascular occlusive disease or totuosity is vital to planning and for dealing with possible complications that may arise during or after the procedure [13]. The recommended graft delivery sheath size for thoracic stent grafts (Table 1) should be adhered to judiciously to avoid access complications.

**Table 1** Graft and delivery sheath sizes for descending thoracic aortic stent grafts currently available in the United States.

| Endograft | Graft size available (diameter) (mm) | Sheath size required (diameter) |
|---|---|---|
| Gore TAG | 26–40 | 20–24 F (7.6–9.2 mm) |
| Zenith TX1/TX2 | 28–42 | 20–22 F (7.6–8.3 mm) |
| Talent | 22–46 | 22–25 F |

TAG, thoracic aortic graft.

An endovascular technique of balloon angioplasty and iliac stenting for patients with iliofemoral occlusive disease allows passage of a large caliber delivery sheath in an artery that is otherwise stenosed and calcified. Balloon dilatation, however, will often not overcome all difficulties encountered with small vessel size and, in such cases, an iliofemoral conduit is the better option. Self-expanding stents or covered stents can be deployed to repair the vessel wall injuries. The kissing technique should be employed to prevent compromise of the contralateral iliac artery. Use of an "endoconduit" such as a Viabhan covered stent (W.L. Gore & Associates, Flagstaff, AZ) to line the diseased iliofemoral vessel and crack the calcified plaque with an oversized balloon have been used with success resulting in a lower rate of iliofemoral conduits to deliver large sheaths.

In the Gore TAG population of our patients, the 40-mm device was used in 30.8%, 37-mm in 26.8%, 34-mm in 29.1%, 31-mm in 6.6%, 28-mm 5.0%, and 26-mm in 1.7%. A conduit was required in 31 patients (8%) compared to the phase II multicenter study of 15% (Figure 1). Femoral delivery of the sheath was successful in 88% of our patients with 4% undergoing delivery by a bareback technique. The bareback technique is not recommended by the Instructions for Use (W.L. Gore & Associates, Flagstaff, AZ). Delivery of the device in this manner leaves the graft exposed to potential damage by disease in the iliac artery. Our 30-day mortality was 6.2% with at least 7 deaths that can be attributed to complications associated with device delivery. Iliac rupture following removal of sheath occurred in 2 patients (Figure 7).

Use of brachiofemoral access wires can help straighten the most angulated of vessels. The technique requires that a protective guiding catheter be placed over the brachial artery to protect the subclavian artery from injury. It is important to have at least a 260-cm-long wire and constant tension must be placed on both ends of the wire as the delivery sheath is passed into the aorta.

Caution should always be exercised when passing a large sheath in a tortuous, calcified, or small access vessel. The prudent surgeon must always ensure that a guide wire remain in the aorta upon removal of a delivery sheath and an aortic occlusion balloon should always be in the operating room.

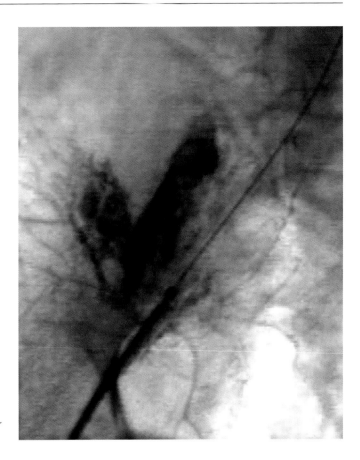

**Figure 7** A retrograde iliac angiogram through the groin sheath demonstrating extravasation of contrast signifying an iliac rupture after removal of a device sheath.

Risk of avulsion or rupture of an iliac artery should always be suspected if the patient becomes hypotensive upon removal of the sheath. A retrograde iliac angiogram should always be performed on removal of a delivery sheath to confirm or exclude an iliac rupture. In cases of rupture, the occlusion balloon should be advanced and inflated. A covered stent can be used to line the area of extravasation or the injured vessel could be exposed and repaired.

In conclusion, proper preparation with adequate imaging should allow successful and safe endovascular repair of the thoracic aorta even in difficult access situations.

## References

1 Coselli JS, LeMaire SA, Miller CC *et al.* Mortality and paraplegia after thoracoabdominal aortic aneurysm repair (a risk factor analysis). *Ann Thorac Surg* 2000; **69**: 409–414.

2 Brandt M, Hussel K, Walluscheck KP, Boning A, Rahimi A, Cremer J. Early and long-term results of replacement of the descending aorta. *Eur J Vasc Endovasc Surg* 2005; **30**: 365–369.

3 Dake MD, Miller DC, Semba CP, Mitchell RS, Walker PJ, Liddell RP. Transluminal placement of endovascular stent-grafts for the treatment of descending thoracic aortic aneurysms. *N Engl J Med* 1994; **331**: 1729–1734.

4 Gaines PA, Gerrard DJ, Reidy JF, Beard JB, Taylor PR. The endovascular management of thoracic aortic disease— some controversial issues. *Eur J Vasc Endovasc Surg* 2002; **23**: 162–164.

5 Wheatley GH III, Gurbuz AT, Rodriguez-Lopez JA *et al.* Midterm outcome in 158 consecutive Gore TAG thoracic endoprostheses: single center experience. *Ann Thorac Surg* 2006; **81**(5): 1570-1577; discussion 1577.

6 Greenberg RK, O'Neill S, Walker E *et al.* Endovascular repair of thoracic aortic lesions with the Zenith TX1 and TX2 thoracic grafts (intermediate-term results). *J Vasc Surg* 2005; **41**: 589–596.

7 Bavaria JE, Appoo JJ, Makaroun MS, Verter J, Zi-Fan Yu, Scott Mitchell RS. Endovascular stent grafting versus open

surgical repair of descending thoracic aortic aneurysms in low-risk patients: a multicenter comparative trial. *J Thorac Cardiovasc Surg* 2007; **133**: 369–377.

8 Makaroun MS, Dillavou ED, Kee ST *et al.* Endovascular treatment of thoracic aortic aneurysms (results of the phase II multicenter trial of the GORE TAG thoracic endoprosthesis). *J Vasc Surg* 2005; **41**: 1–9.

9 Gore TAG Thoracic Endoprosthesis Annual Clinical Update, September 2006.

10 Fairman RM, Velazquez O, Baum R *et al.* Endovascular repair of aortic aneurysms (critical events and adjunctive procedures). *J Vasc Surg* 2001; **33**: 1226–1232.

11 Yano OJ, Faries PL, Morrissey N, Teodorescu V, Hollier LH, Marin ML. Ancillary techniques to facilitate endovascular repair of aortic aneurysms. *J Vasc Surg* 2001; **34**: 69–75.

12 Carpenter JP, Baum RA, Barker CF *et al.* Impact of exclusion criteria on patient selection for endovascular abdominal aortic aneurysm repair. *J Vasc Surg* 2001; **34**: 1050–1054.

13 Lal BK, Cerveira JJ, Seidman C *et al.* Observer variability of iliac artery measurements in endovascular repair of abdominal aortic aneurysms. *Ann Vasc Surg* 2004; **18**: 644–652.

# CASE 6

# Endovascular management of a thoracic aortic aneurysm with small tortuous calcified iliac vessels (retroperitoneal conduit)

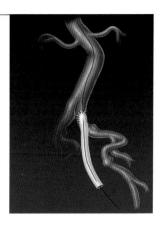

## Introduction

Problems related to vascular access for stent grafts occur in up to 28% of cases and are related to iliofemoral occlusive disease, small vessel size, and excessive iliofemoral tortuosity [1, 2]. Many patients are not able to be candidates for endoluminal graft therapy due to suboptimal vascular access, aortic arch angulation, and landing zone inadequacies. Currently, available endografts in the United States require delivery sheaths ranging from 20 to 25-F (French) depending on the size of the graft required to treat the aorta (Table 1).

Patients with calcified, tortuous, and small vessel size may not be candidates for delivery of large sheaths through femoral access and are at an increased risk of iliac artery rupture or the "artery on a stick" phenomenon. Retroperitoneal exposure with construction of a 10-mm iliofemoral conduit is a technique that permits delivery of large sheaths in patients with tortuous, calcified, and small iliac vessels or vessels with severe iliofemoral vascular occlusive disease.

## Case scenario

An 81-year-old female was admitted to the hospital for chest and abdominal pain. She had a past

medical history significant for diverticulitis, chronic bronchitis with steroid dependence, history of a small abdominal aortic aneurysm, and a strong history of smoking. A CT scan of the chest abdomen and pelvis was ordered for evaluation of her pain and a 6.0-cm descending thoracic aortic aneurysm in association with a 3.2-cm infrarenal abdominal aortic aneurysm was identified (Figure 1). She was noted to have small tortuous and calcified iliac arteries on her CT scan (Figure 2). Due to her comorbidities she was felt to be a high-risk surgical candidate and enrolled in a single-site investigational device exemption study for endoluminal graft placement.

## Recommendations

The presence of small, tortuous, or calcified iliac arteries increases the risk of rupture if a large sheath is introduced for the delivery of an endoluminal graft into the thoracic aorta. Current recommendations for the Gore TAG device delivery through a Gore sheath are resummarized in Table 2.

## Endovascular procedure

Under general anesthesia, open exposure of the right common femoral artery was performed. The

**Table 1** Graft and delivery sheath sizes for descending thoracic aortic stent grafts currently available in the United States.

| Endograft | Graft size available (diameter) (mm) | Sheath size required (diameter) |
|---|---|---|
| Gore TAG | 26–40 | 20–24 F (7.6–9.2 mm) |
| Zenith TX1/TX2 | 28–42 | 20–22 F (7.6–8.3 mm) |
| Talent | 22–46 | 22–25 F |

right common femoral artery was noted to be small and heavily calcified. Open retrograde puncture of the right common femoral artery was performed with an 18-G (Cook Inc., Bloomington, IN) needle and attempts to cannulate the right common iliac artery with a 0.035-in. soft-tip angled glide wire under fluoroscopic guidance beyond the external iliac

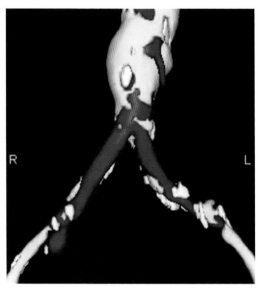

**Figure 2** A reconstructed CT scan demonstrating small-sized iliac vessels with diffuse calcification and stenosis of bilateral external iliac arteries.

artery was met with resistance with an area of dissection created from the wire.

Percutaneous access of the left common femoral artery was performed with an 18-G needle and a 0.035-in. soft-tip angled glide wire could not be advanced. A retrograde percutaneous left brachial approach was performed with a 6-F sheath. Using a 5-F guiding catheter, a 0.035-in. soft-tip angled glide wire was advanced into a very tortuous aorta with two curvatures. A 5-F pigtail angiographic catheter was exchanged for the guiding catheter and an aortogram demonstrated a very tortuous aorta, a large thoracic aortic aneurysm, and small bilateral common iliac arteries with near total occlusion of both external iliac arteries (Figure 3). The right common iliac artery was measured to be 7.0 mm with 6.5 mm on the left side. It was evident that the both iliac

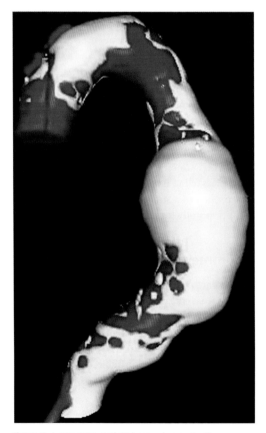

**Figure 1** A reconstructed CT image demonstrating a descending thoracic aortic aneurysm of 6.0 cm in diameter.

**Table 2** Recommended iliac diameters for the introduction of Gore sheaths.

| Size (F) | ID (mm) | OD (mm) |
|---|---|---|
| 20 | 6.7 | 7.6 |
| 22 | 7.3 | 8.3 |
| 24 | 8.1 | 9.1 |

ID, inner diameter; OD, outer diameter.

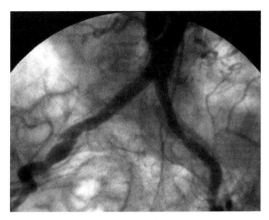

**Figure 3** An angiogram demonstrating small, tortuous iliac vessels.

arteries were prohibitive in nature for the delivery of the device sheath. A retroperitoneal conduit was the only way to deliver an endograft into the thoracic aorta in this patient.

## Retroperitoneal conduit with deployment of endograft

A 15-cm semilunar right flank incision was made four finger breaths above the right groin crease. Division of the external oblique, internal oblique, and transversus abdominus muscle was performed. The peritoneum was identified and gently retracted medially with the help of a retractor. The right common iliac artery along with the hypogastric and the external iliac artery was identified and mobilized. Care was taken to spare the right urether which crossed the common iliac artery before diving into the pelvis. Rummel tourniquets were applied at the proximal right common iliac artery, right external iliac artery, and origin of the hypogastric artery. Five thousand units of heparin were given to the patient. An arteriotomy was made on the right common iliac artery close to the bifurcation with the hypogastric artery and a 10-mm Dacron conduit sewn in an end-to-side fashion using 5-0 Prolene suture. The 10-mm graft was subsequently tunneled through the retroperitoneal space beneath the inguinal ligament and brought out through the right groin incision that had been performed to expose the right common femoral artery. The graft was flashed and clamped at the right groin incision

and the rummel tourniquets released from the right common iliac artery, external iliac artery, and hypogastric artery. The 10-mm conduit was looped with a rummel tourniquet and punctured with an 18-G Cook (Cook Inc., Bloomington, IN) needle; a 0.035-in. glide wire was advanced under fluoroscopic guidance into the thoracic arch and the needle exchanged for a 9-F sheath. A pigtail catheter was advanced up the thoracic arch and an oblique thoracic aortogram was performed and saved as a road map for deployment of endograft (Figure 4). An intravascular ultrasound (IVUS) 8.2-F probe was advanced through the conduit sheath again to confirm the measurements of the neck diameter. A Lunderquist wire (Cook Inc., Bloomington, IN) was exchanged through the IVUS catether. A 22-F sheath was exchanged for the 9-F sheath through the 10-mm conduit, and under fluoroscopic guidance deployment of 34 mm × 20 cm Gore TAG thoracic endoluminal grafts (W.L. Gore & Associates, Flagstaff, AZ) was deployed distal to the left subclavian artery excluding the thoracic aortic aneurysm (Figure 5). Completion angiogram demonstrated complete exclusion of the thoracic aortic aneurysm with no endoleak (Figure 6). Wires and sheaths were removed from the 10-mm conduit. The conduit was clamped. Adequate exposure of the left common femoral artery was performed, proximal

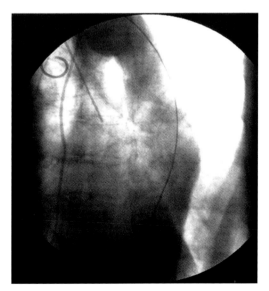

**Figure 4** An angiogram demonstrating a thoracic aortic aneurysm measuring 6.0 cm in diameter.

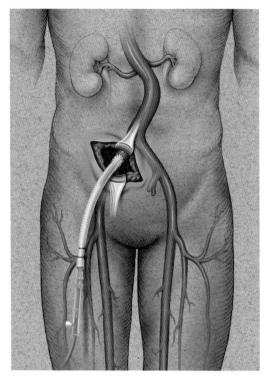

**Figure 5** A right retroperitoneal incision with a 10-mm conduit sewn to the right common iliac artery and connected to a device delivery sheath for deployment of endoluminal graft to the thoracic aorta.

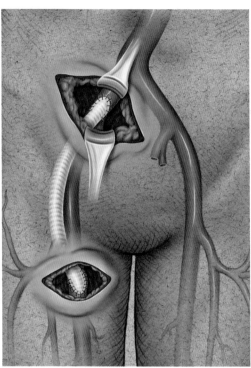

**Figure 7** A retroperitoneal iliac conduit sewn as an end-to-side bypass graft to the right common femoral artery as an iliofemoral bypass graft.

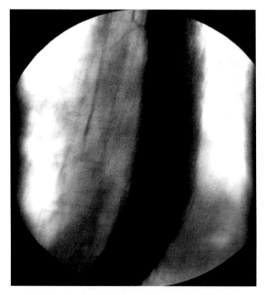

**Figure 6** A completion angiogram demonstrating satisfactory exclusion of thoracic aortic aneurysm with no endoleak.

and distal control of the right common femoral artery was achieved, and an arteriotomy was made with the right 10-mm iliac limb conduit sewn as an end-to-side anastomosis on the right common femoral artery (Figure 7). Adequate flushing maneuvers were performed prior to completion of the anastomosis. The right groin incision was approximated. The right sheath was removed and a closure device used to achieve hemostasis. The right flank incision was irrigated; a 10-F Jackson Pratt drain was placed and the incision closed in layers. The patient was returned to the recovery room, extubated and pulses palpable in both lower extremities. A postoperative CT scan demonstrated satisfactory exclusion of thoracic aneurysm with no endoleak (Figure 8a and 8b).

## Discussion

A retroperitoneal, iliofemoral conduit is the most widely used bypass technique for access during

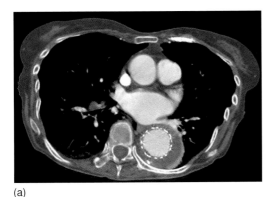

(a)

(b)

**Figure 8** (a and b) Postoperative CT scan demonstrating exclusion of the thoracic aneurysm with no identifiable endoleak.

endovascular repair of descending thoracic aortic aneurysms. Retroperitoneal conduits have been used in up to 22% of reported series [3–6]. In the phase II multicenter Gore TAG trial [4] access

using retroperitoneal conduits were used in 15% of cases of endovascular repair of thoracic aortic aneurysms. At our institution, retroperitoneal conduit was used in 8% of cases for sheath delivery [7]. Indications for use of retroperitoneal conduit include small vessel size, diseased access vessels, and tortuosity of access vessels. Currently, there does not exist a grading system to determine which patients would require a retroperitoneal conduit and, as such, clinical judgment along with careful preoperative imaging of access vessels should be taken into account. Tunneling of the conduit from the abdominal wall to the groin through a separate incision is recommended in obese patients to allow for optimal working angles. We recommend that the conduit be tunneled through separate groin incisions and sewed to the femoral artery as an iliofemoral bypass rather than oversewing the graft in patients with diseased iliac arteries who in future may need access for another procedure requiring sheath delivery.

## References

1 Fairman RM, Velazquez O, Baum R *et al.* Endovascular repair of aortic aneurysms (critical events and adjunctive procedures). *J Vasc Surg* 2001; **33**: 1226–1232.

2 Yano OJ, Faries PL, Morrissey N, Teodorescu V, Hollier LH, Marin ML. Ancillary techniques to facilitate endovascular repair of aortic aneurysms. *J Vasc Surg* 2001; **34**: 69–75.

3 Greenberg RK, O'Neill S, Walker E *et al.* Endovascular repair of thoracic aortic lesions with the Zenith TX1 and TX2 thoracic grafts (intermediate-term results). *J Vasc Surg* 2005; **41**: 589–596.

4 Makaroun MS, Dillavou ED, Kee ST *et al.* Endovascular treatment of thoracic aortic aneurysms (results of the phase II multicenter trial of the GORE TAG thoracic endoprosthesis). *J Vasc Surg* 2005; **41**: 1–9.

5 Fairman RM, Velazquez O, Baum R *et al.* Endovascular repair of aortic aneurysms (critical events and adjunctive procedures). *J Vasc Surg* 2001; **33**: 1226–1232.

6 Wellons ED, Milner R, Solis M, Levitt A, Rosenthal D. Stent-graft repair of traumatic thoracic aortic disruptions. *J Vasc Surg* 2004; **40**: 1095–1100.

7 Wheatley GH, III, Gurbuz AT, Rodriguez-Lopez JA *et al.* Midterm outcome in 158 consecutive Gore TAG thoracic endoprostheses: single center experience. *Ann Thorac Surg* 2006; **81**(5): 1570–1577; discussion 1577.

# Endovascular management of a ruptured thoracic aortic aneurysm

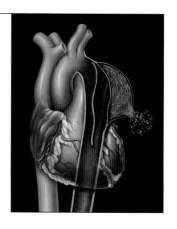

## Introduction

Thoracic aortic rupture is a lethal condition associated with high mortality. The most common cause of thoracic aortic rupture is from trauma. Other less common causes include rupture from acute type B and type A dissections, penetrating aortic ulcers, intramural hematomas, degenerative aortic thoracic aortic aneurysms, and pseudoaneurysms from coarctation of the aorta. Thoracic aortic rupture may be contained resulting in an unstable patient with hypotension or may present as free rupture into the chest cavity, mediastinum resulting in ultimate death if not managed emergently. Endovascular management with an endoluminal graft offers a minimal invasive option with a decrease in morbidity and mortality in a group of patients with a very high risk for any open surgical repair.

## Case scenario

An 89-year-old female with past medical history significant for arthritis and abdominal aortic aneurysm presented with severe abdominal and back pain, and on physical examination she was found to be hypotensive with a drop in hemoglobin count. A CT scan of the chest and abdomen revealed a thoracoabdominal aneurysm measuring 7.0 cm in diameter with an area of rupture with extravasation of contrast into the left chest. An associated moderate pleural left effusion was present. She was resuscitated with blood products and was at high risk for any open surgical repair and

therefore considered a candidate for endoluminal graft under an investigational device exemption protocol.

## Endovascular approach

Under general anesthesia open retrograde cannulation of both common femoral arteries was performed with an 18-G Cook (Cook Inc., Bloomington, IN) needle and 0.035-in. soft-tip angled glide wire were advanced into the thoracic aortic arch. Nine-French (F) sheaths were advanced through both groins. Heparin was given to the patient to keep the activated clotting time greater than 200 seconds. A 5-F pigtail angiographic catheter was advanced through the left groin 9-F sheath to the thoracic aortic arch for an angiogram. An oblique thoracic aortogram Figure 1 demonstrated thoracic aortic aneurysm with site of rupture distal to the left subclavian artery. An intravascular ultrasound (IVUS) 8.2-F probe (Volcano Therapeutics, Inc., Rancho Cordova, CA) was advanced through the right groin sheath to the thoracic aorta, and the diameter of the proximal neck at the level of the left common carotid artery was measured at 34 mm. Distal neck diameter at the level of the celiac artery was measured at 36 mm in diameter. The length of aorta to be covered measured 35 cm in length. Based on the measurements a 37 mm × 20 cm Gore TAG excluder graft (W.L. Gore & Associates, Flagstaff, AZ) was chosen for deployment in the proximal thoracic aorta with a 40 mm × 20 cm Gore TAG graft to be deployed in

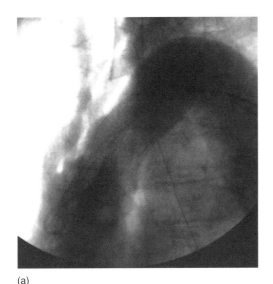

(a)

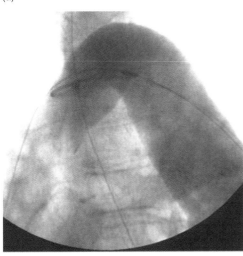

(b)

**Figure 1** (a and b) Thoracic aortogram demonstrating thoracic aortic aneurysm with mild extrvasation of contrast suggestive of thoracic aortic rupture.

tained from the IVUS and the angiogram. A second device 40 mm × 20 cm was deployed distal to the first endograft making sure we had adequate overlap between the endografts and had covered the area of aneurysm rupture. A completion angiogram (Figure 2) showed exclusion of the aneurysm with no endoleak. All wires and sheaths were removed; both common femoral arteries were closed in a transverse fashion with restoration of flow. Patient had bilateral palpable pulses at the end of the procedure and was extubated and transferred to recovery room. A postoperative CT scan (Figure 3a and 3b) performed demonstrated satisfactory exclusion of the area of thoracic aortic rupture with no identifiable endoleak.

## Discussion

Thoracic aortic rupture has been associated mostly with trauma victims with the majority dying at the site of the accident. The patients that do make it to the hospital are often hemodynamically unstable. Open surgical repair requires in simple cases use of clamp and sew techniques or left atriofemoral bypass using a centrifugal pump. The risk of paraplegia seems to be higher after clamp and sew techniques than after bypass unless clamp time is less than

the distal aorta. Consideration was given to possible coverage of the left subclavian artery to achieve an adequate landing zone to exclude area of rupture. A stiff Lundiqist wire (Cook Inc., Bloomington, IN) was exchanged through the IVUS catheter. The right 9-F sheath was exchanged for a 24-F Gore sheath and the 37 mm × 20 cm Gore device was advanced through the Gore sheath and subsequently deployed over an extra-stiff wire after marking the exact proximal and distal landing zones on our road map ob-

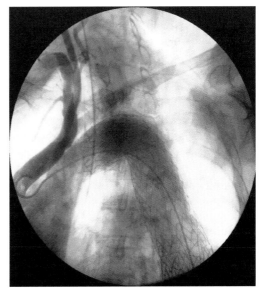

**Figure 2** Completion angiogram demonstrating satisfactory exclusion of thoracic aortic rupture. No endoleak is noted.

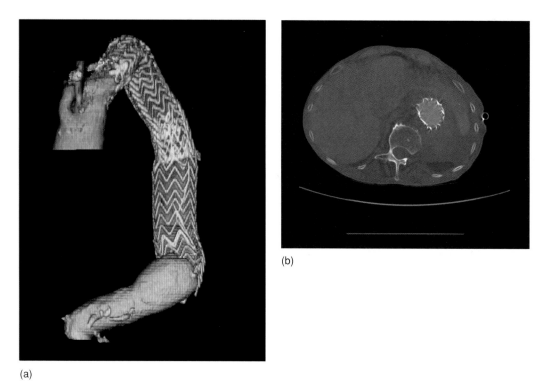

(b)

(a)

**Figure 3** (a and b) CT scan of the chest demonstrating exclusion of thoracic aortic aneurysm rupture with no identifiable endoleak.

30 minutes [1]. Endovascular stent grafts have been approved in the United States for the management of thoracic aortic aneurysms with decreased morbidity, mortality, and risk of paraplegia [2, 3] and avoids a thoracotomy with aortic cross clamping with heperinization.

Traumatic aortic rupture disruption often involves the aortic isthmus immediately distal to the left subclavian artery requiring mandatory coverage of the left subclavian artery to achieve adequate length of proximal neck. Although coverage of the left subclavian artery is generally well tolerated and does not cause complications, cerebral problems and upper extremity claudication have been described [4]. Aortic ruptures associated with thoracic aortic aneurysms are related to the size of the aorta [5] with ruptures-associated fatalities in 33–50% of the patients with comorbidities related to the remaining deaths [6, 7]. Endovascular stent-graft application to thoracic aortic rupture should be tailored to the aortic pathology. In traumatic thoracic aortic rupture the aorta is often normal proximally and distal to the area of pathology, which means short-length stent grafts can be used to exclude the area of rupture which may result in a low risk of paraplegia. Challenges associated with trauma patients include small thoracic aortas which sometimes require customizing off-the-shelf abdominal endoluminal graft components and problems with small access sites. Coverage of the left subclavian artery is almost always required since the pathology tends to be confined to the aortic isthmus. Thoracic aortic ruptures from thoracic aortic aneurysms, aortic penetrating ulcers, and type B dissections may require longer length of aorta to be covered with a possible increase in risk of paraplegia.

In conclusion, the endovascular management of patients with thoracic aortic rupture from various etiologies can be successfully managed with an endoluminal graft with acceptable procedural morbidity and mortality.

## References

1 Fabian TC, Richardson JD, Groce MD *et al*. Prospective study of blunt aortic injury. Multicenter trial of the American association for the surgery of trauma. *J Trauma* 1997; **42**: 374–383.

2 Makaroun MS, Dillavou ED, Kes ST *et al.* Endovascular treatment of thoracic aortic aneurysms: results of the phase II multicenter trial of the Gore TAG thoracic endoprosthesis. *J Vasc Surg* 2005; **41**: 1–9.

3 Bavaria JE, Appoo JJ, Makaroun MS, Verter J, Zi-Fan Yu, Scott Mitchell RS. Endovascular stent grafting versus open surgical repair of descending thoracic aortic aneurysms in low-risk patients: a multicenter comparative trial. *J Thorac Cardiovasc Surg* 2007; **133**: 369–377.

4 Orend KH, Pamler R, Kapfer X, Liewald F, Gorich J, Sunder-Plassmann L. Endovascular repair of traumatic descending aortic transection. *J Endovasc Ther* 2002; **9**: 573–578.

5 Juvonen T, Ergin A, Galla JD *et al.* Prospective study of the natural history of thoracic aortic aneurysms. *Ann Thorac Surg* 1997; **63**: 1533–1545.

6 Bickerstaff LK, Paireloro PC, Hollier LH *et al.* Thoracic aortic aneurysms: a population based study. *Surgery* 1982; **92**: 1103–1108.

7 McNamara JJ, Pressler VM. Natural history of arteriosclerotic thoracic aortic aneurysms. *Ann Thorac Surg* 1978; **26**: 468–473.

# Total percutaneous endovascular management of a thoracic aneurysm with severe iliofemoral occlusive disease: use of an endoconduit in a high-risk patient

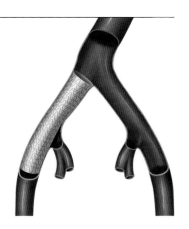

## Introduction

Management of thoracic aortic aneurysms (TAAs) with a thoracic endograft requires patients to have access vessels able to tolerate sheath sizes of 20–25 F (French).

Many patients with multiple comorbidities and diseased iliac vessels are often denied access to endoluminal graft therapy. The use of percutaeous techniques for the access and delivery of endoluminal grafts in patients with iliofemoral vascular occlusive disease may offer such high-risk patients the possibility of being managed with an endoluminal graft without requiring general anesthesia.

## Case scenario

An 80-year-old gentleman with a history of coronary artery bypass graft surgery, hypertension, iliofemoral vascular occlusive disease, and chronic obstructive pulmonary disease requiring home oxygen presented with increasing back pain. His physical examination was notable for decreased femoral pulses and a decreased ankle brachial index. On further evaluation, a CT scan of the chest and abdomen, he was found to have a thoracoabdominal aneurysm with the thoracic component measuring 7.0 cm and the infrarenal component measuring 3.0 cm (Figure 1). The thoracic arch was very tortuous and the proximal neck diameter was measured at 29 mm with a short distal neck component measured at 31 mm. Due to his numerous comorbidities, concerns about diseased vessel access he was felt not to be an open surgical candidate. He was offered the possibility of an endoluminal graft under local/sedation with a percutaneous approach and the possibility of an endoconduit.

## Endovascular procedure

Under local anesthesia with mild sedation, percutaneous cannulation of the right common femoral artery was performed with an 18-G needle and a 0.035-in. soft-tip angled glide wire (Medi-tech/Boston Scientific, Natick, MA) was passed in the thoracic aorta and exchanged to a 9-F sheath under fluoroscopic visualization. Percutaneous access of the left common femoral artery was similarly performed and a 5-F sheath introduced. A retrograde iliac angiogram performed demonstrated diffuse

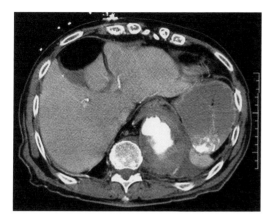

**Figure 1** A CT scan of the chest demonstrating a 7.0-cm TAA.

bilateral iliac disease (Figure 2). There was a focal segment of disease in the left iliac artery that could be amenable to balloon angioplasty. A Prostar Perclose device was chosen for delivery of endoluminal graft. The left groin 9-F (sheath) was exchanged for a single, monorail, 10-F Prostar XL device (Perclose, an Abbott Laboratory Company, Redwood City, CA). The two Perclose sutures were placed before the arteriotomy was enlarged by the endograft deployment sheaths. After confirmation of arterial flow through the marker lumen, the barrel was aligned and the ring withdrawn. The proper amount of tension was maintained on the shaft so

that the artery was not compressed when the needles were deployed. This technique ensured that the sutures were placed adjacent to the arteriotomy and only in the anterior arterial wall. The two Perclose 3-0 braided polyester sutures (one device) were deployed through the artery wall when the ring was pulled back completely. The needles were removed from the back end of the Perclose housing and each needle cut from the suture. The closure device was partially withdrawn from the artery and the four suture ends retrieved. The two Perclose sutures (four suture ends) were left, untied, to rest upon the patient in radial orientation until after the endograft deployment had been completed. We then gave 5000 units of heparin to keep the activated clotted time greater than 200 seconds. A Lunderquist guide wire (Cook Inc., Bloomington, IN) access was regained through the monorail side port on the shaft of the closure device and a 12-F groin sheath passed into the aorta over a stiff wire and through the untied sutures. Balloon angioplasty of the left common iliac artery was performed with an OPTA Pro 9 mm × 4 cm balloon with angiographic resolution of the focal area of stenosis as demonstrated by a retrograde left iliac angiogram (Figure 3). A 5-F pigtail angiographic catheter was advanced through the right groin sheath into the thoracic aorta. The fluoroscopic C-arm was positioned in a left

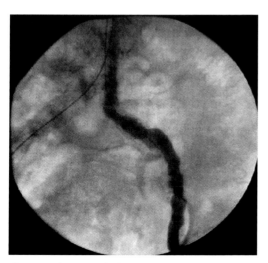

**Figure 2** Left retrograde iliac angiogram demonstrating a diseased iliac vessel.

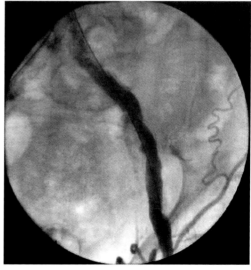

**Figure 3** Retrograde left iliac angiogram after postballoon angioplasty.

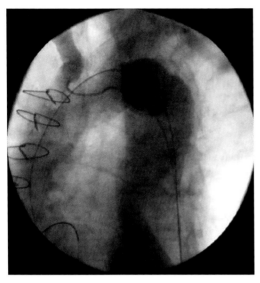

**Figure 4** An angiogram demonstrating a TAA measuring 7.0 cm in diameter.

anterior oblique angle and an oblique thoracic arch aortogram was performed to visualize the orifices of the arch vessels and the descending TAA (Figure 4). Intravascular ultrasound (IVUS) was

performed using an 8.2-F probe (Volcano Therapeutics, Inc., Rancho Cordova, CA). The IVUS catheter was advanced through the left groin sheath to confirm the size of aneurysm, presence or absence of thrombus, proximal neck diameter and length, distal neck diameter and length. The IVUS measurements were similar to those measured on the CT scan. Based on the measurements a 34 mm × 15 cm TAG stent graft was chosen. The IVUS catheter was exchanged for an extra-stiff 260-cm Lunderquist wire (Cook Inc., Bloomington, IN). Attempt to deliver the 22-F Gore sheath up the left common iliac artery was met with resistance. A decision was made to use an endoconduit for delivery of the thoracic endograft instead of the conventional iliofemoral conduit due to high-risk comorbidities that precluded open surgical techniques under general anesthesia. The 22-F sheath was exchanged to a 9-F sheath and a 13 mm × 10 cm Gore Viahbahn endoluminal graft was deployed across the left common iliac and external iliac artery covering the hypogastric vessels (Figure 5). Postdeployment balloon angioplasty was performed with a 12 mm × 4 cm Synergy balloon to the left common

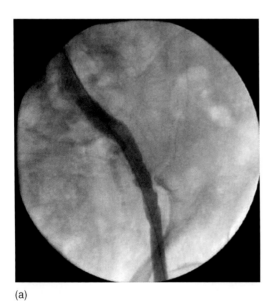

(a)

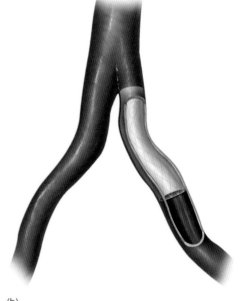

(b)

**Figure 5** (a) Retrograde left iliac angiogram after successful deployment of an endoconduit. (b) Illustration demonstrating a deployment of an endoluminal graft to

the left common iliac and external iliac artery to be used as an endoconduit for delivery of 22-F Gore delivery sheath.

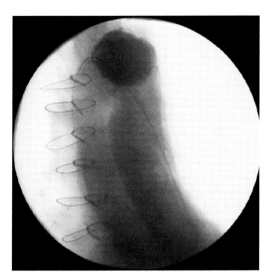

**Figure 6** A completion angiogram demonstrating complete exclusion of TAA with an endoluminal graft.

iliac endoluminal graft. The 9-F sheath was subsequently exchanged to a 22-F Gore delivery sheath that tracked pretty smoothly up to the descending thoracic aorta. A 34 mm × 15 cm TAG stentgraft device (W.L. Gore & Associates, Flagstaff, AZ) was advanced through the Gore sheath and subsequently deployed over an extra-stiff wire after marking the exact proximal and distal landing zones on our road map angiogram. A Gore trilobe balloon was used to perform postdeployment balloon angioplasty to the proximal and distal segments of the graft for good fixation. A completion angiogram demonstrated exclusion of the aneurysm with no endoleak (Figure 6). All wires and sheaths were removed from the left common femoral artery; the sutures were generously soaked with heparinized saline and wiped free of any thrombus and then subsequently tied with a slipknot or a standard surgeon's knot while an assistant maintained proximal manual pressure. A 6/5 Boomerang closure device was deployed to the right common femoral artery. Patient had bilateral palpable pulses at the end of the procedure and was extubated and transferred to recovery room. Patient was discharged on postoperative day 2 in satisfactory condition, and CT scan of the chest prior to discharge showed exclusion of the 6-cm aneurysm with no endoleak noted (Figure 7).

## Discussion

All the devices developed to date for endograft repair of abdominal and thoracic aortic aneurysms are deployed through relatively large (12–25 F) sheaths. They must be positioned appropriately within the aorta after the sheaths are passed through access sites in the common femoral or iliac vessels. Traditionally, and with few exceptions, this access has required arterial exposure via cut down skin incisions. In general, this process is safe but it does require practitioners experienced in open surgical technique, and in many institutions, a cut down mandates operating room availability with general or spinal anesthesia. In addition, open arterial access does have a well-defined set of potential complications.

Potential advantages to percutaneous endograft deployment include shorter procedure time, improved patient acceptance, earlier ambulation, and reduced risk for wound complication [1–4]. Percutaneous sheath placement has its own unique set of risks, and practitioners must be comfortable with

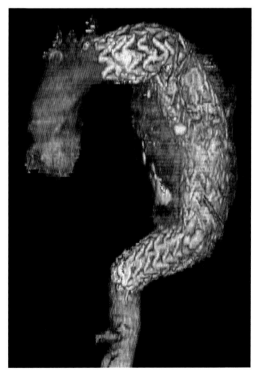

**Figure 7** Postoperative CT scan demonstrating satisfactory exclusion of TAA with no identifiable endoleak.

the technique for the benefits to outweigh these risks.

Device entrapment, acute arterial thrombosis with limb ischemia, arterial injury, suture breaks resulting in hemorrhage, arterial dissection, suture infection, and pseudoaneurysm or arteriovenous fistula formation have all been described after use of this closure technique [5–11].

The use of an endoluminal conduit for managing patients with thoracic aortic pathologies offers a percutaneous technique for delivering an endograft in a small-calcified iliac vessel that alternatively would require an iliofemoral bypass conduit. The endoluminal conduit technique allows aggressive balloon dilation of long segments of iliofemoral stenosis without the risk of vessel rupture. The endoluminal graft conduit can be custom-assembled using grafts diameters of at least 8 mm and preferably 10 mm and can be back-loaded into a delivery sheath and deployed via a femoral arteriotomy into the common iliac artery covering the origin of the internal iliac artery. Alternatively, commercially available endoluminal grafts of appropriated diameters such as the Gore Viahbahn, Atrium iCast, and Fluency grafts can be used as an endoconduit. A noncompliant balloon is used to dilate the iliac artery to diameters of 8–10 mm from within the endoluminal conduit. The aortic endograft can then be placed through the conduit into the aorta. Upon completion, the distal end of the graft can be trimmed and sutured to the common femoral artery from within the existing arteriotomy. Although this technique has the advantage of requiring only femoral access, the increased risk of dislodging the endograft when larger delivery systems are used will likely limit its use with larger-profile thoracic stent-graft systems. Furthermore, covering the internal iliac artery risks the development of colonic ischemia, especially in the presence of inferior mesenteric artery occlusion.

In summary, the use of an endoconduit and a total percutaneous approach offers a minimal invasive approach to the treatment of thoracic aortic pathologies.

## References

1  Rachel ES, Bergamini TM, Kinney EV, Jung MT, Kaebnick HW, Mitchell RA. Percutaneous endovascular abdominal aortic aneurysm repair. *Ann Vasc Surg* 2002; **16**: 43–49.

2  Howell M, Villareal R, Krajcer Z. Percutaneous access and closure of femoral artery access sites associated with endoluminal repair of abdominal aortic aneurysms. *J Endovasc Ther* 2001; **8**: 68–74.

3  Traul DK, Clair DG, Gray B, O'Hara PJ, Ouriel K. Percutaneous endovascular repair of infrarenal abdominal aortic aneurysms (a feasibility study). *J Vasc Surg* 2000; **32**: 770–776.

4  Kibbe MR, Evans ME, Morasch MD. Percutaneous repair of abdominal aortic aneurysms. In: Yao J, Pearce W, & Matsumura J, eds. *Trends in Vascular Surgery*. Precept Press, Chicago, 2003: 225–232.

5  Morasch MD, Kibbe MR, Evans ME *et al*. Percutaneous repair of abdominal aortic aneurysm. *J Vasc Surg* 2004; **40**: 12–16.

6  Duffin DC, Muhlestein JB, Allisson SB *et al*. Femoral arterial puncture management after percutaneous coronary procedures (a comparison of clinical outcomes and patient satisfaction between manual compression and two different vascular closure devices). *J Invasive Cardiol* 2001; **13**: 354–362.

7  Sesana M, Vaghetti M, Albiero R *et al*. Effectiveness and complications of vascular access closure devices after interventional procedures. *J Invasive Cardiol* 2000; **12**: 395–399.

8  Falstrom JK, Goodman NC, Ates G, Abbott RD, Powers ER, Spotnitz WD. Reduction of femoral artery bleeding post catheterization using a collagen enhanced fibrin sealant. *Cathet Cardiovasc Diagn* 1997; **41**: 79–84.

9  Illi OE, Meier B, Paravicini G. First clinical evaluation of a new concept for puncture-site occlusion in interventional cardiology and angioplasty. *Eur J Pediatr Surg* 1998; **8**: 220–223.

10  Kornowski R, Brandes S, Teplitsky I *et al*. Safety and efficacy of a 6 French Perclose arterial suturing device following percutaneous coronary interventions (a pilot evaluation). *J Invasive Cardiol* 2002; **14**: 741–745.

11  Mehta H, Fleisch M, Chatterjee T *et al*. Novel femoral artery puncture closure device in patients undergoing interventional and diagnostic cardiac procedures. *J Invasive Cardiol* 2002; **14**: 9–12.

# Complete endovascular management of a patient with multilevel aortic disease

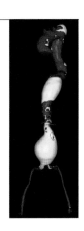

## Introduction

Patients with multilevel aortic disease are at an increased risk of paraplegia when both a thoracic and an abdominal aneurysm need to be excluded. A mortality of close to 40% was reported by Crawford [1, 2] when repair was carried out at the same setting. Staged repair is associated with improved survival but a risk of rupture still exists while waiting for the second part of the operation. The risk of paraplegia is increased when a patient with a previous abdominal aneurysm repair requires thoracic aortic aneurysm repair. A prophylactic spinal drain prior to the repair of a thoracic aneurysm may decrease the risk of paraplegia.

## Case scenario

A 76-year-old gentleman developed abdominal pain and was found to have both an infrarenal aortic aneurysm measuring 6.8 cm in diameter and a thoracic aortic aneurysm measuring 6.4 cm in diameter (Figure 1). His past medical history was notable for hypertension, pontine cerebrovascular accident, three-vessel coronary artery bypass graft, and bilateral carotid endarterectomies. From a medical standpoint, he was on proper preventative including a β-blocker, aspirin, and a lipid-lowering agent. Of the two aneurysms identified, the abdominal aneurysm was given priority due to its larger size and more prone to rupture. The thoracic aneurysm was to be repaired approximately 6 weeks after the abdominal surgery to allow the patient to recover and

encourage the collateralization of his spinal cord. Once the abdominal endoluminal graft (ELG) had been performed, a new CT scan was obtained to evaluate how the new endoprosthesis will change the surgical plan for the thoracic aorta (Figure 2a and 2b). It demonstrated a 6.4 cm × 5.4 cm thoracic aortic aneurysm in the mid-descending thoracic aorta with an adequate proximal and distal neck. The principal concern going into the procedure was that the legs of the abdominal ELG would make access a difficulty. When the patient presented for the thoracic portion of his staged procedure, his neurological function was protected aggressively with the placement of a spinal drain and a conservative coverage of the thoracic aorta with an endoluminal graft.

## Technical details

The patient was placed in a sitting position and the spinal drain was placed with the opening pressures measured at 10 cm water. The drain was then taped in place after connecting to a transducer and a drain bag. Once the patient was in the supine position, he was intubated and placed under general anesthesia. The right groin was exposed and an incision made to accommodate the advancement of the delivery sheath. The left groin was punctured for percutaneous access and used for concurrent imaging.

A 5-F (French) angiographic pigtail catheter was advanced through the left groin 5-F sheath to the thoracic aortic arch for an angiogram. Oblique thoracic aortic angiogram demonstrated a thoracic

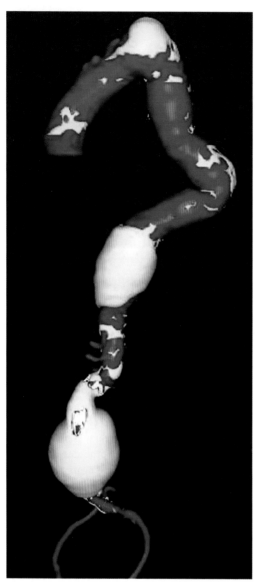

**Figure 1** A 3-D reconstruction of the chest, abdomen, and pelvis demonstrating a 6.8-cm abdominal aneurysm and a 6.4-cm thoracic aneurysm.

common femoral artery 9-F sheath. Two areas of dilatation were identified. One area was near the thoracic arch with a diameter of less than 5.0 cm and the previously described aneurysm in the distal thoracic aorta. The diameter of the proximal neck in the medial thoracic aorta was measured at 32 mm with a distal neck diameter measured at 32 mm in diameter and the length of aorta to be covered measured at 15 cm in length. Based on the measurements, a 37 mm × 15 cm Gore TAG graft (W.L. Gore & Associates, Flagstaff, AZ) was chosen for deployment in the proximal aorta. A stiff Lunderquist wire (Cook Inc., Bloomington, IN) was exchanged through the IVUS catheter and the right 9-F sheath was exchanged for a 24-F Gore. Significant resistance was encountered while trying to advance the sheath through the iliac vessels. With this difficulty, the two remaining options were the creation of a retroperitoneal 10-mm conduit to the right common iliac artery or to deliver the graft in a bareback fashion with no sheath. The bareback method is not endorsed by the manufacturer. The exact position of the celiac artery was ascertained and the graft was deployed just proximal that mark. A postdeployment angiogram showed that the graft had landed in area of tortuosity with some contrast able to get into the aneurysm sac. We decided to deploy a second endoluminal graft measuring 40 mm × 10 cm, also using the bareback technique, proximal to the first endograft making sure we had an adequate overlap with the first graft. Postdeployment balloon angioplasty was carried out with a 40-mm Coda balloon (Cook Inc., Bloomington, IN). A second aortogram demonstrated adequate exclusion of the thoracic aneurysm with no endoleak (Figure 5). Immediately after the second device deployment, the patient's blood pressure was raised to a systolic of 140–160s to encourage blood flow to the spinal cord. A retrograde iliac angiogram performed prior to removal of wires and sheaths demonstrated a dissection of the right external iliac artery (Figure 6a). Balloon angioplasty of the right external iliac artery was performed with an 8 mm × 60 mm OPTA Pro (Cordis) balloon, followed by the deployment of an iliac limb from a Gore excluder abdominal endoluminal graft measuring 16 mm × 14.5 mm × 12 cm. Satisfactory management of the dissection and brisk flow of contrast was obtained with the repair (Figure 6b). In closing the access sites,

aortic aneurysm with adequate proximal and distal landing zones for deployment of an endograft (Figure 3). Due to concerns about iliac access, bilateral retrograde iliac angiograms were performed which demonstrated tortuous iliac vessels with small external iliac arteries (Figure 4). An 8.2-F (Volcano Therapeutics, Inc., Rancho Cordova, CA) intravascular ultrasound (IVUS) catheter was advanced to the thoracic aorta through the right

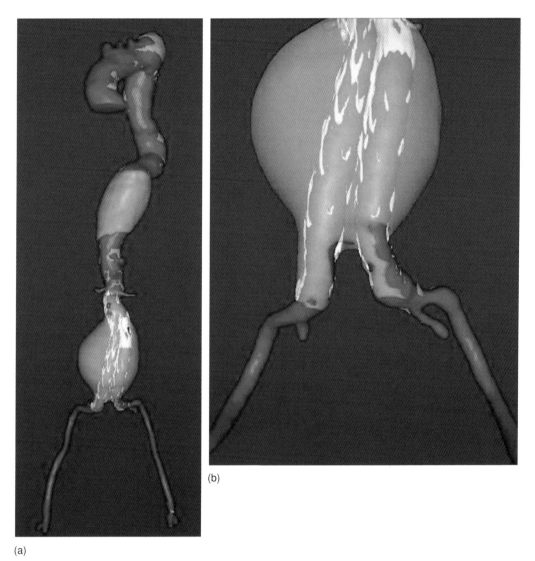

**Figure 2** (a and b) 3-D reconstruction models showing the presence of an abdominal ELG with thrombus (transparent yellow).

a closure device was deployed to the left groin site with the right groin arteriotomy closed in a standard method. Immediately after the procedure, a quick neurological examination was done in the operating room to check on his movement and sensation in all extremities. The spinal drain was kept in for 48 hours. A CT scan conducted prior to discharge showed that the distal thoracic aneurysm was excluded and that the abdominal endoluminal graft was still in good position with aneurysm exclusion (Figure 7a and 7b).

## Discussion

Open surgical repair of patients with multilevel aortic disease is associated with a relatively high surgical morbidity and mortality. When dealing with multilevel aneurysmal disease, a staged approach would seem to be favored. Many patients are not able to undergo the second stage either because of complications associated with the first stage operation or from rupture of the aorta while awaiting treatment for the second stage. Paraplegia is a dreaded

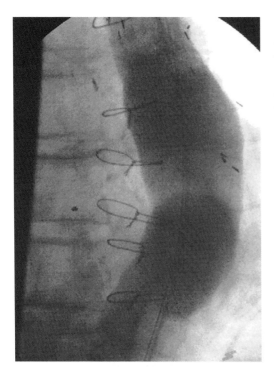

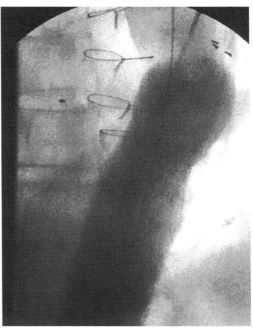

**Figure 5** Exclusion of the lower descending thoracic aneurysm is accomplished with a thoracic endoluminal graft.

**Figure 3** An angiogram demonstrating a 6.4 cm × 5.4 cm thoracic aortic aneurysm.

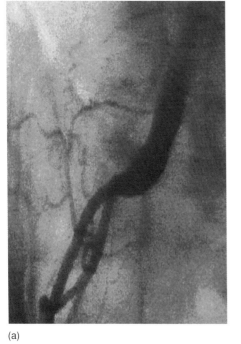

(a)

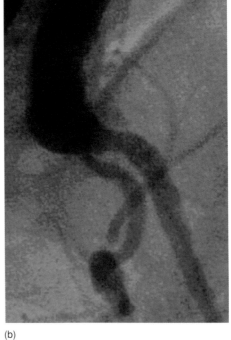

(b)

**Figure 4** (a and b) Bilateral iliac angiograms demonstrating severe tortuosity and small external iliac arteries with atherosclerotic disease.

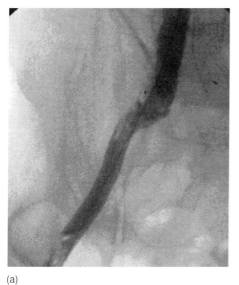

(a)

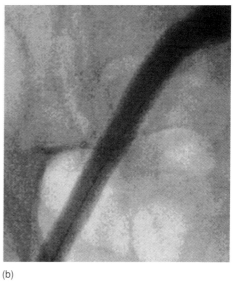

(b)

**Figure 6**   (a) A retrograde right iliac angiogram demonstrating a right iliac artery dissection from the initial attempt to advance a 24-F sheath through the right common iliac artery. (b) The same iliac artery after treatment with a covered stent to seal the iliac dissection.

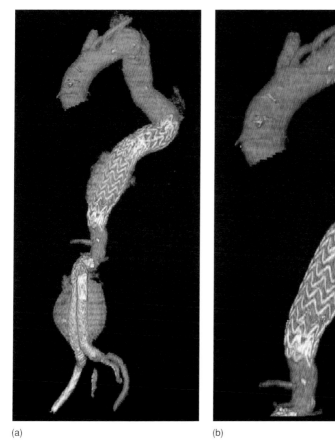

(a)                                               (b)

**Figure 7**   (a and b) 3-D models showing the extent of coverage of the aorta with endoluminal grafts.

complication of extensive replacement of the thoracic and abdominal aorta with paraplegia rates of 5–10% [3–7].

The rapid evolution of stent grafting has permitted many patients to be treated with a decreased morbidity and mortality. Potential risks of paraplegia exist with coverage of long segment of the aorta that can potentially compromise the collateral blood supply to the spine. The coverage of the hypogastric arteries and the left subclavian artery are known to affect circulation to the spine and should be spared at all costs. Despite coverage of the entire thoracic and abdominal aorta in 14% of our patients, our site did not have any those patients develop paraplegia. In our series, the two highest risk factors in paraplegia were the female gender and complicated access. Most patients who suffered paraplegia in our site experience either suffered an iliac rupture or had undergone a retroperitoneal conduit. It remains unclear what the etiological factors for paraplegia are but we are of the opinion that collateral pathways from the left subclavian artery and the hypogastric artery may play a critical role in supplying the spinal cord once extensive coverage of the aorta is undertaken. Staged repair may also allow collateral circulation to develop to supply the spinal cord.

In summary, extensive coverage of the thoracoabdominal aorta can be performed with acceptable morbidity and mortality using a totally endovascular approach. The use of prophylactic spinal drain should be entertained when extensive coverage of the aorta is to be performed.

## References

1 Crawford ES, Walker HSJ, Saleh SA, Norman MA. Graft replacement of aneurysm in descending thoracic aorta: results with bypass or shunting. *Surgery* 1981; **89**: 73–85.

2 Crawford ES. Aortic aneurysm: a multifocal disease. *Arch Surg* 1982; **117**: 1393–1400.

3 Svenson LG, Crawford ES, Hess KR *et al.* Experience with 1509 patients undergoing thoracoabdominal aortic operations. *J Vasc Surg* 1993; **17**: 357–368.

4 Coselli JS, LeMaire SA, Conklin LD, Koksoy C, Schmittling ZC. Morbidity and mortality after extent II thoracoabdominal aortic aneurysm repair. *Ann Thorac Surg* 2002; **73**: 1107–1115; discussion 1115–1116.

5 Coselli JS, LeMaire SA, Miller CC *et al.* Mortality and paraplegia after thoracoabdominal aortic aneurysm repair (a risk factor analysis). *Ann Thorac Surg* 2000; **69**: 409–414.

6 Safi HJ, Winnerkvist A, Miller CC *et al.* Effect of extended cross-clamp time during thoracoabdominal aortic aneurysm repair. *Ann Thorac Surg* 1998; **66**: 1204–1209.

7 Cambria RP, Giglia JS. Prevention of spinal cord ischemic complications after thoracoabdominal aortic surgery. *Eur J Vasc Endovasc Surg* 1998; **15**: 96–109.

## CASE 10

# Endovascular repair of a descending thoracic aneurysm with previous open resection of abdominal aortic aneurysm

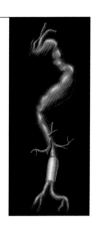

## Introduction

Sequential open surgical repair of patients with multilevel aortic disease is associated with a high morbidity and mortality. Patients who undergo an open surgical repair are exposed to a laparotomy and a thoracotomy either simultaneously or sequentially. Endovascular repair is associated with a decreased morbidity, mortality, and decreased risk of paraplegia.

## Case scenario

This is a 79-year-old male with a prior history of an open abdominal aortic aneurysm (AAA) repair conducted 9 years ago along with multiple back surgeries. Her medical history consisted of cancer of the prostate status postradiation therapy, carotid artery disease status post left internal carotid stent as well as chronic obstructive pulmonary disease. The patient was admitted with chest pain. CT scan of the chest and abdomen revealed a 6.0 cm × 5.5 cm descending thoracic aneurysm (DTA) starting from the mid-descending aorta approximately 3-cm above the celiac axis as well as a previous abdominal aortic graft replacement (Figure 1a–1d). Due to the increased risks associated with multiple redo procedures, the patient was referred to an endovascular center for DTA repair using an

endoluminal graft. The patient was evaluated by anesthesia prior to surgery for spinal cord drainage but due to his multiple back surgeries they were unable to place a spinal cord drain. The device was placed in a successful fashion with no permanent adverse events.

## Technical details

The patient was brought to the operating room and placed supine on the operating table. An oblique incision was made into the right groin to access the right common femoral artery. An 18-G needle was used to directly access the right common femoral artery and a 0.035-in. soft-tip angled glide wire inserted under direct fluoroscopy visualization into the thoracic aorta and a 9-F (French) groin sheath inserted. Percutaneous cannulation of the left common femoral artery was performed and a 6-F groin sheath was introduced. A 5-F pigtail angiographic catheter was inserted through the left groin sheath and an oblique thoracic angiogram and a distal abdominal angiogram (Figure 2) were performed that showed tortuosity of the thoracic aortic arch, DTA, and tortuous iliac vessels. Intravascular ultrasound (IVUS) was performed through a 9-F sheath in the right groin. The proximal landing zone diameter was approximately 35 mm and the distal landing zone diameter was 35 mm. The distance between the proximal and the distal landing zones was 25 cm. It was decided to use two endoluminal grafts, 40 mm × 20 cm and 40 mm × 10 cm, to exclude the thoracic aortic aneurysm thereby achieving a minimum of 2 cm of proximal and distal neck. The soft-tip angled glide wire was exchanged to a stiff Lunderquist wire (Cook Inc., Bloomington, IN) using the IVUS catheter as an exchange catheter. The 9-F sheath was replaced with a 24-F Gore sheath. The 40 mm × 20 cm Gore TAG excluder endoluminal graft (W.L. Gore & Associates, Flagstaff, AZ) was first deployed followed by a 40 mm × 10 cm Gore TAG excluder endoluminal graft. We then exchanged the Gore sheath to a 14-F sheath and performed balloon angioplasty of the proximal and distal neck as well as the zone of overlap between the endografts using the Coda balloon (Cook Inc., Bloomington, IN). Through a 5-F pigtail catheter a completion thoracic angiogram performed showed (Figure 3) no evidence of endoleak and the exclusion of the DTA. The right common femoral artery was closed with primary closure using 5-0 Prolene. The patient tolerated the procedure well and went to the recovery room in stable condition. A postoperative

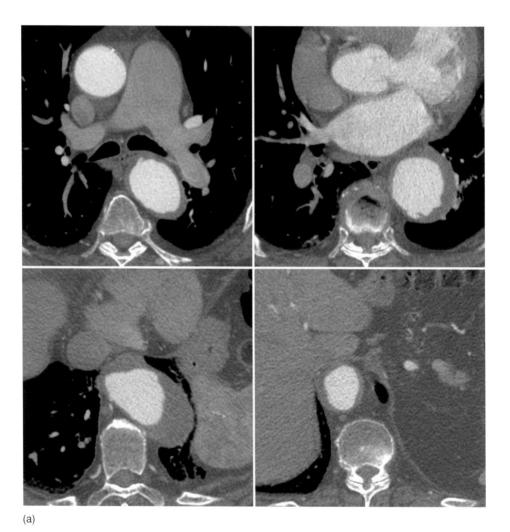

(a)

**Figure 1** (a) CT scan axial images demonstrating a 6.0 × 6.5 cm DTA. (b) A 64-slice CT scan demonstrating the thrombus within an aneurysm sac. (c) A 64-slice CT scan demonstrating a previous infrarenal aortic aneurysm repair with an abdominal aortic graft (arrow). (d) A 64-slice 3-D reconstruction with an emphasis on the presence of intercostal arteries.

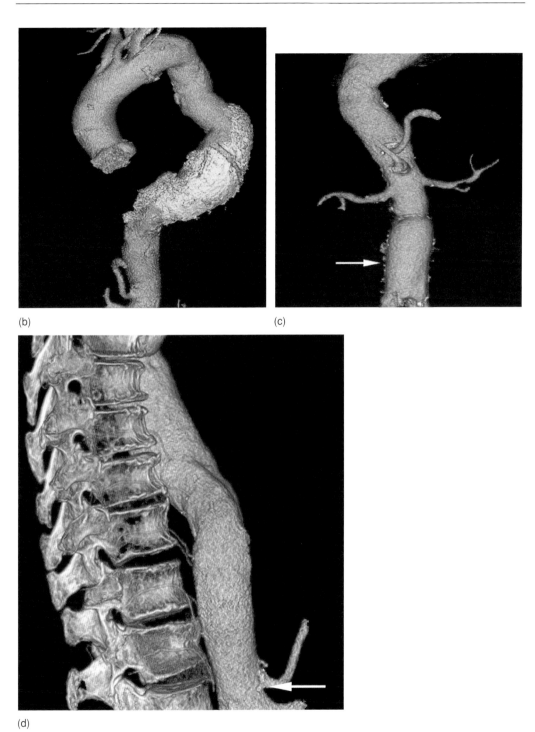

(b)

(c)

(d)

**Figure 1** (*Cont.*)

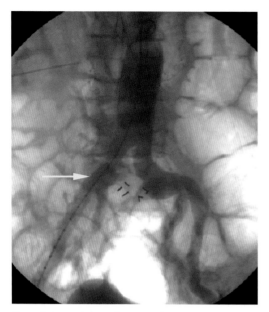

**Figure 2** An angiogram demonstrating tortuous arteries and an abdominal graft (yellow arrow).

CT scan demonstrated adequate deployment of the endograft with no endoleak detected (Figure 4).

## Discussion

The mortality rate of surgical repair in patients with multilevel aortic disease can be substantial. Five percent of patients with an AAA have a DTA [1] and 3–29% of patients with a DTA have an AAA [2]. Endovascular stent grafts have recently been developed for repair of thoracic aortic aneurysm with encouraging results [3]. The operative mortality rate for patients undergoing elective open surgical repair for isolated DTA was 11.7% in the US multicenter trial compared to 2.1% with the endovascular approach [3]. The mortality for conventional AAA is 2–5% [4]. The risk of paraplegia with abdominal aortic replacement is minimal 0–0.2% [5, 6] with paraplegia from open repair of DTA averaging 4% (range 0–18%). In chronic thoracic aneurysms thrombosis of the intercostals occur within the diseases segment, leaving the spinal cord dependent on proximal and distal collateral vessels. Endovascular repair of DTA is associated with low mortality of 2.1% and a paraplegia rate lower than that of open surgical repair. Paraplegia rates have been noted to

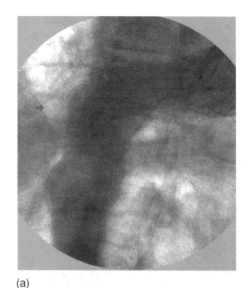

(a)

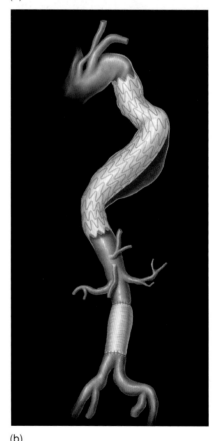

(b)

**Figure 3** (a and b) Angiogram (a) and illustration (b) demonstrating exclusion of thoracic aortic aneurysm with endoluminal graft (red arrow) and no demonstrable endoleak.

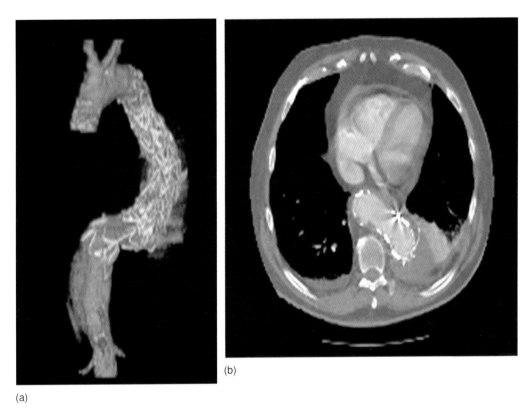

(a)

(b)

**Figure 4** (a and b) Postoperative CT scan showing exclusion of thoracic aortic aneurysm with no identifiable endoleak.

be higher in patients with multilevel aortic disease that have had previous AAA repair and undergo endovascular stent-graft therapy to treat a DTA. Possible etiologies to an increased rate of paraplegia in these group of patients is believed to be due to some of the lumbar arteries which may provide some collaterals to the spinal cord are sacrificed in AAA open surgical repair leaving few collaterals supplying the spinal cord. Excess distal coverage of the DTA should be avoided in order not to cover many intercostals arteries which supply the spinal cord.

## References

1 Wright IS, Urdaneta E, Wright B. Re-opening of the case of the abdominal aortic aneurysm. *Circulation* 956; **13**: 754–768.

2 Preeler V, McNamara JJ. Thoracic aortic aneurysm: natural history and treatment. *J Thorac Cardiovasc Surg* 1980; **79**: 489–498.

3 Makaroun MS, Dillavou ED, Kes ST *et al.* Endovascular treatment of thoracic aortic aneurysms: results of the phase II multicenter trial of the Gore TAG thoracic endoprosthesis. *J Vasc Surg* 2005; **41**: 1–9.

4 Abu Rahma AF, Robinson PA, Boland JP *et al.* Elective resection of 332 abdominal aortic aneurysms in a southern Western Virginia community during a rcent 5-year period. *Surgery* 1991: **109**; 244–251.

5 Johnston KW. Multicenter prospective study of no ruptured abdominal aortic aneurysms. Part II: Variables predicting morbidity and mortality. *J Vasc Surg* 989; 437–447.

6 Borst HG, Jurmann M, Buhner B, Laas J. Risk of replacement of descending thoracic aorta with a standardized left heart bypass technique. *J Thorac Cardiovasc Surg* 994; **107**: 126–133.

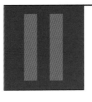

# SECTION II

# Penetrating aortic ulcers

# CASE 11

# Endovascular management of penetrating aortic ulcer

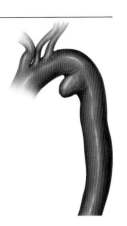

## Introduction

Penetrating thoracic ulcers most commonly result from a disruption in the aortic wall. Such a disruption can be limited to the media resulting in a dissection, adventitia resulting in a pseudoaneurysm, or transmural resulting in free rupture. The natural history of asymptomatic thoracic aortic ulcers remains unknown, although when the ulcers are symptomatic, they can be associated with more than 50% risk of rupture [1]. Patients with penetrating aortic ulcers often have cardiovascular related comorbidities and open surgical repair, especially in emergency circumstances, is associated with a high morbidity and mortality. Endovascular techniques offer a less invasive approach in this group of patients with cardiovascular comorbidities.

## Case scenario

An 85-year-old frail man with a history of diabetes, hyperlipedemia presented with new onset back pain and a recent history of hoarseness. His cardiovascular work-up was negative for coronary artery disease. His blood pressure was well controlled with a β-blocker. A CT scan performed demonstrated a penetrating aortic ulcer with a focal 2-cm pseudoaneurysm-containing mural thrombus involving the lesser curve of the distal aortic arch (Figures 1 and 2). The mass effect of the penetrating aortic ulcer and pseudoaneurysm on the recurrent laryngeal nerve could be responsible for the recent change in voice. The presence of back pain is often associated with the increased risk of rupture. Taking into account all the symptoms and comorbidities, there was a significant indication for endovascular management with an endoluminal graft. Endoluminal graft therapy for the management of symptomatic penetrating aortic ulcers is a less invasive approach which does not require cross clamping of the aorta and a thoracic incision.

## Endovascular procedure

Under general anesthesia, a cut down incision was made in the right groin with percutaneous access obtained in the opposite groin. The patient was heparininzed for the entire duration of the procedure. A 5-F (French) pigtail catheter was advanced through the left groin sheath into the thoracic aorta. An oblique thoracic arch aortogram was performed which demonstrated the penetrating aortic ulcer just distal to the left subclavian artery (Figure 3). For cases involving the proximal thoracic aorta, the C-arm apparatus is usually angled 50–70° so that the views are perpendicular to the target arch. This makes the ability to deliver the device in an accurate fashion more achievable. Due to the ulcer coming off the lateral wall of the aorta, visualization using angiography would be difficult. An intravascular ultrasound (IVUS) probe was introduced to evaluate the proximal neck to validate the measurements taken from the CT scan and confirm that a proximal neck of 2 cm was available to seat the graft properly. The CT measurements were confirmed and a treatment length of 8 cm was determined by a wire "pullback" method. The IVUS probe was exchanged for a Lunderquist

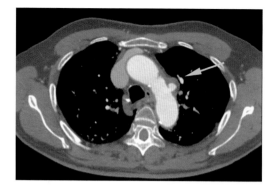

**Figure 1** A CT scan image showing the penetrating ulcer with surrounding hematoma.

wire (Cook Inc., Bloomington, IN). Based on the measurements, a 37 mm × 10 cm Gore TAG graft (W.L. Gore & Associates, Flagstaff, AZ) was chosen to be deployed to exclude the aortic pathology.

The right 9-F sheath was exchanged for a 24-F sheath and the 37 mm × 10 cm Gore device was advanced through the Gore sheath. An anterior–posterior thoracic aortogram was performed and a road map obtained with a guiding needle placed at the proximal and distal landing zone. After ensuring

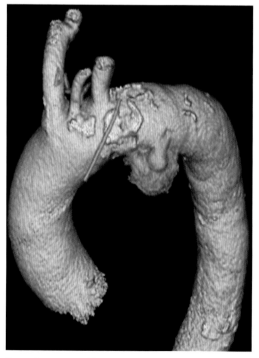

**Figure 2** A 3-D model demonstrating the ulcer in relation to the supra-aortic arch vessels.

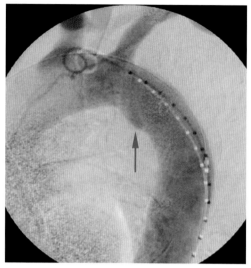

**Figure 3** An angiogram demonstrating a penetrating ulcer (blue arrow) on the lesser curvature of the aortic arch.

the mean blood pressure was lower than 90 mm Hg, a 37 mm × 10 cm Gore TAG graft was deployed successfully excluding the ulcer. The 24-F sheath was exchanged to a 14-F sheath and a 40-mm Coda balloon (Cook Inc., Bloomington, IN) was advanced into the endoluminal graft. Balloon angioplasty of both the proximal and distal neck was performed to ensure proper aortic wall apposition of the endoluminal graft. A completion angiogram showed exclusion of the aortic penetrating ulcer with no endoleak (Figure 4). All wires and sheaths

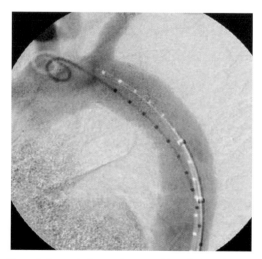

**Figure 4** A completion angiogram with exclusion of penetrating ulcer with an endograft.

were removed; the right common femoral artery was closed in a transverse fashion with restoration of flow. A vascular closure device was deployed to the left common femoral artery. Patient had bilateral palpable pulses at the end of the procedure was extubated and transferred to recovery room. A discharge CT scan demonstrated successful exclusion of the ulcer (Figure 5). He was discharged from the hospital within 3 days and placed on a surveil-lance program that mirrors the recommendations from the manufacturer. At the 1-month follow-up, the patient's hoarseness was markedly improved with the back pain resolved. His most recent annual examination notes an endoluminal graft in proper position with continued exclusion of his penetrating aortic ulcer.

## Discussion

Penetrating aortic ulcers usually arise in atheromatous plaques located in the descending thoracic aorta that can burrow through the internal elastic lamina into the media. This can lead to a variable amount of intramural hematoma formation, and may be complicated by aortic dissection, progressive aneurysmal dilatation, pseudoaneurysm formation, or rupture [2, 3]. The typical patient with a penetrating aortic ulcer is elderly with multiple cardiac risk factors and diffuse atherosclerosis of the aorta who presents with acute onset of chest and back pain. Diagnosis is generally confirmed by CT, MRA, or arteriography and IVUS. Symptomatic penetrating aortic ulcers have an increased risk of rupture. Open surgical repair in emergency situations requires thoracotomy, aortic cross clamping, and extracorporeal circulation and can be associated with significant morbidity of spinal cord ischemia (8%), myocardial infarction (20%), respiratory complications (33%), renal complications (15%), and death (60%) [4].

Endovascular techniques have been applied to the treatment of aneurysms [5, 6], dissections [7], and ulcers [8, 9], all of which have led to a marked decrease in the morbidity, mortality, and paraplegia. In a recent report by Brinster *et al.* [10], technical success in the deployment of endoluminal grafts was achieved in patients. There was no 30-day mortality and no paraplegia in his series of 21 patients.

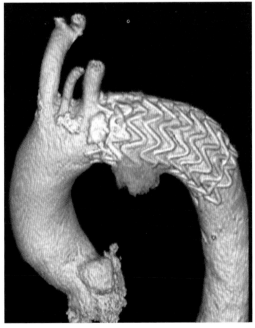

(a)

(b)

**Figure 5** (a) An axial CT scan demonstrating exclusion of penetrating aortic ulcer and thrombosed pseudoaneurysm sac. (b) A 64-slice 3-D image showing a thrombosed penetrating ulcer.

## References

1 Tittle SL, Lynch RJ, Cole PE *et al.* Midterm follow-up of penetrating ulcer and intramural hematoma of the aorta. *J Thorac Cardiovasc Surg* 2002; **123**: 1051–1059.

2 Coady MA, Rizzo JA, Hammond GL *et al.* Penetrating ulcer of the thoracic aorta: what is it? how do we recognize it? how do we manage it? *J Vasc Surg* 1998; **27**: 1006–1016.

3 Stanson AW, Kazmier FJ, Hollier LH *et al.* Penetrating atherosclerotic ulcer of the thoracic aorta: natural history

and clinicopathological correlations. *Ann Vasc Surg* 1986; **1**: 15–23.

4 Svensson LG, Crawford ES, Hess KR *et al*. Variables predictive of outcome in 832 patients undergoing repairs of the descending thoracic aorta. *Chest* 1993; **104**: 1248–1253.

5 Ellozy SH, Carroccio A, Minor M *et al*. Challenges of endovascular tube graft repair of thoracic aortic aneurysms: midterm follow-up and lessons learned. *J Vasc Surg* 2003; **38**: 676–683.

6 Criado FJ, Clark CS, Barnatan MF. Stent graft repair in aortic arch and descending thoracic aorta: a 4-year experience. *J Vasc Surg* 2002; **36**: 1121–1128.

7 Dake MD, Kato N, Mitchell RS *et al*. Endovascular stent grafts placement for the treatment of acute aortic dissection. *N Engl J Med* 1999; **340**: 1546–1552.

8 Brittenden J, McBride K, McInnes G *et al*. The use of endovascular stents in the treatment of penetrating ulcers of the thoracic aorta. *J Vasc Surg* 1999; **30**: 946–949.

9 Schoder M, Grabenwoger M, Holzenbein T *et al*. Endovascular stent-graft repair of complicated penetrating atherosclerotic ulcers of the descending thoracic aorta. *J Vasc Surg* 2002; **36**: 720–726.

10 Brinster DR, Wheatley GH, Williams J, Ramaiah VG, Diethrich EB, Rodriguez-Lopez JA. Are penetrating aortic ulcers best treated using an endovascular approach? *Ann Thorac Surg* 2006; **82**: 1688–1691.

# CASE 12

# Endovascular management of a penetrating aortic ulcer with rupture

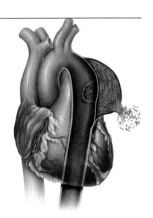

## Introduction

Penetrating atherosclerotic ulcers (PAUs) were originally described in 1934 by Shennan, who described a pathologic entity in which ulceration penetrates the internal elastic lamina into the media and can be associated with a variable amount of hematoma within the aortic wall [1]. Penetrating ulcers of the thoracic aorta arise when atherosclerotic lesions rupture through the internal elastic lamina of the aortic wall with subsequent hematoma formation between the media and the adventitia. The ulcers are most often found in the distal descending thoracic aorta but can occur throughout the thoracic and abdominal aorta and have a characteristic appearance on computed tomography (CT) and magnetic resonance imaging. PAUs may represent one pathology in the spectrum of acute aortic diseases but it may be associated with aortic dissection and aneurysm formation, although it is distinct from those conditions.

The clinical presentation of penetrating ulcers are similar to that of a classic aortic dissection but the risk of aortic rupture has been higher among patients with PAU (40%) when compared to patients with type A (7.0%) or type B (3.6%) aortic dissection [2, 3]. The natural history of untreated patients with PAU would seem to include an eventual enlargement of the defect with the formation of a saccular or fusiform aneurysm. This would not discount the possibility of intramural thrombus with late aortic rupture [4]. The criterion for offering a patient a surgical intervention should include age,

gender, location of the ulcer, and a perceived rate of growth or rupture.

## Case scenario 1

An 80-year-old woman with multiple comorbidities developed a sudden onset of severe back pain. As part of her work-up, she underwent a contrast-enhanced CT scan of her chest that showed a penetrating ulcer with a contained rupture complete with periaortic hematoma (Figure 1a and 1b). Due to her high risk for open surgical repair, she was evaluated for endovascular graft repair under an investigational protocol.

## Procedure

Under general anesthesia, open retrograde cannulation of the right common femoral artery was performed and a 9-F (French) sheath was introduced. Percutaneous access of the left common femoral artery was similarly performed and a 5-F sheath was introduced. The patient was then heparinized. An oblique thoracic arch aortogram was performed with a 5-F pigtail catheter advanced through the left groin sheath. The angiogram demonstrated a penetrating aortic ulcer in the descending thoracic aorta with rupture (Figure 2a). Intravascular ultrasound (IVUS) was then performed using an 8.2-F probe (Volcano Therapeutics, Inc., Rancho Cordova, CA) through the right groin sheath. IVUS was used to identify the penetrating aortic ulcer, the site of rupture, proximal neck diameter/length, and the distal

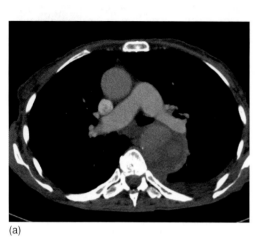

(a)

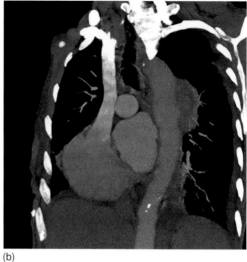

(b)

**Figure 1** (a) An axial CT image demonstrating PAU with contained rupture. (b) An oblique CT image demonstrating a penetrating ulcer with contained rupture.

neck diameter/length. Based on the CT scan measurements, a 34 mm × 15 cm Gore TAG graft (W.L. Gore & Associates, Flagstaff, AZ) was selected.

Based on the initial angiogram of the intended landing site, both the proximal and distal landing zones were identified and marked to aid in the precise deployment of the device. The right 9-F sheath was exchanged for a 22-F sheath and the 34 mm ×

15 cm Gore TAG device was then deployed over a 260-cm extra-stiff Lunderquist wire (Cook Inc., Bloomington, IN). A Gore trilobe balloon was used to perform postdeployment balloon angioplasty to both landing zones to ensure complete apposition to the aortic wall. A postdeployment angiogram showed complete exclusion of the penetrating aortic ulcer with no identifiable endoleak

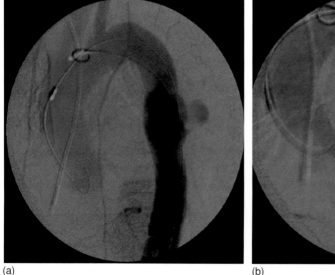

(a)

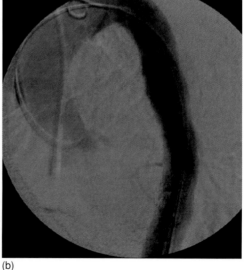

(b)

**Figure 2** (a) An angiogram demonstrating the penetrating aortic ulcer. (b) An angiogram showing the postdeployment exclusion of the ulcer.

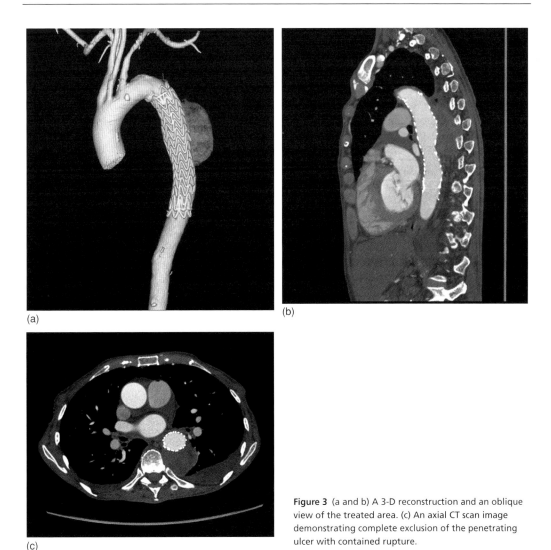

(a)

(b)

(c)

**Figure 3** (a and b) A 3-D reconstruction and an oblique view of the treated area. (c) An axial CT scan image demonstrating complete exclusion of the penetrating ulcer with contained rupture.

(Figure 2b). All wires and sheaths were removed and the right common femoral artery was closed in a transverse fashion. A 5-F angioseal vascular closure device (St. Jude Medical, Inc., St. Paul, MN) was deployed to the left common femoral artery. The restoration of flow in the peripheral arterial system was verified by pulse examination prior to leaving the operating room. In addition, the patient was extubated and transferred to the recovery room in stable condition. A CT scan conducted prior to discharge indicated that total exclusion had been achieved with no signs of device migration or defects (Figure 3a–3c).

## Case scenario 2

A 66-year-old male with a history of coronary artery disease, hypertension, type II diabetes mellitus, and morbid obesity had been experiencing back pain for a period of a month. He developed worsening back pain and reported to the emergency room. His vitals were stable at the time and physical examination was otherwise unremarkable apart. He underwent a CT scan of the chest which demonstrated a contained rupture of the distal arch of the thoracic aorta with extravasation of contrast most likely from a ruptured penetrating ulcer (Figure 4).

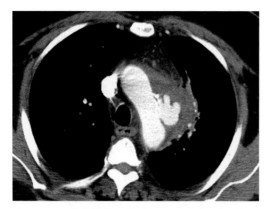

**Figure 4** An axial CT image demonstrating a contained rupture of the descending thoracic aorta.

He was subsequently taken to the operating room for endoluminal graft therapy due to high surgical risk factors for open surgical repair.

## Technical details

Open retrograde cannulation of the right common femoral artery was performed, under general anesthesia and a 9-F sheath was introduced. Percutaneous access of the left common femoral artery was similarly performed and a 5-F sheath was introduced. Heparinization was initiated. Thoracic arch aortogram was performed through the left sheath via a pigtail catheter to delineate the arch and the descending thoracic aorta and revealed a penetrating ulcer with rupture just distal to the left subclavian artery (Figure 5). IVUS was performed using an 8.2-F probe (Volcano Therapeutics, Inc., Rancho Cordova, CA). Based on the measurements a 34 mm × 15 cm Gore TAG graft (W.L. Gore & Associates, Flagstaff, AZ) was chosen. Right 9-F sheath was exchanged for a 22-F Gore sheath and a 34 mm × 15 cm Gore TAG device was deployed over an extra-stiff wire after marking the exact proximal and distal landing zones on our road map at the level of the subclavian artery. A Gore trilobe balloon was used to perform balloon angioplasty to the proximal and distal outflow segments of the graft. A completion angiogram showed presence of a type I endoleak despite exclusion of the rupture site. Retrograde cannulation of the left brachial artery with a 5-F sheath was performed (Figure 6). A JB-2 catheter was advanced over a soft-tip angled glide wire into the left carotid artery to serve as a guide when deploying

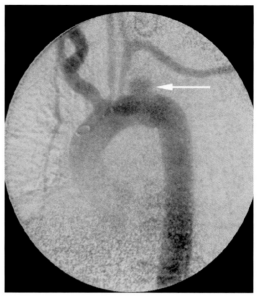

**Figure 5** Thoracic aortogram with arrow demonstrating site of rupture.

the proximal extension. A 37 mm × 10 cm endoluminal graft was deployed just distal to the marked left carotid artery after exchanging the Gore sheath to a 24-F sheath just distal to the left carotid artery followed by balloon angioplasty. Coil embolization of the left subclavian artery using Tornado coils (Cook Inc., Bloomington, IN) was performed to prevent the possibility of type II endoleak from the left subclavian artery. Completion angiogram demonstrated resolution of endoleak with exclusion of rupture (Figure 7). All wires and sheaths were removed and the right common femoral artery was closed in a transverse fashion with restoration of flow. A vascular closure device was deployed to the left common femoral artery. The patient had bilateral palpable pulses at the end of the procedure was extubated and transferred to recovery room. Postoperative CT scan demonstrated satisfactory exclusion of penetrating aortic ulcer with no identifiable endoleak (Figure 8a–c).

## Discussion

PAU is a disease process of a typically elderly population who often has extensive comorbidities that include coronary artery disease, hypertension, and chronic pulmonary obstructive disease. Diffusely

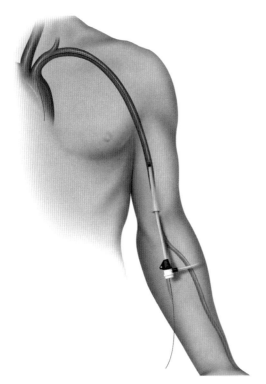

**Figure 6** Left percutaneous brachial approach for coil embolization of the left subclavian artery.

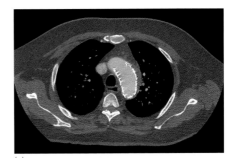

(a)

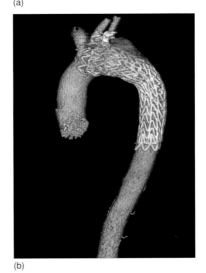

(b)

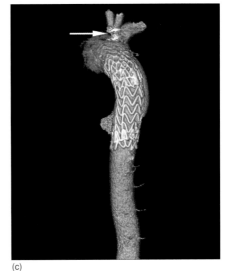

(c)

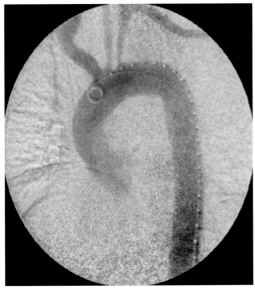

**Figure 7** A completion angiogram taken postendoluminal graft deployment demonstrating complete exclusion of penetrating aortic ulcer.

**Figure 8** (a) An axial CT scan postprocedure with exclusion of rupture and no endoleak. (b) A 64-slice CT scan with coil embolization of left subclavian artery and endoluminal graft coverage. (c) A CT scan chest (arrow) demonstrating coils in the ostium of the left subclavian artery.

diseased aortas, as commonly exhibited in PAUs, can present significant challenges for conventional repair. Poor tissue integrity combined with a high likelihood for intraoperative thromboembolism is a prime setting for severe complications. The natural etiology of PAUs is unknown as all such patients need close follow-up with serial imaging studies to document any progression of disease or complications. Aortic ulcers may break through the adventitia to form a pseudoaneurysm [4, 5] or may rupture to form a contained rupture [6, 7] or free rupture with immediate death or may precipitate an aortic dissection. The entry tears for the dissection subset of PAUs are the ulcer crater and, in contradistinction to type B dissections, the dissections are localized in nature. Additional distinctions from type B dissection entry tears include the size of the true lumen not compromised to the same extent and the flap having a thicker, calcified composition that is less fluidic. Therapeutic principles of management in the symptomatic patient include strict control of blood pressure with β-blockers to decrease the chance of rupture and pain management. Surgical intervention is advocated for patients who present with uncontrollable pain, pleural effusions, or ulcers that are large in size with deep penetration. The mortality associated with replacement of the descending aorta varies from 5 to 20% with certain specialized centers reporting 30-day mortalities as low as 6%.

Penetrating ulcers perhaps present one of the most appealing clinical indications for this stent-graft technology [8–10]. Simple stent-graft coverage of the penetrating ulcer can limit the progression of dissection and exclude areas of adventitial interruption allowing healing to occur. Even with successful stent-graft implantation, retrograde aortic dissections, and new ulcer formation have been noted in a significant percentage of patients. The incidence of these events demonstrates the diffuse and severe nature of this disease process and the need for serial evaluation following an endovascular procedure.

In a recent report of 21 patients who underwent endovascular treatment for PAU at the Arizona Heart Institute [11], the average age was 73 ± 12 years. Patients presented with acute symptoms (<14 days; 16/21, 76.2%) and chronic symptoms (5/21, 23.8%). Successful delivery and deployment were achieved in all cases. The 30-day mortality was 0% with an overall mortality of 4.8% at 14 ± 18 months. No death was related to the device or procedure. There were no endoleaks detected in our case series and no incidents of paraplegia.

Based on our experience with the use of endoluminal grafts to treat PAU [11, 12], we are of the opinion that patients with evidence of intimal tear, who are symptomatic and not responding to medical management, are ideal candidates for this type of surgery. This recommendation is dependent on the patient being properly assessed for arterial access, landing zone evaluation, desired length of the treatment area, and its location in respect to vital blood vessels.

We conclude that endovascular stent grafting is a safe treatment modality for the management of PAU although it remains unclear what the long-term data will indicate. However, the short- and mid-term data seem to be very encouraging.

# References

1 Shennan T. Dissecting aneurysms. Medical Research Council, Special Report Series, No. 193, 1934.

2 Coady MA, Rizzo JA, Elefteriades JA. Pathologic variants of thoracic aorticdissections: penetrating atherosclerotic ulcers and intramural hematomas. *Cardiol Clin* 1999; **17**: 637–657.

3 Cooley DA. The history of surgery of the thoracic aorta. *Cardiol Clin* 1999; **17**: 609–613.

4 Sundt TM. Intramural hematomas and penetrating ulcer of the descending aorta. *Ann Thorac Surg* 2007; **83**: S835–S841.

5 Vilacosta I, San Roman JA, Aragoncillo P *et al.* Penetrating atherosclerotic aortic ulcer: documentation by transesophageal echocardiography. *J Am Coll Cardiol* 1998; **32**: 83–89.

6 Von Kodolitsch Y, Csosz SK, Koschyk DH *et al.* Intramural hematoma of the aorta: predictors to dissection and rupture. *Circulation* 2003; **107**: 1158–1163.

7 Stanson AW, Kazmier FJ, Hollier LH *et al.* Penetrating atherosclerotic ulcers of the thoracic aorta: natural history and clinicopathologic correlations. *Ann Vasc Surg* 1986; **1**: 15–23.

8 Demers P, Miller C, Mitchell RS, Kee ST, Chagonjian L, Dake M. Stent graft repair of penetrating atherosclerotic ulcers in the descending thoracic aorta: mid-term results. *Ann Thorac Surg* 2004; **77**: 81–86.

9 Sailer J, Peloschek P, Rand T, Grabenwoger M, Thunher S, Lammer J. Endovascular treatment of aortic type B dissection and penetrating ulcer using commercially

available stent grafts. *AJR AM J Roentgenol* 2001; **177**: 1365–1369.

10 Schoder M, Grabenwoger M, Holzenbein T *et al.* Endovascular stent graft repair of penetrating atherosclerotic ulcers of the descending aorta. *J Vasc Surg* 2002; **36**: 720–726.

11 Brinster DR, Wheatley GH, Williams J, Ramaiah VG, Diethrich EB, Rodriguez-Lopez JA. Are penetrating aortic ulcers best treated using an endovascular approach? *Ann Thorac Surg* 2006; **82**: 1688–1691.

12 Wheatley GH, III, Gurbuz AT, Rodriguez-Lopez JA *et al.* Midterm outcome in 158 consecutive Gore TAG thoracic endoprostheses: single center experience. *Ann Thorac Surg* 2006; **81**(5): 1570–1577; discussion 1577.

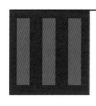

# SECTION III
# Traumatic aortic injuries

# CASE 13

# Endovascular management of thoracic aortic disruption

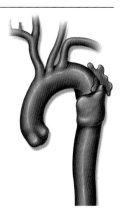

## Introduction

Blunt thoracic injury is the second cause of death after head injury. It accounts for about 20% of fatal motor accidents with high prehospital mortality of 80–90%. Thirty percent of survivors who make it to the hospital die within 6 hours [1, 2]; 90% of traumatic aortic disruption occurs at the isthmus. Open surgical repair using thoracotomy, aortic cross clamping, and partial or full use of extracorporeal circulation is the standard treatment. Operative mortality after surgical repair ranges from 15 to 30% [2, 3] with paraplegia rates up to 19% when the cross clamp and sew technique is used [4]. Endovascular repair of blunt thoracic disruption avoids cross clamping, systemic heparinization, extracorporeal circulation and thoracotomy and is associated with a mortality ranging from 0 to 6% [5]. Most traumatic transections occur at the isthmus; very few intercostals are covered decreasing the risk of paraplegia. The thoracic aorta in the trauma patient is often normal and has a smaller aortic radius of aortic curvature in contrast to older patients with aortic aneurysms or various aortic pathologies that have wider aortic curvature. Aortic disruption often occurs close to the aortic isthmus requiring coverage of the subclavian artery to achieve a satisfactory proximal neck for fixation. Consideration also must be given to small iliac vessels for access which may require retroperitoneal exposure to deliver the endoluminal grafts. Endovascular repair of young patients with traumatic aortic disruption poses a surgical challenge because of lack of commercially available thoracic endografts to treat the small thoracic aorta requiring customization with off-the-shelf abdominal endoluminal components to treat the small thoracic aorta.

## Case scenario

A 49-year-old male suffered a traumatic aortic transection of the aorta after been involved in a parachute accident. Failure of the parachute to deploy resulted in a vertical fall with multiple injuries. He arrived at the trauma center intubated with a Glasgow coma scale of 7. Diagnostic studies revealed multiple left rib fractures, a left hemopneumothorax, right subarachnoid hemorrhage, a left temporal contusion, a left iliac wing fracture, and humeral fracture. Chest X-ray revealed loss of aortic knob with mediasinal widening. CT scan of the chest (Figure 1) identified a transection of the descending thoracic aorta 2-cm distal to the left subclavian artery. Patient was stabilized and transferred to our facility for possible endovascular repair of the thoracic aortic transection.

## Endovascular procedure

Under general anesthesia open retrograde cannulation of the right common femoral artery was performed with an 18-G Cook needle and 0.035-in. soft-tip angled glide wire was passed in the aorta and exchanged to a 6-F (French) sheath after 5000 units of heparin were given.

Percutaneous access of the left common femoral artery was similarly performed and a 9-F sheath was introduced. Oblique thoracic arch aortogram

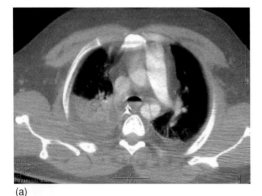

(a)

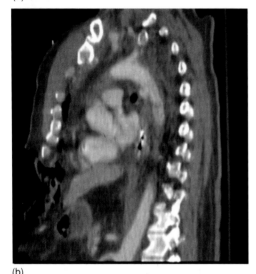

(b)

**Figure 1** (a and b) Axial and sagittal CT scan demonstrates thoracic aortic transection with mediastinal hematoma and pulmonary contusion.

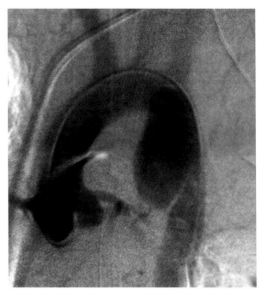

**Figure 2** An angiogram demonstrating transection of the descending thoracic aorta distal to the left subclavian artery.

deployed over an extra-stiff wire after marking the exact proximal and distal landing zones on our road map. A Gore trilobe balloon was used to perform postdeployment balloon angioplasty to the proximal and distal segments of the graft for good aortic fixation. A completion angiogram (Figure 3)

was performed through the left sheath via a pigtail catheter to delineate the arch and the descending thoracic aorta and aneurysm (Figure 2). Intravascular ultrasound (IVUS) was performed using an 8.2-F probe (Volcano Therapeutics, Inc., Rancho Cordova, CA) through the right groin sheath. The area of transection was identified close to the left subclavian artery. The proximal and distal neck diameter and length of aorta to be covered was determined. Based on the measurements a 34 mm × 15 cm Gore TAG excluder graft (W.L. Gore & Associates, Flagstaff, AZ) was chosen.

Right groin 9-F sheath was exchanged for a 22-F sheath and the Gore 34 mm × 15 cm device was advanced through the Gore sheath and subsequently

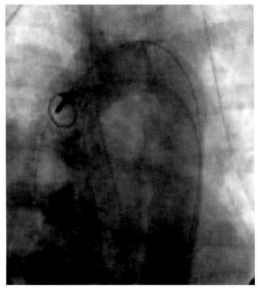

**Figure 3** A completion angiogram demonstrates exclusion of thoracic aortic disruption with an endoluminal graft.

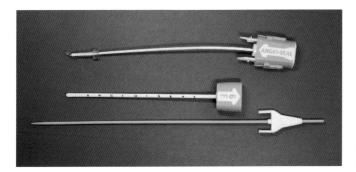

**Figure 4** Angioseal vascular closure device used to achieve hemostasis.

demonstrated exclusion of the area of transection with no endoleak. All wires and sheaths were removed; the right common femoral artery was closed in a transverse fashion with restoration of flow. A 6-F angioseal (St. Jude Medical, Inc., St. Paul, MN) vascular closure device (Figure 4) was deployed to the left common femoral artery. Patient had bilateral palpable pulses at the end of the procedure; he was transferred back to the trauma hospital for further management of his other injuries. Postoperative CT scan (Figure 5) demonstrated no endoleak with exclusion of area of transection.

## Discussion

Traumatic disruption of the thoracic aorta (TDTA) arises as a result of a lesion involving the aortic wall from the intima to the adventitia as a result of blunt trauma. Blunt traumatic aortic injury is the second most common cause of death from blunt trauma after head injury [2]. Most patients with TDTA are victims of motor vehicle accidents with 80–90% dying at the scene of accident from free rupture and exsanguinations into the chest. In those that live the aortic adventitia continuity is maintained and

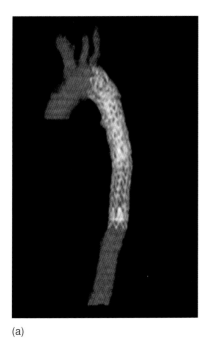

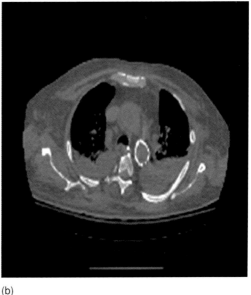

(a)                                    (b)

**Figure 5** (a) Postoperative CT scan demonstrating exclusion of thoracic aortic transection with no identifiable endoleak. (b) Postoperative CT scan demonstrating endoluminal graft in satisfactory position with bilateral loculated effusions.

hemorrhage is contained by the surrounding mediastinal structures resulting in a contained rupture. The most common injury mechanism of blunt thoracic aorta is related to the combination of sudden deceleration and traction at the relative immobile aortic isthmus. The aortic isthmus is the principal area ruptured in 80% of cases in pathological series and 90–95% of cases in clinical series [6, 7] followed by the ascending aorta, or aortic arch 18% and the distal aorta 14%. Making the diagnosis requires a high index of suspicion and most patients have other more obvious injuries. Symptoms may include dyspnoea; chest and or back pain and up to 75% of patients have rib or sternal fractures. Commonly associated injuries may include extremity, pelvic fractures, head injury, intra-abdominal injury. Chest radiograph may show evidence of mediastinal bleeding in over 90% of cases with other associated findings of widened mediastinum, obliteration of aortic knob, rightward deviation of trachea, depression of left main bronchus, and left apical cap. Gold standard for diagnosing TDTA remains the aortogram. Other diagnostic modalities includes CT scan of chest, transesophageal echocardiogram, IVUS, and magnetic resonance imaging. Pathological classification [1] include (i) intimal hemorrhage, (ii) intimal hemorrhage with laceration, (iii) medial wall laceration, (iv) complete laceration of the aorta, (v) false aneurysm formation, and (vi) periaortic hemorrhage. Complete transection leads to death although Parmley et al. [1] described 9 patients out of 38 who survived temporarily from a transection due to a contained hematoma in the periaortic and mediastinal tissues. Operative intervention is the standard of care with an operative mortality of 15–28% for open surgical repair. The mortality correlates with preoperative patient factors such as age, type and severity of associated injuries, duration of diagnosis and operative repair. Delayed open surgical repair has been advocated by some authors for those that survive and are stable [8, 9]. They found that delaying repair and treating comorbidities in a stable patient with blunt thoracic aortic injury decreased overall morbidity without increasing mortality. Paraplegia is a potential complication of descending thoracic aortic surgery. The risk increases with increase clamp time greater than 30 minutes. Fabian et al. [2] reported paraplegia

rates of 4.5% with partial bypass and 16.4% with clamp and sew techniques.

Endovascular endograft has recently been approved to treat thoracic aortic aneurysms with decrease morbidity and mortality compared to open surgical repair [10].

Endovascular management of traumatic aortic transection confers an advantage over open surgical repair by avoiding thoracotomy, cross clamping, single lung ventilation, reduced blood loss, heparinization and reduced ischemic events relating spinal cord, viscera, and kidneys [11–14]. The endoluminal graft can be deployed with minimal operative intervention via the common femoral artery. Potential shortcomings include endoleaks. Endograft migration, device infection caused by fistula formation and not all patients has adequate aortic morphology to undergo repair. Experience with endoluminal grafts for traumatic aortic transection is limited to a few case reports by various authors. Ott et al. [15] compared the treatment of thoracic aortic transection using open surgical and endovascular techniques and reported that in 18 patients followed over 11 years the mortality was 17% and a paraplegia rate of 16% in the open surgical group compared to no mortality and paraplegia in the endovascular group. Similarly, in a series of 5 patients reported by Kasirajan et al. [16] the mortality was 20% compared to 50% for open surgical repair. The injury severity score (ISS) was higher ($42 \pm 9$ vs $32 \pm 11$) for those patients that had endovascular treatment. Technical success was achieved in all 5 patients and no endoleak was reported. No case of paraplegia has been reported to date with endovascular management of traumatic aortic transection. Rousseau et al. [17] reported a mortality and paraplegia rate of 21 and 7% for 35 patients who had open surgical repair for the management of blunt thoracic injury and a 0% mortality and paraplegia rate for 29 patients managed using endografts at a mean follow-up of 46 months (range 13–90 mo) [18]. Younger patients have a tapering luminal aortic diameter as well as a higher aortic pulsatile compliance than elderly patients. The smallest commercially available endoluminal graft 26 mm in a thoracic aorta less than 22 mm may result in gross oversizing. This may result in suboptimal conformability along the inner curve of the aortic arch, which can lead to device fracture, endoleaks, migration, and device collapse which have been estimated to be about 3% in the traumatic aortic disruptions.

In conclusion, endoluminal graft for the management of disruption of the thoracic provides a minimal invasive way to treat such lethal injuries with acceptable morbidity and mortality. Device refinements such as a more flexible shaft to accommodate the aortic curvature may be needed in young patients who have a sharp aortic angulation juxtadistal to the subclavian artery reducing the need for coverage of left subclavian artery. Sometimes abdominal endoluminal grafts cuffs or iliac limbs may need to be custom assembled as thoracic endoluminal grafts to accommodate the small aortic diameter.

## References

1 Parmley LF, Mattingly TW, Manion WC, Jahnke EJ, Jr. Nonpenetrating traumatic injury of the aorta. *Circulation* 1958; **17**: 1086–1101.

2 Fabian TC, Richardson JD, Groce MA *et al*. Prospective study of blunt aortic injury: multicenter trial of the American Association for the Surgery of Trauma. *J Trauma* 1997; **42**: 374–383.

3 Turney SZ, Attar S, Ayella R, Cowley RA, Mclaughlin J. Traumatic rupture of the aorta: a five year experience. *J Thorac Cardiovasc Surg* 1976; **7**: 727–732.

4 Von Oppell UO, Dune TT, De Groot MK *et al*. Traumatic rupture: a 20 year meta-analysis of mortality and risk of paraplegia. *Ann Thorac Surg* 1994; **58**: 585–593.

5 Avery JE, Hall DP, Adams JE, Headrick JR, Nipp RE. Traumatic rupture of the aorta. *South Med J* 1979; **72**: 1238, 1240, 1245.

6 Hunt JP, Baker CC, Lentz CW *et al*. Thoracic aorta injuries: management and outcome in 144 patients. *J Trauma* 1996; **40**: 547–556.

7 Kodalis, Jiameson WRE, Leia-Stephens M, Miyagishima RT, Janusz MT, Tyers GFO. Traumatic rupture of the thoracic aorta. A 20 year review: 1969–1989. *Circulation* 1991; **84**(Supp lIII): III40–III46.

8 Maggisano R, Cina C. Traumatic rupture of the thoracic aorta. In: McMurtry RY & McLellan BA, eds. *Management of Blunt Trauma*. Williams and Wilkins, Baltimore, 1990: 206–226.

9 Maggisano R, Nathens A, Alexandrova NA *et al*. Traumatic rupture of the thoracic aorta: should one always operate immediately? *Ann Vasc Surg* 1995; **9**: 44–52.

10 Makaroun MS, Dillavou ED, Kes ST *et al*. Endovascular treatment of thoracic aortic aneurysms: results of the phase II multicenter trial of the Gore TAG thoracic endoprosthesis. *J Vasc Surg* 2005; **41**: 1–9.

11 Fujikawa T, Yukioka T, Ishimaru S *et al*. Endovascular stent grafting for the treatment of blunt thoracic aortic injury. *J Trauma* 2001; **50**: 223–229.

12 Lachat M, Pfammatter T, Witzke H *et al*. Acute traumatic aortic rupture: early stent graft repair. *Eu J Cardiothorac Surg* 2003; **21**: 959–963.

13 Lawlor DK, Ott M, Forbes TL, Kribs S, Harris KA, De Rose G. Endovascular management of traumatic thoracic injuries. *Can J Surg* 2005; **48**(4): 293–297.

14 Thompson CS, Rodriguez JA, Ramaiah VG *et al*. Acute traumatic rupture of the thoracic aorta treated with endoluminal stent grafts. *J Trauma* 2002; **52**: 1173–1177.

15 Ott MC, Stewart TC, Lawlor DK, Gray DK, Forbes TL. Management of blunt thoracic aortic injuries: endovascular stent versus open repair. *J Trauma* 2004; **56**: 565–570.

16 Kasirajan K, Heffernan D, Langsfield D. Acute thoracic aortic trauma: a comparison of endoluminal stent grafts with open repair and nonoperative management. *Ann Vasc Surg* 2003; **17**(6): 589–595.

17 Rousseau H, Dambrin C, Marcheix B *et al*. Acute traumatic aortic rupture: a comparison of surgical or stent graft repair. *J Thorac Surg* 2005; **129**: 1050–1055.

18 Verhoye JP, Bertrand DL, Kakon C, Rousseau H, Verhoye JP, Heautot JF. Classification and design algorithm of post traumatic chronic lesions of the isthmus and the descending thoracic aorta. *Thoracic Aortic Diseases* 345–349.

# Endovascular management of a traumatic pseudoaneurysm postcoarctation repair

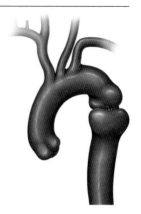

## Introduction

Traumatic aortic transection is associated with a 80–90% mortality at the site of the accident with a 32% mortality for those that make it to the hospital [1–3]. Patients with thoracic aortic transections often have multiple injuries including chest, abdomen, and head injuries. Operative mortality for the repair of traumatic aortic transection varies from 0–54% with a paraplegia rate of 0–36.4% [4]. Endovascular treatment of traumatic thoracic aortic transection avoids aortic cross clamping and the need for a thoracotomy in patients with chest injuries and compromised respiratory status.

## Case scenario

A 33-year-old male with three previous surgeries for coarctation repair, the last repair at 16 years old, was involved in a high-speed motor vehicle accident. He sustained significant chest, facial, and thoracic aortic transection with a pseudoaneurysm formation requiring an urgent trip to the operating room for repair of the thoracic aortic injury. The planned repair of his thoracic aortic injury had to be abandoned due to dense adhesions encountered making the procedure very hazardous. He was transferred to our facility for an alternative less invasive approach. CT scan of the chest (Figure 1a) performed revealed he had a small thoracic aorta which was not suitable for any of the readily available commercial thoracic endoluminal grafts. The traumatic pseudoaneurysm was identified immediately distal to the

takeoff of the left subclavian artery. After enrolling the patient in an investigational device exemption study, an endovascular approach which consisted of deployment of off-the-shelf abdominal endoluminal graft components was customized to treat the thoracic aortic pathology.

## Endovascular procedure

Under general anesthesia percutaneous access of the left common femoral artery was performed with an 18-G needle. A 260-cm, 0.035-in. soft-tip angled glide wire was advanced into the thoracic aorta and a 5-F Cordis sheath placed. Open retrograde cannulation of the right common femoral artery was performed with an 18-G needle under fluoroscopic visualization; a 0.035-in. soft-tip angled glide wire was advanced and a 9-F sheath was exchanged. A 5-F pigtail angiographic catheter was advanced through the left groin sheath, and after positioning the C-arm in a left anterior oblique view an oblique thoracic aortogram was performed. The arch aortogram (Figure 2) demonstrated a small thoracic aorta with the area of postcoarctation pseudoaneurysm from trauma to the thoracic aorta immediately distal to the left subclavian artery. An intravascular ultrasound (IVUS) 8.2-F probe (Volcano Therapeutics, Inc., Rancho Cordova, CA) was advanced over the glide wire and the diameter of the proximal neck at the level of the left carotid artery was measured to be 15 mm × 18 mm; the distal neck was measured at 22 mm. The length of

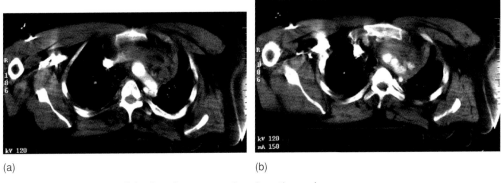

(a)                                              (b)

**Figure 1** (a and b) A CT scan of the chest demonstrates thoracic aortic pseudoaneurysm.

aorta to be covered was measured at 10 cm. Due to concerns about size discrepancy, it was of the opinion that the smallest commercially available thoracic endoluminal graft 26 mm would represent a greater than 20% oversizing of the aorta. A plan was made to use a 22 mm × 5.5 cm Cook Zenith (Cook Inc., Bloomington, IN) iliac limb for the proximal neck and a 26-mm Gore TAG thoracic endograft for the distal neck. A 260-cm extra-stiff Lunderquist wire (Cook Inc., Bloomington, IN) was exchanged through the IVUS probe.

Since the delivery catheter for deploying an abdominal endoluminal graft would not be long enough to reach the thoracic aorta, an iliac limb extension 22 mm × 55 mm was deployed on the back table and reloaded into a 20-F Cook Keller-Timmermans (Cook Inc., Bloomington, IN) sheath and after exchanging it for the right groin 9-F sheath was advanced into the thoracic aorta. Proximal and distal landing zones were marked on our road map angiogram and the endograft was successfully deployed to the target area covering the stump of the left subclavian artery. The device was then exchanged for a 26 mm × 10 cm Gore TAG endograft (W.L. Gore & Associates, Flagstaff, AZ) and deployed distally to cover the area of transection and pseudoaneurysm making sure we had the proximal aspect into the customized iliac limb with 5 cm of overlap between the endoluminal grafts. Completion angiogram (Figure 3) demonstrated

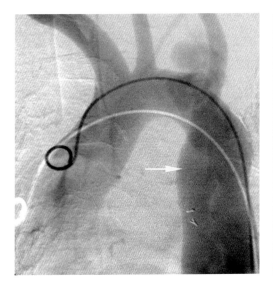

**Figure 2** Thoracic aortogram demonstrating a small thoracic aorta with area of transection and a contained pseudoaneurysm (yellow arrow).

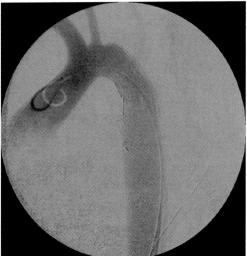

**Figure 3** A completion angiogram with satisfactory exclusion of transection and pseudoaneurysm with no endoleak identified.

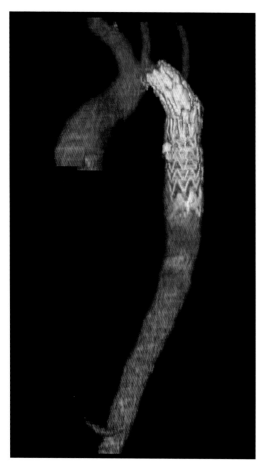

**Figure 4** Postoperative CT scan demonstrating satisfactory exclusion of transection without any endoleak.

exclusion of the area of transection with no endoleak identified. All wires and sheaths were removed; the right common femoral artery was closed in a transverse fashion with restoration of flow. An 8-F angioseal (Medtronic) closure device was deployed to the left common femoral artery. A postoperative CT scan (Figure 4) was obtained the following day with satisfactory exclusion of the area of transection with no visualized endoleak.

## Discussion

Endovascular management of traumatic thoracic aortic disruption offers a minimal invasive approach to managing critically ill patients while avoiding aortic cross clamping and extracorporeal circulation [5]. Younger patients are particularly challenging because their thoracic aorta is often small, narrow with tighter radius angle of the thoracic arch. Other critical issues include small iliac vessels which may be problematic for delivery of the endograft. The smallest thoracic endograft currently available commercially in the United States is the 26-mm-diameter Gore TAG device. Attempts to place this device in aorta 23 mm in diameter can create a situation of significant oversizing which have been associated with numerous instances of device collapse [6].

The use of customized off-the-shelf abdominal components like iliac extender cuffs and aortic cuffs permit management of the small thoracic aorta in traumatic transections without the need for graft oversizing. One shortcoming of the abdominal cuffs is obviously their short length, requiring the use of multiple devices and creating the potential for device separation and potential endoleak. This could be a particular problem in situations involving a large defect. Another issue with respect to the abdominal cuffs is the relatively short delivery system requiring deployment of the endoluminal graft on the back table with custom assembly of the abdominal components in longer delivery sheaths able to reach the thoracic aortic arch.

Device collapse has been reported in cases of graft oversizing in the small thoracic aorta and also when endoluminal grafts are deployed in horizontal arches. Deployment of endografts in horizontal arches subjects the device to extreme tangential forces that causes collapse with a fair degree of predictability. Options for treatment of device collapse include explantation with open repair or insertion of a second stent-graft device or balloon-expandable stent within the collapsed device [6, 7]. Most transections do occur at or near the aortic isthmus which may require coverage of the left subclavian artery to achieve adequate proximal fixation. Coverage of the left subclavian artery is fairly well tolerated but occasionally symptoms of left hand ischemia may result which may require an elective left carotid artery to left subclavian bypass. Elective left carotid to left subclavian bypass operations should be performed prior to coverage of the left subclavian in patients with an internal mammary bypass graft to the left anterior descending artery and patients with a dominant left vertebral artery.

With advances in graft technology, devices designed specifically to address the small thoracic and the horizontal aorta will decrease the incidence of graft oversizing and collapse associated with current commercially available endografts. A broader range of diameters and lengths as well as more flexible endografts should be designed to fully appose to the inner curve of the thoracic aorta. Until such grafts are available the treatment of patients with traumatic transection should be individualized and patients should be enrolled in study protocols with routine clinical and imaging surveillance.

## References

1 Pierangeli A, Turinetto B, Galli R, Caldarera L, Fattori R, Gavelli G. Delayed treatment of isthmic aortic rupture. *Cardiovasc Surg* 2000; **8**: 280–282.

2 Gammie JS, Shah AS, Hattler BG *et al.* Traumatic aortic rupture: diagnosis and management. *Ann Thorac Surg* 1998; **66**: 1295–1300.

3 Galli R, Pacini D, Di Bartolomeo R *et al.* Surgical indications and timing of repair of traumatic ruptures of the thoracic aorta. *Ann Thorac Surg* 1998; **65**: 461–464.

4 von Oppell UO, Dunne TT, De Groot MK, Zilla P. Traumatic aortic rupture: twenty-year meta-analysis of mortality and risk of paraplegia. *Ann Thorac Surg* 1994; **58**: 585–593.

5 Szwerc MF, Benckart DH, Lin JC *et al.* Recent clinical experience with left heart bypasses using a centrifugal pump for repair of traumatic aortic transection. *Ann Surg* 1999; **230**: 484–490; discussion 490–492.

6 Idu MM, Reekers JA, Balm R, Ponsen KJ, de Mol BA, Legemate DA. Collapse of a stent-graft following treatment of a traumatic thoracic aortic rupture. *J Endovasc Ther* 2005; **12**: 503–507.

7 Steinbauer MG, Stehr A, Pfister K *et al.* Endovascular repair of proximal endograft collapse after treatment for thoracic aortic disease. *J Vasc Surg* 2006; **43**: 609–612.

## CASE 15

# Endovascular management of a traumatic pseudoaneurysm of the thoracic aorta

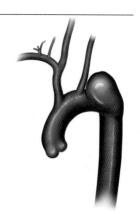

## Introduction

Posttraumatic false aneurysms arise from intimal tears more or less circumferential and often misdiagnosed at the initial stage. The tears evolve into a saccular aneurysm and most often are picked up on routine thoracic imaging studies performed for other reasons. Occasionally, the pseudoaneurysm may become symptomatic by mechanical compression on surrounding structures like the tracheobronchial tree or recurrent laryngeal nerve. The gold standard for the diagnosis of pseudoaneurysm is angiography; however, newer noninvasive imaging techniques, such as magnetic resonance angiography, computed tomography with 3-D reconstruction, and transesophageal echocardiography [1] are currently used more frequently. They provide information not only about the lumen but also about the vascular wall.

Most posttraumatic pseudoaneurysms occur at the aortic isthmus and often enlarge to encompass the left subclavian artery. The high morbidity and mortality associated with thoracic aortic injury in a polytrauma patient has resulted in the delayed repair of the acute thoracic aortic injury to a consciously delayed repair. Occasionally, such lesions have resulted in an aortic rupture during the period of watchful waiting.

Elective surgical repair of posttraumatic pseudoaneurysm involves a thoracotomy, partial cardiopulmonary support, aortic cross clamping and is associated with acceptable low mortality, low renal and pulmononary complications in the best series [2, 3]. Patients at high risk for open surgical repair and elderly patients benefit from a minimal invasive approach using endovascular stent grafts. Results from recent studies with the use of stent graft in the management of the patients with thoracic aortic injuries have been associated with even lower morbidity and mortality with very low incidence of paraplegia, respiratory, and renal complications [4–7].

## Case scenario

A pleasant 61-year-old female, who recently underwent a diagnostic evaluation for an unrelated event, was found to have a distal arch aneurysm. She had a remote history of being involved in a motor vehicle accident a couple of decades prior. She denied any history of compressive symptoms relating to the recently discovered pseudoaneurysm. She was referred for further management. Axial CT scan images demonstrated a pseudoaneurysm which involved the ostium of left subclavian artery with close proximity to the left carotid artery (Figure 1). Due to concerns of the proximity to the left carotid artery, the patient was referred for a catheterization including an intravascular ultrasound (IVUS) study to see if the anatomy would allow for a conventional endoluminal graft repair or if a hybrid procedure would be required.

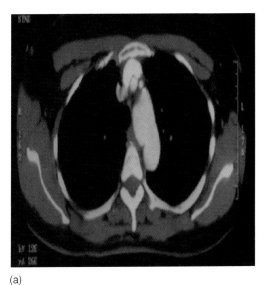

(a)

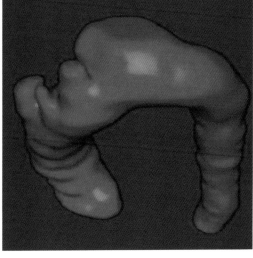

(b)

**Figure 1** (a and b) Axial and reconstructed CT images of a patient with a pseudoaneurysm of the arch aorta from previous trauma involving the ostium of the left subclavian artery.

## Intravascular ultrasound procedure

Percutaneous access of the left common femoral artery was performed with an 18-G needle and a 0.035-in. soft-tip angled glide wire was advanced into the thoracic aorta under fluoroscopic guidance and a 9-F (French) sheath was introduced. A thoracic arch aortogram was performed through the left groin sheath with a 5-F pigtail angiographic catheter to delineate the arch, the descending thoracic aorta, and the pseudoaneurysm. An IVUS 8.2-F probe (Volcano Therapeutics, Inc., Rancho Cordova, CA) was then advanced into the arch to confirm the size of the pseudoaneurysm, the presence or absence of significant thrombus, the proximal thoracic aortic neck diameter and length, and the distal thoracic aortic neck diameter and length. We identified a 4-cm distance between the innominate artery and the left common carotid artery. The distance between the left common carotid artery and left subclavian artery was 1 cm. Due to the close proximity of the pseudoaneurysm to the left carotid artery, the patient was not an anatomical candidate for the conventional procedure but would require a vessel rerouting procedure to create sufficient space so that an endoluminal graft could be safely deployed.

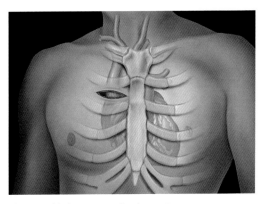

**Figure 2** Third space anterior thoracotomy.

## Open surgery

A right anterior transverse thoracotomy incision was made over the right third intercostal space to expose the ascending aorta (Figure 2). Similarly, a left neck incision was made, division of the platysma was achieved, and the sternocleidomastoid muscle was retracted laterally to expose the carotid sheath. The left common carotid artery was identified. Five thousand units of heparin were given and a side-biting clamp was used (Figure 3). The proximal end of an 8-mm Hemashield vascular graft was sewn to the aorta (Figure 4). The clamp was released and the

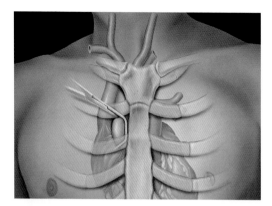

**Figure 3** Partial aortic clamp applied.

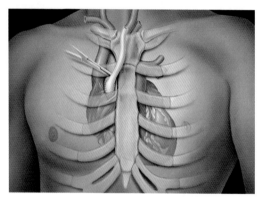

**Figure 4** 10-mm conduit sewn to aorta.

graft was flushed and then clamped. It was then tunneled up to the left neck (Figure 5). The left common carotid artery was clamped proximally and distally and an end-to-side anastomosis was performed in a standard fashion using running 5-0 Prolene suture (Figure 6). There was a palpable pulse in the graft as well as distally in the carotid artery. The neck incision and the thoracotomy incision were closed in a layered fashion.

## Endovascular approach

Under general anesthesia, open retrograde cannulation of the right common femoral artery was performed with an 18-G Cook (Cook Inc., Bloomington, IN) needle and 0.035-in. soft-tip angled glide wire was passed in the aorta and exchanged to a 9-F sheath. Five thousand units of heparin were given.

Through the existing left groin 5-F sheath, an oblique thoracic arch aortogram was performed

through the left sheath via a pigtail catheter to delineate the arch and the descending thoracic aorta and pseudoaneurysm (Figure 7). An IVUS probe was advanced into the thoracic aortic arch to measure the proximal neck diameter. Based on our neck diameter the measurement 34 mm × 20 cm Gore TAG graft was selected.

The right 9-F sheath was exchanged for a 22-F sheath and the Gore TAG device (W.L. Gore & Associates, Flagstaff, AZ) was advanced through the sheath and subsequently deployed over an extra-stiff wire to cover the ostium of the left common carotid and left subclavian artery after marking the exact proximal and distal landing zones on our road map (Figure 8). A Gore trilobe balloon was used to perform postdeployment balloon angioplasty to both the proximal and distal segments of the graft to ensure complete apposition. A completion angiogram showed late retrograde filling of the left subclavian pseudoaneurysm with a type II endoleak. Percutaneous access of the left brachial

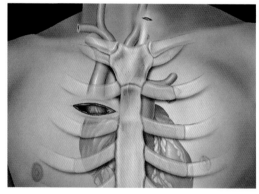

**Figure 5** 10-mm conduit tunneled to neck.

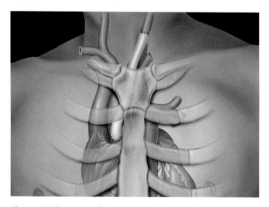

**Figure 6** 10-mm conduit sewn to left carotid artery.

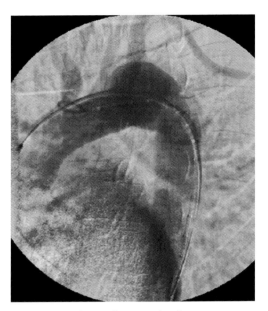

**Figure 7** An angiogram demonstrating the pseudoaneurysm.

artery was performed with an 18-G needle and a 0.035-in. glide wire was advanced into the left sub-clavian artery and exchanged to a 6-F sheath. An angiogram performed through the left brachial access demonstrated filling of the pseudoaneurysm. We then advanced a 5-F guiding catheter and coil embolized the left subclavian artery using 5 mm × 10 cm Cook (Cook Inc., Bloomington, IN) embolization coils. A repeat completion angiogram showed resolution of the type II endoleak. All wires and sheaths were removed; the right common femoral artery was closed in a transverse fashion with restoration of flow. A 6-F angioseal vascular closure device (St. Jude Medical, Inc., St. Paul, MN) was deployed to the left common femoral artery. The left brachial sheath was pulled and manual compression was performed to achieve hemostasis. A postoperative CT scan demonstrated satisfactory exclusion of pseudoaneurysm with no evidence of endoleak. She continues to do well more then 2 years after the procedure. Annual imaging with a CT scan showed no endoleak, a patent bypass graft, and the device in proper position (Figure 9).

## Discussion

With the arrival of routine imaging protocols and the introduction of advanced medical imaging soft-

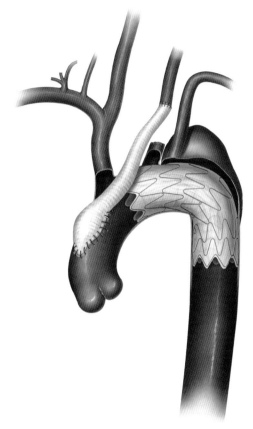

**Figure 8** An artist's rendition of the complete procedure.

ware, many posttraumatic false aneurysms have been discovered. These lesions are mostly intimal tears more or less circumferentially misdiagnosed at an initial stage. Most false aneurysms are discovered incidentally with imaging techniques or because of targeted imaging due to symptoms of compression on the tracheobronchial tree or recurrent laryngeal nerve palsy. Patients with traumatic pseudoaneurysms, unlike those with acute traumatic injury, are usually older with a remote history of a motor vehicle accident decades prior. Patients are mostly asymptomatic with the pseudoaneurysm picked up incidentally on routine imaging study or from compressive symptoms. The risk of rupture of the pseudoaneurysm is hard to qualify.

Open surgical repair has proven its long-term efficacy with a low morbidity and mortality in patients younger than 70 years. The goal of stent-graft therapy would be to get the polytrauma patients out of

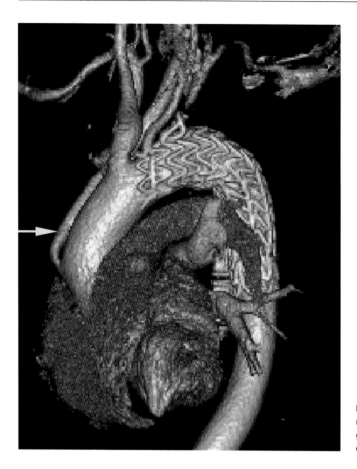

**Figure 9** A 2-year follow-up CT scan reconstruction shows a patent bypass graft (yellow arrow) with satisfactory exclusion of the pseudoaneurysm.

an acute phase by preventing thoracic aortic rupture. It could also be used in the management of patients older than 70 years old in which open surgical repair carries a significantly higher risk. In a multicenter study [8] conducted in France for patients with traumatic pseudoaneurysms, stent-graft deployment was successful in all 47 patients. There was one late paraparesis, with one patient developing a type I endoleak and another type II endoleak which spontaneously resolved at 6 months. Actuarial survival was at 1 and 3 years 97.7% ± 2.3 and 87.9 ± 9.5 years, respectively. The actuarial freedom from reintervention was 100% and 90.9 ± 8.7% at 3 years, respectively. The mean diameter of the pseudoaneurysm was 44 ± 18 mm before treatment and decreased significantly to 40 ± 18 mm ( $p < .0001$ ) after treatment.

The presence of an adequate neck and single long-length endografts are essential to prevent endoleaks. Frequently, posttraumatic pseudoaneurysms become large and occasionally involve the origins of the arch vessels. Vessel bypasses now provide a way to create enough space to land an endoluminal graft and to spare a patient a complicated open procedure. Various hybrid techniques including extra-anatomic extrathoracic debranching and thoracic aortic debranching procedures can be readily performed with less morbidity and mortality than open surgical replacement of the aortic arch.

Currently, fenestrated and branched endografts are being developed and, in the not to distant future, these technologies will allow for a complete percutaneous approach in treating extensive posttraumatic pseudoaneuryms involving the supra-aortic vessels.

## References

1 Coselli JS, Moreno PL. Descending and thoracoabdominal aneurysm. In: Cohn LH & Edmunds LH, Jr, eds. *Cardiac*

*Surgery in the Adult.* McGraw-Hill, New York, 2003: 1169–1190.

2 Finkelmeier BA, Mentzer RM, Kaiser DL, Tegtmeyer CJ, Nolan SP. Chronictraumatic thoracic aneurysm. Influence of operative treatment on natural history: an analysis of reported cases 1950–1980. *J Thorac Cardiovasc Surg* 1982; **84**: 257–266.

3 McCollum CH, Graham JM, Noon GP, DeBakey MC. Chronic traumaticaneurysms of the thoracic aorta: an analysis of 50 patients. *J Trauma* 1979; **19**: 248–252.

4 Rousseau H, Dambrin C, Marcheix B *et al.* Acute traumatic aortic rupture: a comparison of surgical or stent graft repair. *J Thorac Surg* 2005; **129**: 1050–1055.

5 Demers P, Miller C, Scott Mitchell R, Kee ST, Lynn Chagonjian RN, Dake MD. Chronic traumatic aneurysms of the descending thoracic aorta: midterm results of endovascular repair using first and second generation stent grafts. *Eur J Cardiothorac Surg* 2004; **25**: 394–400.

6 Rousseau H, Soula P, Perreault P *et al.* Delayed treatment of traumatic rupture of the thoracic aorta with endoluminal covered stent. *Circulation* 1999; **99**: 498–504.

7 Kato N, Dake MD, Miller DC *et al.* Traumatic thoracic aorta aneurysm: treatment with endovascular stent-grafts. *Radiology* 1997; **205**: 657–662.

8 Verhoye JP, Bertrand DL, Kakon C, Heautot JF. Classification and decision algorithm of posttraumatic chronic lesions of the isthmus and the descending thoracic aorta. *Thoracic Aortic Diseases*, 2006: 345–349.

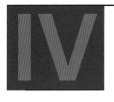

## SECTION IV

# Thoracic aortic dissections

# CASE 16

# Endovascular management of acute Stanford type B dissection

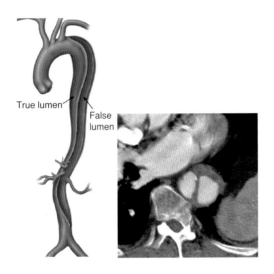

True lumen
False lumen

## Introduction

Acute aortic dissections are one of the most common catastrophic events that can affect the aorta. The pathognomonic aortic dissection lesion usually begins with a transverse tear in the aortic intima. The intima's medial layer is cleaved both longitudinally and circumferentially for a variable distance allowing access for the surging blood column to the aortic intramural space [1]. The flow of blood is usually antegrade within the aortic wall; however, retrograde flow and dissection may occur. Sixty-five percent of intimal tears occur in the ascending aorta, 20% in the descending aorta, 10% in the aortic arc, and 5% in the abdominal aorta [2].

An aortic dissection diagnosed within 2 weeks of the onset of symptoms is considered as acute dissection. Stanford type B dissections are confined to the descending thoracic aorta with entry tears at or distal to the left subclavian artery.

In the International Registry of Acute Aortic Dissection (IRAD) study, the most reported symptom was pain in greater than 93% of patients with 85% of those patients specifying an abrupt onset [2, 3]. Hypertension was present in 70% of type B dissections. Syncope complicated the presentation of dissection in 5–10% of patients with spinal cord ischemia occurring in 2–3% of type B aortic dissections. The sensitivity of transesophageal echocardiography (TEE) in the diagnosis of aortic dissection has been reported to be as high as 98% with the specificity ranging from 63 to 96% [4]. TEE is able to detect entry tear sites, false lumen flow thrombus formation, involvement of the arch or coronary arteries, degrees of aortic valvular regurgitation, and pericardial effusions. Its limitations are the anatomic blind spot in the distal ascending aorta, the arch secondary to the air-filled trachea, the left main stem bronchus, and the inability to document dissection extension beyond the diaphragm. CT scanning has reported a sensitivity of 83–95% with a specificity of 87–100% for the diagnosis of acute aortic dissection [5]. The chief limitation is in the ascending aorta where the sensitivity may drop to less than 80%, but adjunctive imagery such as TEE can compensate for this decreased sensitivity. Compared with other modalities, a CT scan tends to be the least subjective of the modalities. Intravascular ultrasound (IVUS) is particularly useful in the identification of entry and reentry tears in aortic dissections and the verification of patient's eligibility in terms of endovascular graft treatment. IVUS can be used to identify the origin of branch vessels, determine the proximal point of fixation related to the brachiocephalic vessels, and the successful reperfusion of the true lumen upon deployment of the endoluminal graft. It can also identify the location of critical visceral vessels related to reentry sites and assess pulsatility in both the true and the false lumen before and after deployment. IVUS enables observation of the false lumen after coverage of entry or reentry sites by demonstrating the return of systolic pulsatile flow to the true lumen and the concomitant decrease/stagnation of flow in the false lumen.

Until recently, acute uncomplicated Stanford type B dissections were preferably managed by conservative medical treatment. Complications including rupture, visceral or lower limb ischemia, refractory hypertension, continuing pain, and aortic diameter progression occur in 5–20% of patients during the acute phase [6–9]. A considerable number of patients without acute complications experienced dissection-related adverse events during the chronic phase that remain a treatment challenge [7, 8]. Fourteen to twenty percent of patients with type B dissections develop false aneurysms at 4-year follow-up despite aggressive medical therapy. The failure of medical therapy will require aortic replacement by open surgery to prevent a rupture of the false lumen [9]. Despite advances in the diagnosis and the various types of management of aortic dissection, morbidity and mortality remain significant, with an overall mortality of 27% reported in the IRAD study [2].

The current indications for intervention in acute type B dissections involve rupture or signs of impending rupture, rapid diameter progression

malperfusion of abdominal or peripheral vessels, persisting pain, and uncontrollable hypertension. The effectiveness of surgical or endovascular repair for aortic dissection is dependent on closure of the entry tear, re-expansion of the true lumen, and the depressurization of the false lumen. The surgical mortality rate in complicated, acute dissections remains 14–31% with a remarkable increase in patients with end-organ ischemia [2, 10–15].

Closure of the primary entry tear by endovascular repair may lead to thrombosis of the false lumen with remodeling of the true lumen in both the acute and the chronic setting. Furthermore, lowering the pressure in the false lumen may restore perfusion in any compromised aortic branch vessels.

## Case scenario

A 56-year-old male with no previous significant medical history developed severe interscapular back pain while working. The pain persisted for 24 hours despite a visit to his chiropractor. At the recommendation of the chiropractor, he presented to the emergency room. Upon arrival, he was diaphoretic with normal blood pressure, weakened pulses in the extremities, and possessed an elevated creatinine suggestive of impaired renal function. Cardiac work-up was negative for myocardial infarction. Due to impaired renal function, a magnetic resonance angiography (MRA) of his chest was performed which revealed an acute type B dissection with contained rupture into the right chest (Figure 1a and 1b). There was also evidence of malperfusion from a compressed true lumen. Despite measures to aggressively control his blood pressure and pain with intravenous medication, he continued to have unrelenting pain. The presence of unrelenting pain, malperfusion, and acute thoracic aortic rupture prompted surgical management. To limit the invasiveness of the procedure, he was consented for treatment by endoluminal graft implantation.

## Endovascular procedure

Under general anesthesia, open retrograde cannulation of the right common femoral artery was performed using an 18-G needle. A 9-F (French) sheath was introduced over a 0.035-in. soft-tip

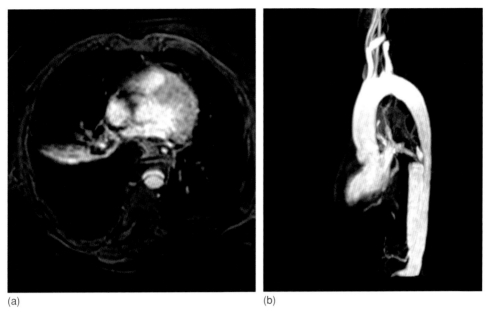

(a)                                                    (b)

**Figure 1** (a and b) MRA with axial cuts that demonstrates a type B dissection with compressed true lumen and rupture of blood into the right hemithorax.

angled glide wire. Percutaneous retrograde access of the left common femoral artery was similarly performed and a 5-F sheath was introduced. Heparin was given to achieve an activated clotting time of 200 seconds. An oblique arch aortogram was performed using a 5-F pigtail angiographic catheter that was advanced through the left groin sheath. Aortogram demonstrated a type B dissection with extravasation of contrast from the acute thoracic aortic rupture (Figure 2). An IVUS was performed through the right groin 9-F sheath using an 8.2-F probe (Volcano Therapeutics, Inc., Rancho Cordova, CA) to identify the true lumen, false lumen, and entry point of the dissection which was identified at the level of the left subclavian artery (Figure 3). The proximal neck and distal neck diameter and the length of aorta to be covered were measured in preparation for the selection of the endograft. Entry points were identified at the level of the subclavian artery and at the level of the celiac artery. The IVUS probe was exchanged for a 260-cm Lundequist stiff wire (Cook Inc., Bloomington, IN). The right groin 9-F sheath in the right common femoral artery was exchanged to a 22-F Gore sheath. Two Gore TAG devices measuring 34 mm × 20 cm (W.L. Gore & Associates, Flagstaff,

AZ) were deployed at the level of the left subclavian artery to exclude the entry point all the way down to the celiac axis where another entry point was identified. The deployment of the thoracic

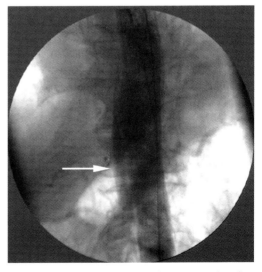

**Figure 2** An angiogram demonstrating extravasation of contrast from an acute rupture from a type B dissection (yellow arrow).

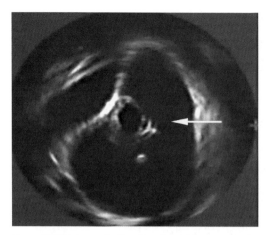

**Figure 3** IVUS demonstrating dissection with compressed true lumen (white arrow).

endograft resulted in the collapse of the false lumen and an expansion of the true lumen upon completion aortogram (Figure 4). Wires and sheaths were removed after retrograde iliac angiograms demonstrated no evidence of dissection or rupture. The right common femoral artery was repaired and a closure device deployed to the left common femoral artery. Postoperative CT scans demonstrated the thrombosis of the false lumen and an exclusion of left subclavian artery entry point (Figure 5a, 5b, and 5c).

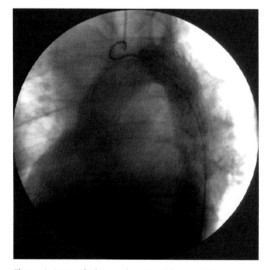

**Figure 4** A completion angiogram with true lumen expansion and exclusion of site of rupture.

## Discussion

Stanford type B dissections are a lethal disease which continues to be associated with an overall high morbidity and mortality of 27.4% regardless of which treatment modality is pursued as initially reported by the IRAD study [2]. The standard of care for the management of (Stanford type B) aortic dissections is medical therapy with open surgical repair indicated for life-threatening complications such as uncontrolled hypertension, ongoing chest pain despite medical therapy, progression of dissection, aneurysmal enlargement, rupture, and visceral or extremity ischemia [16–19]. However, several studies have showed that adverse events during the clinical course were strongly correlated with a patent false lumen and a maximal thoracic aortic diameter of 40 mm or more [6, 7, 9].

Surgery for aortic dissection requires open thoracotomy, aortic cross clamping, extracorporeal circulation, and graft interposition. There is a predictably high rate of complications associated with this surgery in these patients who are frequently poor candidates with an in-house mortality rate reported as high as 29.3% when intervention is required. The merits of early versus late intervention continue to be argued in the literature 40 years after the first publication of superior results with medical management. The continued debate on the appropriate treatment reflects the situation that neither approach is ideal.

Management of thoracic aortic disease has evolved ever since the first report of endovascular stent-graft repair for the treatment of thoracic aortic aneurysm was first performed in 1992 [20]. Lately, numerous reports exist detailing the initial technical success of thoracic endograft deployment for type B dissections [20–22]. Despite the lack of any long-term data to support definitive evidence, endovascular treatment of thoracic aortic dissections have been proposed as an alternative therapy to medical management and surgery in patients with Stanford type B dissection. The ideal candidates for this surgery are people who have severe comorbidities and are poor candidates for any form of surgical therapy. These devices have the ability to successfully exclude a proximal entry point with resulting thrombosis of false lumen as the best indicator of a successful outcome. Our treatment strategy for

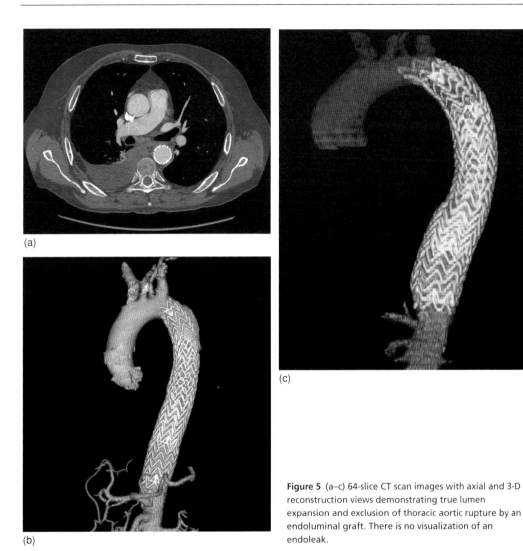

(a)

(b)

(c)

**Figure 5** (a–c) 64-slice CT scan images with axial and 3-D reconstruction views demonstrating true lumen expansion and exclusion of thoracic aortic rupture by an endoluminal graft. There is no visualization of an endoleak.

stent grafting for type B dissection has been to exclude the entry point of the dissection from the systemic circulation so as to cause thrombosis of the false lumen despite the possibility of reentry sites in the distal aorta. The remaining patent false lumen in the distal aorta served by other multiple reentry points provides flow to the major arteries emanating from the false lumen preventing malperfusion syndrome. Debate still continues as to whether the presence of an appropriately positioned endograft excluding the proximal tear is enough to alter the natural history of this disease.

The natural history of patients with chronic thoracic dissecting aneurysm is to experience chronic expansion of the thoracic aorta that could poten-

tially lead to rupture [23]. Patency of a false lumen as a result of a persistent entry and an initial aortic diameter of more than 4 cm and a persistent entry into the false lumen have been identified as determinants for chronic expansion of the aorta as well as independent risk factors for dissection-related death and for a dissection-related event [24]. There are multiple reports suggesting that thoracic endografts perform suboptimally when employed in an attempt to correct distal malperfusion once this has occurred [19, 25]. Our aggressive approach to the treatment of type B dissections with endoluminal grafts is based partly on the difficulty in predicting which patients are prone to aortic dilation and subsequent rupture.

**Table 1** Patient characteristics and comorbidities.

| Patient characteristic/comorbidity | Number |
|---|---|
| Mean age (yr; range) | 67 [39–91] |
| Male/female ratio | 11/29 |
| Hypertension | 36 (90%) |
| Tobacco abuse | 28 (70%) |
| AAA | 17 (43%) |
| Coronary artery disease | 16 (40%) |
| Chronic renal insufficiency | 15 (38%) |
| COPD | 11 (28%) |
| Diabetes mellitus | 5 (13%) |
| Previous myocardial infarction | 4 (10%) |
| CVA | 4 (10%) |
| ESRD | 1 (3%) |

AAA, abdominal aortic aneurysm; COPD, chronic obstructive pulmonary disease; CVA, cerebrovascular accident; ESRD, end-stage renal disease.

**Table 2** Patient presentation.

| Indication | Number |
|---|---|
| Intractable pain | 22 (55%) |
| Aortic expansion | 9 (23%) |
| Compression of true lumen | 9 (23%) |
| Impending rupture | 6 (15%) |
| Intractable hypertension | 6 (15%) |
| Extension of dissection | 4 (10%) |
| End-organ ischemia | 3 (8%) |

In our series of 40 patients, treated with an endoluminal graft for type B dissections (Tables 1–6), hypertension was the most common presenting sign (90%; Table 1), with pain the most common symptom for intervention (Tables 2 and 3), mean aortic diameter was 5.5 cm (Table 4), and we were able to exclude the entry tear in 100% of cases (Table 6) [26]. No patient suffered from an aortic rupture at the 5-year follow-up. Thrombosis of

**Table 3** Criteria for intervention.

| Characteristic | Number |
|---|---|
| Acute/chronic | 23/17 |
| Symptomatic | 34 (85%) |
| Chest pain | 22 (55%) |
| Back pain | 21 (53%) |
| Abdominal pain | 12 (30%) |

**Table 4** Anatomic characteristics.

| Anatomic characteristics | Number |
|---|---|
| Mean thoracic aortic diameter (cm; range) | 5.5 (2.6–9.0) |
| Distal extent of dissection | |
| Celiac artery | 23 (58%) |
| Renal arteries | 5 (13%) |
| Aortic bifurcation | 1 (3%) |
| Iliac arteries | 9 (23%) |
| Femoral arteries | 2 (5%) |

**Table 5** Morbidity and mortality.

| Complication | Number of events |
|---|---|
| Pleural effusion without respiratory compromise | 8 (20%) |
| Pneumonia/COPD exacerbation with respiratory compromise | 5 (13%) |
| Renal failure | 5 (13%) |
| Hematoma/pseudoaneurysm/lymphocele | 5 (13%) |
| Paraplegia | 1 (3%) |
| 30-day mortality | 1 (3%) |
| Overall 1-yr survival | 85 % |

the false lumen was achieved in 79% of patients with thoracic aortic stability or regression achieved in 97% of patients followed-up. There was only 1 of the 31 patients (3%) followed by postoperative CT scans who had demonstrated expansion of the thoracic aorta 3 years after placement of a thoracic

**Table 6** Follow-up data.

| Mean follow-up period (days; range) | 453 (92–1513) |
|---|---|
| CT scan availability | 31 (78%) |
| Exclusion of proximal entry point | 31 (100%) |
| Persistently patent distal false lumen | 6 (21%) |
| Persistent retrograde flow into proximal false lumen | 4 (14%) |
| Thoracic aortic expansion | 1 (3%) |
| Thoracic aortic stability | 22 (71%) |
| Thoracic aortic regression | 8 (26%) |
| Rupture | 0 |

endoluminal graft. We believe that the patient may have developed a new reentry site since his aorta had been stable 3 years prior. Communication between the true lumen and the false lumen did not seem to be an adverse factor since none of the patients in the reported series experienced any significant mesenteric, renal, or limb malperfusion due to graft deployment with exclusion of entry point. Our relatively good outcomes reported with the use of endoluminal grafts for the treatment of type B dissection is probably attributed to our early intervention in the course of the disease. Although every one of the patients in the study had one of the indications for intervention as outlined in Table 3, only 3 patients exhibited evidence of distal malperfusion at the time of the procedure. We believe that thoracic aortic stabilization with an endograft may be most effective if the paradigm for treatment is shifted to an earlier intervention.

Achieving proximal anchorage of at least 2 cm is necessary to avoid a proximal type 1 endoleak and seal the entry point of the dissection. The blood pressure and blood velocity in the false lumen are related to the blood volume that enters the false lumen. Conversion of a large entry point to a small one results in a dramatic reduction in blood volume; the drastic drop in blood pressure and velocity in the false lumen results in thrombosis of the false lumen. Coverage of the left subclavian vessel is sometimes necessary to achieve good anchorage and seal from the entry point of the dissection. In our series all proximal type 1 endoleaks were treated with proximal endoluminal graft and coiling of left subclavian artery when indicated. The presence of a distal type 1 endoleak was not associated with adverse outcome.

One of the 40 patients developed spinal cord ischemia and permanent paraplegia. This patient had a previous history of open abdominal aortic aneurysm repair and also underwent repair with two devices for a total coverage length of 30 cm. Long coverage length, perioperative hemodynamic instability, and prior abdominal aortic aneurysm repair have been previously identified as risk factors known to be associated with a spinal cord ischemia, placing this patient in a high-risk group. Our reported result of paraplegia of 2.5% (Table 5) is consistent with other reports [26] and much lower than the paraplegia rate of up to 15% reported for open surgical cases. We do not routinely

perform prophylactic spinal cord protection maneuvers such as cerebrospinal fluid drainage as we feel that randomized data comparing prophylactic cerebrospinal fluid drainage to no drainage at all did not show any difference in paraplegia [27, 28]. We would, however, perform spinal cord drainage in very high-risk patients and also postoperatively should any patient have any evidence of spinal cord ischemia. In our report, this maneuver was not successful in preventing paraplegia in our patient.

A substantial proportion of the dissections we treated did not extend distal to the celiac artery. Examination of this subgroup of patients revealed no significant differences in presentation (acute vs chronic), indication for intervention, or rate of postoperative complication. While this group does include the one patient in whom we detected a significant increase in aortic diameter, it is likely that this was related to the new development of a second distal entry point between 3 and 4 years following the original procedure as we did not notice aortic enlargement during the early years of follow-up. There was no extension of the dissection in any of the other patients in this group of patients treated. We believe that the expeditious deployment of the device in this setting may serve to prevent extension of the dissection and consequent distal malperfusion and could account for those results we reported.

Despite the minimal invasiveness of endoluminal graft for the treatment of type B dissections complications relating to respiratory, renal systems as well as hematomas, lymphocele, and pseudoaneurysms did arise. Our 30-day mortality of 2.5% and 1-year survival of 85% compares favorably to various reports [29–34] (Figure 6). Our results suggest that with a low major morbidity and mortality, exclusion of the proximal entry point with endovascular prosthesis may stabilize the thoracic aorta and aid in the prevention of aneurysm expansion, malperfusion, and ultimately decreasing the incidence of thoracic aortic rupture when endoluminal grafts are used to treat acute type B dissections.

Prospective randomized, controlled studies would be required to definitively address the utility of this therapeutic modality in the prevention of aortic expansion and rupture in the setting of type B dissection as well as comparison to medical therapy. However, the myriad presentations of thoracic

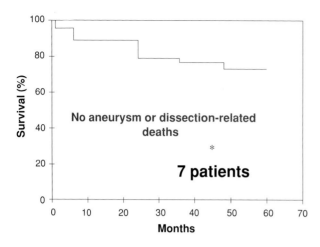

**Figure 6** Kaplan-Meier survival curve 23 ± 18.9 months (12–60 mo).

aortic dissection would make such an initiative difficult. There is certainly room for improvement with regard to traditional therapeutic approaches to aortic dissection. The Gore TAG thoracic endoprosthesis is the only commercial endograft available in the US market. The current instructions for use for the device state that the device is approved only for the use of the treatment of descending thoracic aneurysms. The use of the Gore TAG thoracic endoprosthesis to treat dissections has been mainly restricted to single-center studies at this time. Other novel devices currently under Food and Drug Administration investigation include a covered proximal part and an uncovered distal part may further improve the paraplegia rate as we believe there would be less segments of the descending thoracic aorta subject to a covered endoprosthesis. Our experience indicates that endografting of the thoracic aorta is a beneficial adjunct in the management of this difficult disease entity and is associated with satisfactory short-term and mid-term results. We believe that long-term follow-up of patients, current and future devices are necessary to further define the role of thoracic endografting in the management of type B thoracic dissection.

## References

1 Khan IA, Nair CK. Clinical, diagnostic, and management perspectives of aortic dissection. *Chest* 2002; **122**: 311–328.

2 Hagan PG, Nienaber CA, Isselbacher EM *et al.* The International Registry of Acute Aortic Dissection (IRAD) (new insights into an old disease). *JAMA* 2000; **283**: 897–903.

3 Januzzi JL, Movsowitz HD, Choi J, Abernethy W, Isselbacher E. Significance of recurrent pain in acute type B aortic dissection. *Am J Cardiol* 2001; **87**: 930–933.

4 Hartnell G, Costello P. The diagnosis of thoracic aortic dissection by noninvasive imaging procedures. *N Engl J Med* 1993; **328**: 1637; author reply 1638.

5 LePage MA, Quint LE, Sonnad SS, Deeb GM, Williams DM. Aortic dissection (CT features that distinguish true lumen from false lumen). *AJR Am J Roentgenol* 2001; **177**: 207–211.

6 Sueyoshi E, Sakamoto I, Hayashi K, Yamaguchi T, Imada T. Growth rate of aortic diameter in patients with type B aortic dissection during the chronic phase *Circulation* 2004; **110**: II256–II261.

7 Akutsu K, Nejima J, Kiuchi K *et al.* Effects of the patent false lumen on the long-term outcome of type B acute aortic dissection. *Eur J Cardiothorac Surg* 2004; **26**: 359–366.

8 Onitsuka S, Akashi H, Tayama K *et al.* Long-term outcome and prognostic predictors of medically treated acute type B aortic dissections. *Ann Thorac Surg* 2004; **78**: 1268–1273.

9 Marui A, Mochizuki T, Mitsui N, Koyama T, Kimura F, Horibe M. Toward the best treatment for uncomplicated patients with type B acute aortic dissection. *Circulation* 1999; **100**: II275–II280.

10 Lauterbach SR, Cambria RP, Brewster DC *et al.* Contemporary management of aortic branch compromise resulting from acute aortic dissection. *J Vasc Surg* 2001; **33**: 1185–1192.

11 Eleftteriades JA, Lovoulos CJ, Coady MA, Tellides G, Kopf GS, Rizzo JA. Management of descending aortic dissection. *Ann Thorac Surg* 1999; **67**: 2002–2005.

12 Gysi J, Schaffner T, Mohacsi P, Aeschbacher B, Althaus U, Carrel T. Early and late outcome of operated and

non-operated acute dissection of the descending aorta. *Eur J Cardiothorac Surg* 1997; **11**: 1163–1170.

13 Fann JI, Sarris GE, Mitchell RS *et al*. Treatment of patients with aortic dissection presenting with peripheral vascular complications. *Ann Surg* 1990; **212**: 705–713.

14 Cambria RP, Brewster DC, Gertler J *et al*. Vascular complications associated with spontaneous aortic dissection. *J Vasc Surg* 1988; **7**: 199–209.

15 Laas J, Heinemann M, Schaefers HJ, Daniel W, Borst HG. Management of thoracoabdominal malperfusion in aortic dissection. *Circulation* 1991; **84**: 20–24.

16 Wheat MJ, Jr, Bartley T, Seelman RC. Treatment of dissecting aneurysms of the aorta without surgery. *J Thorac Cardiovasc Surg* 1965; **50**: 364–373.

17 Hata M, Shiono M, Inoue T *et al*. Optimal treatment of type B acute aortic dissection: long-term medical follow-up results. *Ann Thorac Surg* 2003; **75**: 1781–1784.

18 Chirillo F, Marchiori MC, Andriolo L *et al*. Outcome of 290 patients with aortic dissection: a 12-year multicenter experience. *Eur Heart J* 1990; **11**: 311–319.

19 Roseborough G, Burke J, Sperry J, Perler B, Parra J, Williams GM. Twenty-year experience with acute distal thoracic aortic dissections. *J Vasc Surg* 2004; **40**: 235–246.

20 Dake MD, Miller DC, Semba CP *et al*. Transluminal placement of endovascular stent-grafts for the treatment of descending thoracic aortic aneurysms. *N Engl J Med* 1994; **331**: 1729–1734.

21 Herold U, Piotrowski J, Baumgart D *et al*. Endoluminal stent graft repair for acute and chronic type B aortic dissection and atherosclerotic aneurysm of the thoracic aorta: an interdisciplinary task. *Eur J Cardiothorac Surg* 2002; **22**: 891–897.

22 Czermak BV, Waldenberger P, Fraedrich G *et al*. Treatment of Stanford type B aortic dissection with stent-grafts: preliminary results. *Radiology* 2000; **217**: 544–550.

23 Rodriguez JA, Olsen DM, Diethrich EB. Thoracic aortic dissections: unpredictable lesions that may be treated using endovascular techniques. *J Card Surg* 2003; **18**: 334–350.

24 Suzuki T, Mehta RH, Ince H *et al*. Clinical profiles and outcomes of acute type B aortic dissection in the current era: lessons from the International Registry of Aortic Dissection (IRAD). *Circulation* 2003; **108**: II312–II317.

25 Kato M, Bai H, Sato K *et al*. Determining surgical indications for acute type B dissection based on enlargement of aortic diameter during the chronic phase. *Circulation* 1995; **92**(Suppl): II107–II112.

26 Nathanson DR, Rodriguez-Lopez JA, Ramaiah VG *et al*. Endoluminal stent-graft stabilization for thoracic aortic dissection. *J Endovasc Ther* 2005; **12**: 354–359.

27 Gravereaux EC, Faries PL, Burks JLA *et al*. Risk of spinal cord ischemia after endograft repair of thoracic aortic aneurysms. *J vasc Surg* 2001; **34**: 997–1003.

28 Crawford ES, Svensson LG, Hess KR, Shenaq SS, Coselli JS, Safi HJ. A prospective randomized study of cerebrospinal fluid drainage to prevent paraplegia after high-risk surgery on the thoracoabdominal aorta. *J Vasc Surg* 1991; **13**(1): 36–45.

29 Dake MD, Kato N, Mitchell RS *et al*. Endovascular stent-graft placement for the treatment of acute aortic dissection. *N Engl J Med* 1999; **340**: 1546–1552.

30 Beregi JP, Haulon S, Otal P *et al*. Endovascular treatment of acute complications associated with aortic dissection: midterm results from a multicenter study. *J Endovasc Ther* 2003; **10**: 486–493.

31 Bortone AS, DeCillis E, D'Agostino D, deLuca TSL. Endovascular treatment of thoracic aortic disease: four years of experience. *Circulation* 2004; **110**(11, Suppl 1): II262–II267.

32 Leurs LJ, Bell R, Degrieck Y *et al*. Endovascular treatment of thoracic aortic diseases: combined experience from the EUROSTAR and United Kingdom thoracic endograft registries. *J Vasc Surg* 2004; **40**: 670–680.

33 Duebener LF, Lorenzen P, Richardt G *et al*. Emergency endovascular stent-grafting for life-threatening acute type B aortic dissections. *Ann Thorac Surg* 2004; **78**: 1261–1267.

34 Kato N, Shimono T, Hirano T *et al*. Midterm results of stent-graft repair of acute and chronic aortic dissection with descending tear: the complication-specific approach. *J Thorac Cardiovasc Surg* 2002; **124**: 306–312.

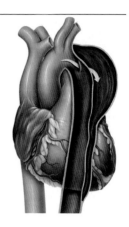

# CASE 17

# Endoluminal graft repair of chronic type B dissections

## Introduction

Acute type B dissections are still associated with a mortality of 10%. The mortality is stabilized once the acute phase has been overcome. Fourteen to twenty percent of patients with an acute type B aortic dissection who are managed conservatively eventually develop false aneurysms during the first 4–5 years of follow-up [1–3]. Surgical aortic replacement is required in these patients to avoid aortic rupture and is still associated with a relatively high mortality of 4–17% [4, 5]. The goal of therapy using the endovascular approach is to avoid aortic rupture or redissection. Inclusion criteria are similar to the surgical indications for repair include:

1. aortic diameter greater than 50 mm on CT scans,
2. aortic diameter greater than 40 mm on CT scan in a dissection less than 1 month,
3. enlargement of an ulcerlike projection during follow-up,
4. persistent back pain despite medical therapy, and
5. findings suggestive of aortic branch ischemia.

The rationale for endovascular treatment of dissections is to close the entry tear, induce thrombosis of the false lumen, and reexpand the true lumen to improve distal perfusion. Complications of endograft therapy include postimplantation syndrome which is characterized by fever and leukocytosis. Paraplegia develops in about 5% of endovascular patients, which is less when compared to open surgical repair. Left arm ischemia can occur when the left subclavian artery is covered by the stent graft to exclude intimal tears close to the left subclavian artery. Remodeling of the aorta can occur at mid-term follow-

up with shrinkage of false lumen and expansion of true lumen. The remodeling of the aorta is not as conspicuous as in acute aortic dissection [6].

## Case scenario

A 63-year-old male presented with a DeBakey 1 thoracic aortic dissection who had previously underwent an ascending aorta replacement and an open infrarenal abdominal aortic aneurysm. He was found to have a 5.7-cm aneurysmal dilatation of a chronic descending thoracic dissection (Figure 1a–1c). His physical examination was otherwise unremarkable. An aortogram and intravascular ultrasound (IVUS) revealed that the aneurysmal expansion of the dissection involved the left subclavian artery. A staged left subclavian to carotid artery bypass was performed after which the deployment of a thoracic endoluminal graft to the thoracic aorta with coverage of the left subclavian artery was accomplished (Figure 2).

## Technical details (left carotid–subclavian bypass)

A left-sided supraclavicular incision was performed (Figure 3). The platysma was divided followed by the clavicular head of the sternocleidomastoid medially to reveal the carotid sheath. The carotid sheath was identified and incised to reveal the common carotid artery and the vagus nerve, which was protected. Next, we divided the omohyoid muscle and identified the scalene fat pad and mobilized it from lateral to medial to reveal the phrenic nerve

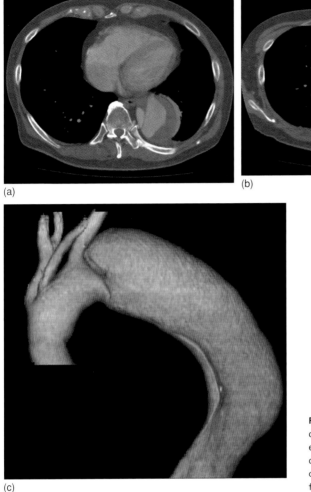

(a)

(b)

(c)

**Figure 1** (a) A CT scan image demonstrating a descending thoracic dissection with aneurysmal expansion. (b) A CT scan with dissection of the distal aortic arch. (c) A 64-slice CT scan with a compressed true lumen and an aneurysmal false lumen.

overlying the scalenus anterior muscle. The phrenic nerve was preserved and the scalenus anterior muscle divided to reveal the aneurysmal ostium of the left subclavian artery. We then divided the left subclavian artery between clamps and proceeded to oversew the proximal subclavian artery with a 4-0 Prolene and sewed the distal end of the subclavian artery to a 10-mm Gore TAG graft (W.L. Gore & Associates, Flagstaff, AZ) in an end-to-end fashion after administering 5000 units of heparin. The graft was tunneled beneath the internal jugular vein and after clamping the left common carotid artery proximally and distally the graft was sewn in an end-to-side fashion with 5-0 Prolene. De-airing maneuvers were performed prior to unclamping the artery to restore flow. The neck incision was closed and patient returned to the recovery room without any complications. An alternative approach of transposition of the left subclavian artery to the left carotid artery (Figure 3) can also be performed alternatively to a left carotid subclavian bypass.

## Technical details of endoluminal graft deployment for dissecting thoracic aneurysm

Access through the left brachial artery with a 5-F (French) sheath was performed in order to access the true lumen. An aortogram performed through an angiographic 5-F pigtail catheter demonstrated

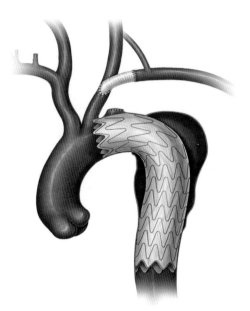

**Figure 2** Illustration of a left carotid artery to left subclavian bypass with coverage of the left subclavian artery with an endoluminal graft.

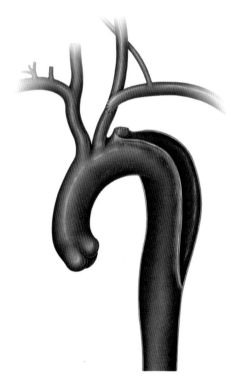

**Figure 3** Left carotid–subclavian transposition.

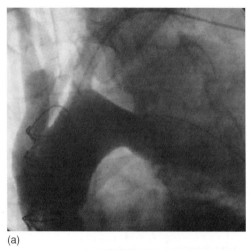

(a)

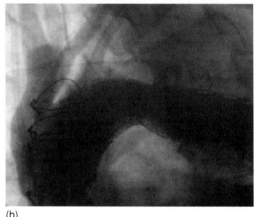

(b)

**Figure 4** (a) An aortogram demonstrating a compressed true lumen. (b) A completion aortogram with expansion of true lumen, with no endoleak visualized.

the aneurysmal dissecting aneurysm with compressed true lumen (Figure 4a). IVUS was performed to determine the size of the dissecting aneurysm as well as to determine the proximal and distal neck diameters for the proper selection of an endoluminal graft. Through the 5-F brachial access, a 0.035-in. soft-tip angled glide wire was advanced from the left brachial artery into the thoracic arch into the true lumen under fluoroscopy; similarly a 0.035-in. soft-tip angled glide wire was advanced through an open retrograde access of the left common femoral artery with introduction of a 9-F sheath. IVUS through the left 9-F sheath was performed that actually confirmed that both the wires from the brachial artery as well as the wire from the left common femoral artery were in the true lumen. The 0.035-in. soft-tip angled glide wire was exchanged to an extra-stiff 260-cm Lunderquist wire (Cook Inc., Bloomington, IN) through the left common femoral artery sheath. Based on our IVUS and aortogram a 40 mm × 20 cm Gore TAG endograft (W.L. Gore & Associates, Flagstaff, AZ) was chosen. An exchange of the 9-F sheath to a 24-F sheath was performed and a 40 mm × 20 cm Gore TAG endograft was delivered through the sheath so that the device was just distal to the left carotid artery. A Gore trilobe balloon was used to balloon the proximal and distal end of the endograft for optimal apposition to the aortic wall. A completion angiogram demonstrated complete exclusion of the aneurysm. All wires and sheaths were removed the left common femoral artery and primarily repaired (Figure 4b).

Patient had a postoperative CT scan which demonstrated satisfactory exclusion of dissecting aneurysm with no identifiable endoleak (Figure 5a and 5b).

## Discussion

The natural history of patients with chronic thoracic dissections is to experience chronic expansion of the thoracic aorta that could potentially lead to rupture [7]. Twenty-five to forty percent of patients with acute type B dissection will progress to develop aneurysmal dilatation of the aorta despite aggressive medical therapy [6, 8].

Patency of a false lumen as a result of a persistent entry [9], poorly controlled hypertension, and an initial aortic diameter of more than 4 cm have been identified as determinants for chronic expansion of the aorta as well as independent risk factors for dissection-related death and dissection-related events [9]. Ten to twenty percent of those patients with a chronic dissection will subsequently experience late rupture of the aneurysm, and conventional surgical repair of such lesions is considerably more complex than with degenerative aneurysms [10].

Marui et al. reported that during the chronic phase, the event-free rate at 1 year was 97% in type B dissections with a thrombosed false lumen and an aortic diameter of less than 40 mm [11]. Conversely, dissections with a patent false lumen and an aortic diameter of 40 mm or more had an event-free rate of only 43% at the same instant. With respect to

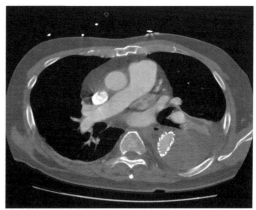

(a)

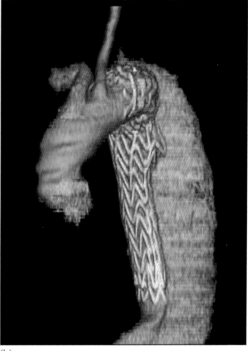

(b)

**Figure 5** (a) An axial CT scan image postendoluminal graft with exclusion of dissecting aneurysm with thrombosis of false lumen and no endoleak. (b) A 64-slice CT scan postendoluminal graft distal to left carotid artery with thrombosis of false lumen and no endoleak.

these findings, the advantage of endovascular treatment of acute type B dissections may not be limited only to treatment of complications, but might also prevent adverse events during the chronic phase [12].

Aneurysms that are the sequelae of chronic dissection tend to be more extensive and occur in younger patients compared with degenerative aneurysms. Treatment with effective $\beta$-blockade is an essential feature of long-term therapy and follow-up. The rationale of such therapy is based on the recognition that patients with aortic dissection have a systemic illness that places their entire aorta at risk for further dissection, aneurysm, or rupture. Guidelines recommend progressive upward titration of $\beta$-blockade to achieve a blood pressure less than 125/80 mm Hg in usual patients and less than 120 in those with Marfan syndrome. In addition, aggressive $\beta$-blockade has been shown to retard the growth of the aortic root in these patients and may have a similar effect on the thoracoabdominal aorta.

Serial imaging is the cornerstone of long-term follow-up in managing patients with type B dissections. Axial imaging modalities as well as 64-slice CT imaging should encompass the entire aorta. The rational for endografting is to exclude the entry tear, induce false lumen thrombosis to prevent the aortic pressure from acting on the aortic wall. Location of entry tear, shape and size of the landing zone, diameter and tortuosity of access route should be obtained by CT scan, IVUS, or angiogram. Sufficient proximal neck length 1.5–2.0 cm must be available to allow sealing of the entry tear. True lumen must be large enough to allow delivery of a device since in chronic dissection the intimal flap is fibrotic and not easily distensible. Due to the nondistensibilty of the true lumen in chronic dissection, stent grafts have to be able to adapt to the shape of the true lumen, which in most circumstances is not circular. Stent grafts with hooks should not be used in dissection due to the possibility of the hooks causing a new intimal tear. Migration is less of an issue since most dissections have a tapering true lumen; hence, tapered graft would be more suitable for the treatment of chronic dissection. Complications of endograft therapy include postimplantation syndrome which is characterized by fever, leukocytosis. Paraplegia develops in about 5% of patients undergoing endografting, which is less than open surgical repair. Left arm ischemia can occur when the left subclavian artery is covered by the stent graft to exclude intimal tears close to the left subclavian artery. Remodeling of the aorta occurs at mid-term follow-up with shrinkage of false lumen and expansion of true lumen; however, this remodeling of the aorta is not as conspicuous as in acute aortic dissection [13].

Two clinical trials to date the EUROSTAR/United Kingdom registry report [14] and the investigation of stent grafts in patients with type B aortic dissection (INSTEAD) trial [15] have been set up to address the use of endoluminal graft therapy in the management of thoracic aortic dissections. The EUROSTAR/United Kingdom registry report [14] is the largest compendium of patients treated with thoracic aortic stent grafts to date. In the combined registry, 131 patients with aortic dissection (5% proximal, 81% distal, 14% not classified) were treated with stent grafts, 57% had symptoms of rupture, aortic expansion, or side branch occlusion. Although no meaningful long-term data are available, primary technical success was achieved in 89% and 30-day mortality was 8.4%. Paraplegia occurred in 0.8% of those treated, and survival at 1 year after treatment was reported in 90% of 67 patients who had such follow-up. The INSTEAD trial which completed recruiting patients in Europe in 2006 is the first randomized trial investigating the role of stent-graft treatment of uncomplicated type B aortic dissection compared with the best medical therapy alone. Inclusion criteria are patients with distal chronic (2–52 wk from the onset of symptoms) dissections without evidence of malperfusion syndrome. Thus, the INSTEAD trial [15] addresses whether patients with chronic, uncomplicated, distal aortic dissection treated with an endovascular stent graft have an improved initial outcome and freedom from late dissection complications. In designing the trial, 80 patients treated by the primary author with stent-graft repair of type B aortic dissection were retrospectively compared with 80 patients managed medically. Two-year survival was 67.5% in the medically treated group and 94.9% in the group managed with endovascular stent-graft treatment.

Currently in the United States, no thoracic endograft devices are specifically approved for the commercial treatment of a descending aortic dissection. These devices are commonly being used in "off-label" procedures for this purpose. To determine the role of endoluminal grafts in the treatment of dissections, both device manufacturers and academic centers are now conducting sanctioned studies to objectively look at the patient outcomes for such a procedure. Looking into the future, endoluminal grafts with designed side-branches that allow for arterial blood flow for critical vessels while covering a diseased area will usher in the next generation of endovascular technologies. The initial experience with endovascular technology in chronic dissections combined with evolving device designs will play an increasingly more important role in the future for dissection management.

## References

1 Acute aortic dissection. *Lancet* 1998; **2**: 827–828.

2 DeBakey ME, McCollum CH, Crawford ES *et al.* Dissection and dissecting aneurysms of the aorta: twenty year follow-up of five hundred and twenty seven patients treated surgically. *Surgery* 2002; **92**: 1118–1134.

3 Juvonen T, Ergin MA, Galla JD *et al.* Risk factors for rupture of chronic type B dissections. *Thorac Cardiovasc Surg* 1999; **117**: 776–786.

4 Miller DC, Mitchell RS, Oyer PE, Stinson EB, Jamieson SW, Shumway NE. Independent determinants of operative mortality for patients with aortic dissections. *Circulation* 1984; **70**(Suppl 1): 1153–1164.

5 Svensson LG, Crawford ES, Hess KR, Coselli JS, Safi HJ. Dissection of the aorta and dissecting aortic aneurysms. *Circulation* 1990; **82**(Suppl IV): IV24–IV 28.

6 Hollier LH, Symmonds JB, Pairolero PC, Cherry KJ, Hallett JW, Gloviczki P. Thoracoabdominal aortic aneurysm repair: analysis of postoperative morbidity. *Arch Surg* 1988; **123**: 871–875.

7 Suzuki T, Mehta RH, Ince H *et al.* Clinical profiles and outcomes of acute type B aortic dissection in the current era: lessons from the International Registry of Aortic Dissection (IRAD). *Circulation* 2003; **108**: II312–II317.

8 Larson EW, Edwards W. Risk factors for aortic dissection (a necropsy study of 161 patients). *Am J Cardiol* 1984; **53**: 849–855.

9 Kato M, Bai H, Sato K *et al.* Determining surgical indications for acute type B dissection based on enlargement of aortic diameter during the chronic phase. *Circulation* 1995; **92**(Suppl): II107–II112.

10 Panneton JM, Hollier LH. Dissecting descending thoracic and thoracoabdominal aortic aneurysms (Part II). Ann Vasc Surg 1995; **9**: 596–605.

11 Marui A, Mochizuki T, Mitsui N, Koyama T, Kimura F, Horibe M. Toward the best treatment for uncomplicated patients with type B acute aortic dissection. *Circulation* 1999; **100**: II275–II280.

12 Akutsu K, Nejima J, Kiuchi K *et al.* Effects of the patent false lumen on the long-term outcome of type B acute aortic dissection. *Eur J Cardiothorac Surg* 2004; **26**: 359–366.

13 Kato N, Shimono T, Hirano T *et al.* Mid-term results of stent graft repair of aortic dissection: comparison between acute and chronic dissection—the complication-specific approach. *J Thorac Cardiovasc Surg* 2002; **124**: 306–312.

14 Leurs L, Bell R, Degrieck Y *et al.* Endovascular treatment of thoracic aortic diseases (combined experience from the EUROSTAR and United Kingdom Thoracic Endograft registries). *J Vasc Surg* 2004; **40**: 670–680.

15 Nienaber CA, Zannetti S, Barbieri B, Kische S, Schareck W, Rehders TC, for the INSTEAD Study Collaborators. Investigation of stent grafts in patients with type B aortic dissection (Design of the INSTEAD trial—a prospective, multicenter, European randomized trial). *Am Heart J* 2005; **149**: 592–599.

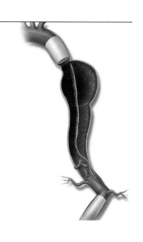

# CASE 18

# Endovascular management of the aneurysmal false lumen distal to an interposition graft placed for ruptured Stanford type B dissection

## Introduction

The natural progression of chronic type B dissection is to dilate over time. Ischemic complications and aortic rupture complicate acute dissections with a mortality of 30% [1] unless successful emergency treatment is rendered. In close to 85% of patients [2] with chronic type B dissection, there is partial to full patency of the false lumen with the risk of progressive dilatation to aneurysmal formation in 35% of patients [3] with cause of late mortality related to rupture. Endoluminal graft treatment of chronic dissection is primarily aimed at covering the entry tear to prevent false lumen flow and subsequent aneurysmal dilatation of the thoracic aorta and for treatment of aneurysmal dilatation of the false lumen to prevent aortic rupture. Fenestration techniques create a communication between the dissecting flaps which allows blood and pressure equilibration between both lumens which is important for reperfusion of compromised branched vessels. The use of endoluminal graft, percutaneous fenestration techniques provides a less invasive approach to managing the high-risk patient with a dissection.

## Case scenario

A 78-year-old male developed a Stanford type B dissection with rupture requiring placement of an interposition graft through a left thoracotomy. He subsequently presented a couple of months later with extension of the dissection into the abdominal aorta, resulting in absence of peripheral pulses and worsening renal function. He underwent an aorto-bifemoral graft with an open fenestration of the dissecting septum with resolution of malperfusion. He had subsequently done well over a period of 12 years when he developed new onset chest and back pain with uncontrolled hypertension. On physical examination his left femoral pulse was stronger than his right femoral pulse. A CT scan of the chest and abdomen performed demonstrated a type B thoracic dissection with aneurysmal dilatation of the descending thoracic aorta at the site of previous repair measured at 8 cm and a dissecting flap extending all the way from the interposition graft to the abdominal graft with a compressed true lumen (Figure 1). He was therefore transferred to our facility for an angiogram/intravascular ultrasound (IVUS) with possibility of an intervention.

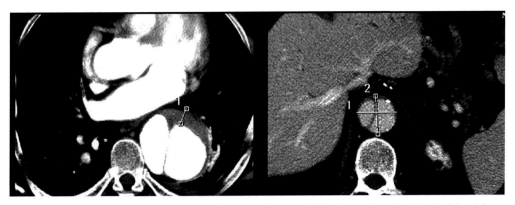

**Figure 1** An axial CT scan demonstrating a type B dissection with true and false lumen flow. At the level of the abdomen, there is true lumen collapse with flow filling both lumens.

## Thoracic aortogram and intravascular ultrasound

The patient was prepped for an open and endovascular repair of his thoracic dissection. The left upper extremity and bilateral groins were prepped. The left brachial artery was accessed with a retrograde puncture and a 6-F (French) short sheath was introduced. Similarly, percutaneous access of both common femoral arteries was performed with an 18-G needle and a 0.035-in. soft-tip angled glide wire was advanced into the distal aorta with sheath exchanged to a 9-F short sheath. A 6-F pigtail angiographic catheter was advanced through both groin sheaths and the left brachial artery sheaths for individual and selective contrast angiograms to identify both true and false lumen dependent flow patterns. The angiographic studies indicated that the visceral branches were supplied by the severely compromised true lumen (Figure 2) with the renal arteries and the distal aortic circulation supplied by the false lumen. There was a communication between both lumens at the proximal descending thoracic aorta just distal to the interposition graft with both lumen separated by a thickened septum extending from the previously placed thoracic interposition graft to the old infrarenal aortic graft (Figure 3). The false lumen aortogram demonstrated the thoracic aortic aneurysm to measure about 8.0 cm in diameter.

Further information to characterize the behavior of the true and false lumen was obtained by IVUS. Exchange of the 6-F angiographic pigtail catheter

for an IVUS 8.2-F probe (Jo-Med, Cardova, CA) was performed. The IVUS probe confirmed that the left brachial pigtail was within the true lumen that the left femoral wire was within the true lumen while the right common femoral artery wire was within the false lumen. The true lumen was markedly compressed from the beginning of the

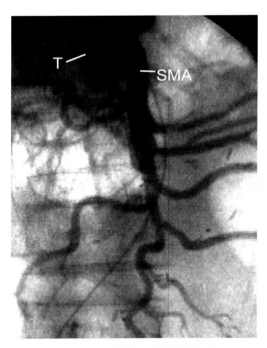

**Figure 2** True lumen angiogram demonstrating a compressed true lumen with flow supplying the superior mesenteric artery (SMA). The renal arteries are supplied by false lumen flow.

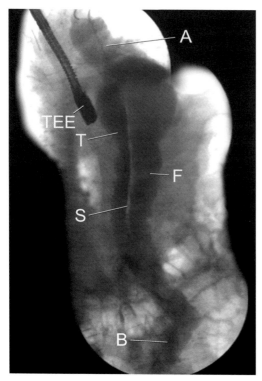

**Figure 3** An angiogram demonstrating a compressed true lumen separated from the false lumen (F) by a thickened septum (S) with an interposition graft in the thoracic aorta (A) and a distal abdominal graft (B).

descending thoracic aortic graft to the superior mesenteric artery with no distal aortic lumen flow coming from the true lumen. The proximal neck diameter was measured at 31 mm and the distal neck diameter at the level of the infrarenal graft measured to be 25 mm. Coverage of the descending thoracic aorta from the distal thoracic aortic graft to the celiac trunk was contemplated with a plan to fenestrate the septum at the level of the renal vessels to supply flow to the renal arteries that was flow de-pendent on the false lumen. The wires were taken out and the sheaths left in place for the procedure.

## Assessment and plan

1. Exclude the symptomatic aneurysmal false lu-men dilatation with deployment of an endolu-minal graft in the true lumen.
2. Seal the upper communication of the two lu-mens, thereby avoiding progression of aortic flow from the true lumen into the false aneurysm sac.
3. Expand the severely compromised distal true lu-men with balloon angioplasty prior to deploy-ment of an endoluminal graft.
4. Establish a communication distal to the superior mesenteric artery after deployment of endolumi-nal graft to collapse the false lumen in order to perfuse the renal vessels and distal aortic circu-lation which were dependent on the false lumen flow.

## Technical details of procedure

A 0.035-in. soft-tip angled glide wire Terumo (Boston Scientific, Natick, MA) was introduced through the true lumen of the left common femoral artery and guided into the proximal thoracic aorta with the help of a RIM catheter (Angiodynamics, Queensbury, NY). Heparin was given to achieve an activated clotting time of greater than 200 sec-onds. Similarly, a 0.035-in. glide wire was advanced through the right groin sheath into the false lu-men. Pressure gradients across both groin sheaths demonstrated a moderate gradient between the groin sheaths. A 12 mm × 4 cm balloon catheter (Cook Inc., Bloomington, IN) was advanced trough the left groin sheath and balloon angioplasty of the distal aorta was performed to expand the true lumen with resolution of the gradient. A straight 0.035-in. stiff wire (Boston Scientific, Natick, MA) along with a support catheter was next used to penetrate and fenestrate the thickened septum at the level of the renal arteries. Serial balloon dilatation of the septum was performed with a 12 mm × 4 cm bal-loon catheter (Cook Inc., Bloomington, IN) and then with a Braun 16 mm × 4 cm balloon catheter (Figure 4). A contrast injection through the true lu-men pigtail catheter showed brisk filling of the renal arteries and distal aorta. Since the device was to be deployed through the true lumen left groin sheath, we advanced our angiographic catheter through the left brachial sheath for true lumen angiogram dur-ing deployment of an endoluminal graft.

We then exchanged the left 9-F sheath to a 22-F Gore sheath and over an extra-stiff wire (Lunderquist) we deployed a 34 mm × 15 cm Gore TAG excluder stent graft (W.L. Gore & Associates, Flagstaff, AZ) distal to the left subclavian artery to

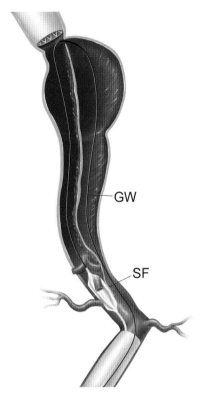

**Figure 4** Illustration demonstrating cannulation of both true and false lumen with a glide wire (GW). Serial balloon angioplasty to create a septal fenestration (SF) at the level of the renal arteries to provide flow to the renal vessels which are false lumen flow dependent prior to deployment of an endoluminal graft to seal false lumen flow supplying the 8-cm thoracic aortic aneurysm.

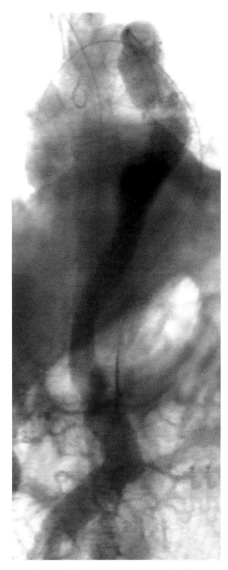

**Figure 5** A completion angiogram demonstrating exclusion of thoracic aortic aneurysm with visceral and renal perfusion.

overlap the distal part of the interposition graft and extended all the way to the celiac trunk by deploying a 34 mm × 10 cm Gore TAG graft distally up to the celiac trunk. An angiogram performed through the left brachial approach demonstrated a proximal type I endoleak which was treated by deploying a 37 mm × 15 cm Gore TAG graft proximally with adequate overlap. Balloon angioplasty of the proximal, distal landing zones, and areas of overlap was performed using the Gore trilobe balloon. A completion angiogram performed demonstrated no endoleak with single true lumen perfusion of the visceral branches with brisk perfusion of the renal arteries from the fenestrated septum with an intact distal circulation (Figure 5).

Postoperative CT scan (Figure 6) demonstrated no endoleak with a reexpanded true lumen. At 36 months post-treatment the patient is well and without any pain and no evidence of endoleak with stabilization of the distal aorta.

## Discussion

The long-term sequelae of type B thoracic dissection with a patent false lumen is to dilate over time with aneurysmal dilatation of the false lumen. Recently,

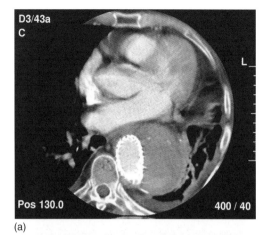

(a)

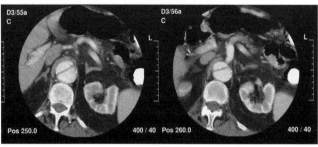

(b)

**Figure 6** (a) Postoperative CT scan demonstrating thrombosis of false aneurysm. (b) Postoperative CT scan with true and false lumen flow to the visceral and renal arteries.

endoluminal grafts have increasingly been applied to the treatment of uncomplicated and complicated dissections [4–6]. Symptomatic type B chronic dissections with thoracic aortic dilatation are at an increased risk of rupture. The use of transesophageal echocardiogram, IVUS, is helpful to determine precise aortic landing zones for the management of dissections with an endoluminal graft.

Percutaneous techniques combining the use of an endoluminal graft and fenestration are sometimes necessary to correct malperfusion syndromes arising from branch vessel occlusion. Dynamic obstruction is the cause of malperfusion in 50% of cases and is appropriately treated with an endoluminal stent graft which results in true lumen expansion with improved blood flow. Static obstruction with resulting occlusion of a branched vessel by a dissecting flap do not improve with an endoluminal graft and in these scenarios fenestration and stent placement should be considered solely as the mode of treatment of the malperfusion. Occasionally,

there is the combination of a static and a dynamic obstruction which requires both the use of an endoluminal graft to improve true lumen flow and fenestration with or without a stent in the branch vessel to improve flow to the branch vessel. In our presentation the deployment of an endoluminal graft was beneficial to firstly exclude the aneurysmal dilated thoracic aorta that was receiving flow from a reentry tear distal to the interposition graft and secondly to expand the collapsed true lumen with collapse of the false lumen resulting improved flow to the visceral branched vessels receiving flow from the true lumen. Fenestration was needed to supply flow to the renal arteries that were flow dependent on the collapsed false lumen resulting from deployment of the endoluminal graft. Preoperative imaging should be performed with CT imaging, contrast angiography, IVUS, and transesophageal echocardiography to determine the dissecting type, location of entry tears, identification of true and false lumen, identification of arteries at risk of malperfusion, and identification of mechanism of obstruction.

In conclusion, the application of endoluminal grafts, fenestration techniques, covered and uncovered stents should be individualized to each patient depending on the understanding of the pathophysiology and mechanism of aortic dissection. Routine surveillance with CT imaging should be performed to evaluate the fate of the false lumen over time.

## References

1 Lindsay J, Hurst JW. Clinical fatures and prognosis in dissecting aneurysm of the aorta: a reappraisal. *Circulation* 1967; **35**: 880–888.

2 Yamaguchi T, Naito H, Ohta M *et al*. False lumens in type III aortic dissections: progress CT study. *Radiology* 1985; **156**: 757–760.

3 Kato M, Bai H, Sato K *et al*. Determined surgical indications for acute type B dissection based on enlargement of aortic diameter during the chronic phase. *Circulation* 1995; **92**(Suppl II): 107–112.

4 Palma JH, Marcondes de Souza JA, Alves CMR, Carvalho AC, Buffolo E. Self-expandable aortic stent grafts for treatment of descending aortic dissections. *Ann Thorac Surg* 2002; **73**: 1138–1142.

5 Nienaber CA, Fattori R, Lund G *et al*. Nonsurgical reconstruction of the thoracic aortic dissection by stent-graft placement. *N Engl J Med* 1999; **340**: 1539–1545.

6 Dake MD, Kato N, Mitchell RS *et al*. Endovascular stent graft placement for the treatment of cute aortic dissection. *N Engl J Med* 1999; **340**: 1546–1552.

# Hybrid management of type A dissection with malperfusion of the lower extremities

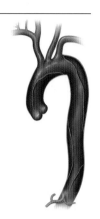

## Introduction

Aortic dissection is defined as the separation of the aortic media with presence of extraluminal blood within the layers of the aortic wall. The presence of one or multiple tears in the aortic intima results in an abnormal communication between the true aortic lumen and the split aortic media. Sixty-five percent of these intimal tears occur in the ascending aorta as a type A dissection, 20% in the descending thoracic aorta, 10% in the transverse arch, and 5% in the abdominal aorta [1]. For patients with Stanford type A dissections, surgical intervention is performed immediately after diagnosis to avert the high risk of death due to various complications such as cardiac tamponade, aortic regurgitation, and myocardial infarction [2, 3]. Untreated type A dissections are associated with a mortality rate of 1–2% per hour during the first 24–48 hours. Many of these patients are frequently too sick to tolerate deep hypothermic circulatory arrest (DHCA) and arch reconstruction, as such are not able to undergo open surgical treatment. The hybrid approach described in this report offers a potentially less morbid and less invasive one-stage approach that could be tolerated in high-risk surgical patients. In cases of limb ischemia, it is sometimes preferable to provide perfusion to the lower limbs to provide an inflow for extracorporeal circulation. Methods of revascularization may include open surgical techniques, percutaneous fenestration techniques, balloon angioplasty, and deployment of stent grafts.

## Case scenario

A 50-year-old man with a family history of aortic dissection presented to an outside facility with a painful, pulseless right lower extremity. An open thrombectomy was attempted, but it failed to restore circulation; angiogram performed demonstrated a type A dissection which was confirmed by CT scan. The aortic dissection was seen extending from the aortic root to the aortic bifurcation extending to the left common iliac artery with an acute occlusion of the right common iliac artery origin (Figure 1). The patient was transferred to our facility for treatment of both the aortic dissection and the ischemic extremity.

## Procedure

At the time of admission, the right limb was cold, and there was loss of sensation and motor function with associated compartment syndrome. A left to right femoral–femoral bypass graft was performed using a 10-mm Hemashield graft to restore flow to the ischemic right limb. A four-compartment below the knee fasciotomy was also performed on the afflicted extremity. The following morning, the patient was taken to the operating room, where a median sternotomy was performed (Figure 2). Upon opening the pericardial sac, the dissection was verified from the ascending aorta across the aortic arch. Cardiopulmonary bypass was established after heparinization using a single right atrial cannula and a

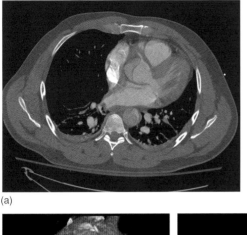

(a)

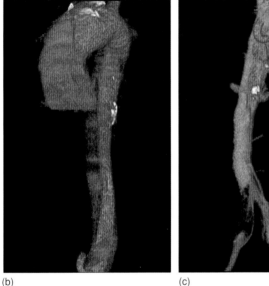

(b)                              (c)

**Figure 1** (a–c) A 64-slice CT scan demonstrating a type A dissection from the ascending aorta with dissection all the way down to the aortic bifurcation and right iliac artery with compressed true lumen resulting in malperfusion of the right lower extremity.

20-F (French) femoral perfusion cannula was inserted proximal to the left femoral–femoral graft (Figure 3). The ascending aorta was cross-clamped at the level of the brachiocephalic artery; cardioplegic solution was administered both retrograde and antegrade, and the patient's body temperature was lowered to 30°C. The entry point of the dissecting aneurysm was visualized in the posterolateral wall of the ascending aorta; the valve leaflets and coronary ostia were examined and found to be spared from the dissection. Two aortic valve commissures were resuspended using a 2-0 Tevdek suture with pledgets. Both the proximal and distal aortic ends were reinforced with strips of felt, and the

vessel layers were reunited before suturing a 30-mm Hemashield graft (Boston Scientific, Natick, MA) in place. The suture lines were reinforced with fibrin glue (Figure 4). The patient was warmed, cardiopulmonary bypass was discontinued, and heparinization was partially reversed. An intraoperative transesophageal echocardiogram showed only minimal residual aortic insufficiency.

After obtaining satisfactory hemostasis, a branched 16 mm × 8 mm woven Dacron graft was sutured to the interposition graft over a partial occluding clamp. A third 10-mm limb was sutured to the bifurcated graft as a conduit for antegrade endoluminal graft delivery (Figure 5). The left common

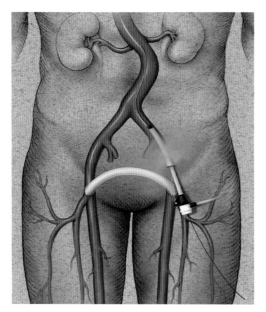

**Figure 2** Illustration of a femoral–femoral bypass graft performed with cannulation of left common femoral artery proximal to bypass graft to place patient on femoral cardiopulmonary bypass.

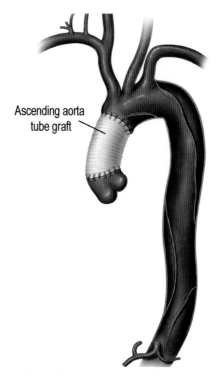

**Figure 4** Illustration of replacement of dissected ascending aorta with a 30-mm Hemashield graft (Boston Scientific, Natick, MA).

carotid was clamped transected at the level of the ostium with a running 4-0 suture. The distal end was sewn in an end-to-end fashion to the 8-mm limb of the bifurcated graft. This was similarly repeated with the innominate artery (Figure 6); the proximal stumps of both the left common carotid and innominate arteries were oversewn prior to removal of clamps. The left arterial perfusion canula was exchanged for a 14-F short sheath under

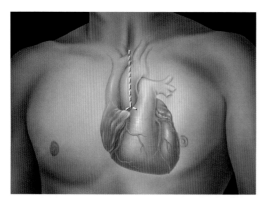

**Figure 3** Illustration of a median sternotomy incision for replacement of ascending aorta.

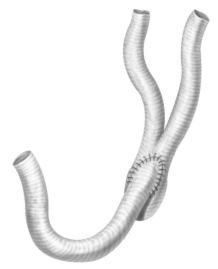

**Figure 5** Illustration of 16 mm × 8 mm woven Dacron graft with a 10-mm side limb sutured for antegrade deployment of endoluminal graft.

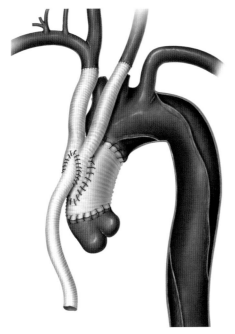

**Figure 6** Illustration of the bifurcated conduit graft anastomosed to the ascending aorta; the common carotid and innominate arteries are transected and anastomosed in an end-to-end to the limbs of the bifurcated graft.

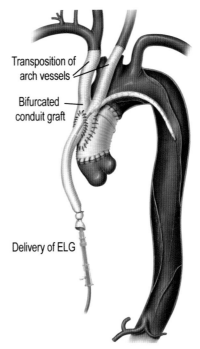

**Figure 8** An illustration of the bifurcated graft and the conduit sutured to the tube graft used to reconstruct the ascending aorta with transposition of arch vessels and antegrade advancement of endoluminal graft for deployment.

fluoroscopic visualization. Percutaneous access of the right common femoral artery was performed with a 9-F sheath. A 9-F sheath was attached to the conduit, and a 0.035-in. angled glide wire (Meditech/Boston Scientific Inc., Natick, MA) was passed through the conduit to the left common iliac artery where it was captured by a snare (Figure 7) that

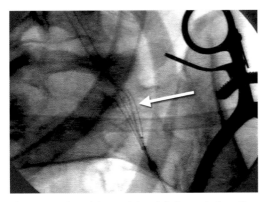

**Figure 7** Snaring of the conduit to left femoral wire with a snare (Microvena).

was delivered through a groin 9-F sheath. A second wire was passed retrograde into the ascending aorta making sure we were in the true lumen and an arch aortogram was performed and stored as a road map. A metal ring was placed around the conduit at its anastomosis to identify the landing zone in the ascending aorta. A 24-F sheath was exchanged for the 9-F sheath attached to the 10-mm limb conduit for delivery of the endoluminal graft through the conduit across the aortic arch (Figure 8); this process was made easier by pulling the ends of the left common femoral–conduit wire simultaneously. A 40 mm × 20 mm TAG stent graft (W.L. Gore & Associates, Flagstaff, AZ) was deployed from the ascending aorta to the mid-descending thoracic aorta after the delivery sheath was retracted (Figure 9). An aortogram showed continued true lumen compromise distally, so a second 40 mm × 20 mm TAG graft was delivered from the left common femoral access through a 24-F sheath exchange (Figure 10). Completion angiogram (Figure 11)

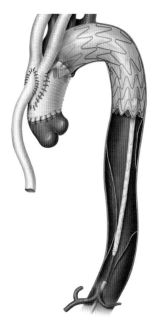

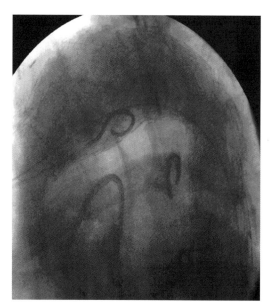

**Figure 11** A completion angiogram with exclusion of dissection flap with true lumen expansion.

**Figure 9** The sheath is withdrawn, and the endoluminal graft is delivered across the aortic arch and into the high descending thoracic aorta with retrograde placement of a second endoluminal graft from the left common femoral artery over the conduit-to-femoral wire.

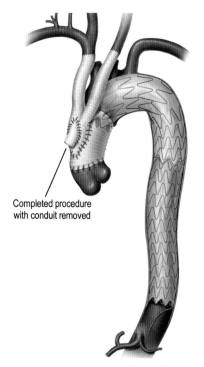

Completed procedure
with conduit removed

**Figure 10** Retrograde deployment of second endoluminal graft to reexpand the compressed true lumen from the left groin sheath.

demonstrated complete exclusion of the dissection flap without true lumen compromise or an identifiable endoleak. The ascending conduit was clamped after sheath retrieval, transected, and then oversewn. A mediastinal drain was placed, hemostasis achieved, and the sternotomy incision closed with sternal wires. The left common femoral artery was repaired after sheath removal. A high-resolution contrast-enhanced CT (Figure 12a, 12b, and 12c) performed prior to hospital discharge showed obliteration of the false channel and no proximal endoleak with a patent femoral–femoral bypass graft and resolution of malperfusion of the lower extremities. At 2-year follow-up CT scan (Figure 13) demonstrated patent debranched grafts to the brachiocephalic and left common carotid arteries were patent, as were the endoluminal grafts in the descending thoracic artery. In the distal abdominal aorta the persistent dissection and a patent femoral–femoral bypass graft were documented.

## Discussion

Despite advance in imaging and surgical techniques, the mortality in the first month of evolution continues to be high 25–30% in patients with type A dissection [4]. The classical treatment for ascending

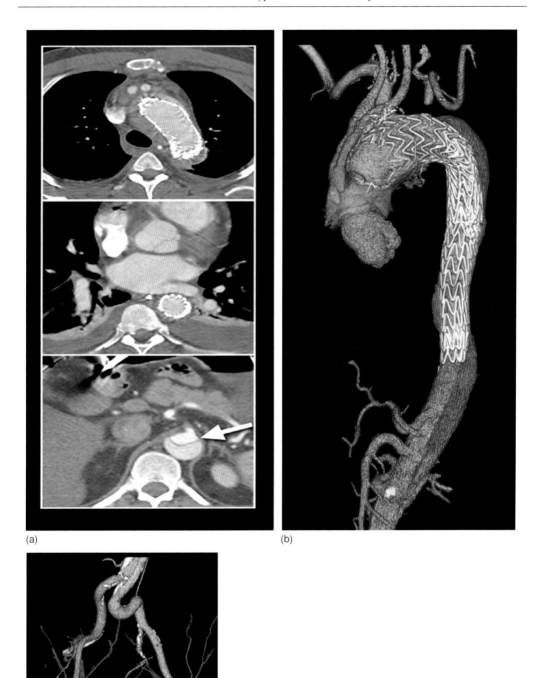

(a)

(b)

(c)

**Figure 12** (a and b) Postoperative 64-slice CT scan examination demonstrating the rerouting of the supra-aortic trunks and exclusion of the dissection in the arch and descending thoracic aorta with true lumen expansion and thrombosis of false lumen (arrow). (c) Postoperative CT scan demonstrating a patent left to right femoral–femoral bypass graft (yellow arrow) with complete resolution of limb ischemia.

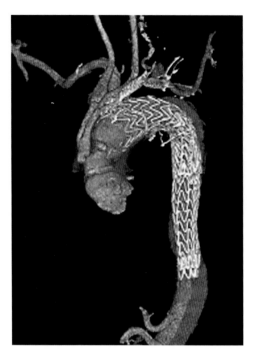

**Figure 13** A 64-slice CT scan at 2 years documenting patency of the ascending tube grafts to the brachiocephalic and left common carotid arteries; the endoluminal grafts were visualized in the descending thoracic aorta.

type A dissection involves the restoration of flow through a reconstructed ascending aorta. Additionally, the nature of the pathological process and its extent present variable requirements for aortic valve replacement or suspension, preservation or reestablishment of coronary blood flow, and the potential to combine these using a valve conduit. Type A dissections often extend across the aortic arch for variable lengths (often below the diaphragm); repair of the ascending component leaves the potential for catastrophic sequelae. Enlarging dissection with aortic rupture, vascular compromise of both visceral and peripheral vasculature are associated with a high morbidity and mortality with neurological deficits more common than appreciated. Ischemia of the lower limbs as a complication of dissection has been described in up to 26% of patients with dissection and may occasionally be isolated with no other clinical data of a suspected dissection [5]. Due to the increased morbidity associated with replacement of the ascending aorta, transverse arch,

and descending aorta to treat a type A dissection, a single-staged procedure combining open surgical and endovascular techniques avoiding DHCA may afford a less morbid operation avoiding the neurological sequalae associated with DHCA. We believe that a more favorable long-term prognosis might be anticipated. Presence of malperfusion syndromes increases the morbidity and mortality of acute dissections to 60%. Prompt revascularization must be achieved either surgically by fenestration or stent-graft deployment to reexpand a collapsed true lumen especially if the malperfusion is a result of a dynamic intimal flap.

In performing the hybrids technique as described [6–11], it is important that the ascending tube graft be of sufficient length to accommodate the conduit. A short graft can complicate the partial occlusion needed when the conduit is sutured. Additionally, a short graft may not provide sufficient overlap between the stent graft and the ascending component.

## References

1 Roberts WC, Honing HS. The spectrum of cardiovascular disease in the Marfan syndrome: a clinico-morphologic study of 18 necropsy patients and comparison to 151 previously reported necropsy patients. *Am Heart J* 1982; **104**: 115–135.

2 Eagle KA, DeSanctis RW. Aortic dissection. *Curr Probl Cardiol* 1989; **14**: 225–278.

3 Cambria RP, Brewster DC, Gertler J *et al.* Vascular complications associated with spontaneous aortic dissection. *J Vasc Surg* 1988; **7**: 199–207.

4 Hagan PG, Nienaber CA, Isselbacher EM *et al.* The international registry of acute aortic dissections (IRAD): new insights into an old disease. *JAMA* 2000; **283**: 897–903.

5 Pacifico L, Spodick D. ILEAD-ischemia of the lower extremities due to aortic dissection: the isolated presentation. *Clin Cardiol* 1999; **22**: 353–356.

6 Diethrich EB, Ghazoul M, Wheatley GH *et al.* Great vessel transposition for antegrade delivery of the TAG endoprosthesis in the proximal aortic arch. *J Endovasc Ther* 2005; **12**: 583–587.

7 Chavan A, Karck M, Hagl C *et al.* Hybrid endograft for one-step treatment of multisegment disease of the thoracic aorta. *J Vasc Interv Radiol* 2005; **16**: 823–829.

8 Greenberg RK, Haddad F, Svensson L *et al.* Hybrid approaches to thoracic aortic aneurysms: the role of endovascular elephant trunk completion. *Circulation* 2005; **112**: 2619–2626.

9  Diethrich EB, Ghazoul M, Wheatley GH, III *et al.* Surgical correction of ascending type A thoracic aortic dissection: simultaneoues endoluminal exclusion of the arch and distal aorta. *J Endovasc Ther* 2005; **12**: 660–666.

10  Zhou W, Reardon M, Peden EK, Lin PH, Lumsden AB. Hybrid approach to complex thoracic aortic aneurysms in high risk patients: surgical challenges and clinical outcomes. *J Vasc Surg* 2006; **44**(4): 688–693.

11  Criado FJ, Clark NS, Barnatan MF. Stent graft repair in the aortic arch and descending thoracic aorta: a 4-year experience. *J Vasc Surg* 2002; **36**: 1121–1128.

# Endovascular management of a type B dissection complicated by renovascular hypertension

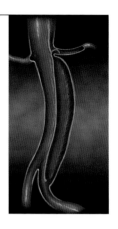

## Introduction

Type B dissection may be complicated by branched vessel occlusion with resulting malperfusion syndromes. The mechanism of branch vessel occlusion may be from a dynamic obstruction in which a flap prolapses across the vessel lumen, a static obstruction in which the dissection flap involves the branch vessel resulting in narrowing of the vessel [1] or a combination of both. Features in a dissected aorta with branch vessel obstruction include equalization of blood pressures in both the true and the false lumen; the compromised branch almost always arises from the true lumen or is perfused by both the true and the false lumen, and false lumen branches rarely show evidence of ongoing obstruction. In dynamic branch occlusion deployment of an endoluminal graft results with reexpansion of the true lumen with improvement in distal blood flow with resolution of malperfusion. Percutaneous fenestration techniques with or without stent deployment is necessary to resolve malperfusion from branch vessel occlusion resulting from a dissecting flap in static obstruction. A thorough familiarity with the mechanism of malperfusion as well as a wide array of endovascular techniques must be available to the cardiovascular specialist who treats patients with aortic dissection.

## Case scenario

A 64-year-old male with past medical history significant for emergent replacement of the ascending aorta for a type A dissection 2 years prior history of controlled hypertension developed a sudden onset of back pain with uncontrolled hypertension and a worsening renal function. CT scan performed (Figure 1a and 1b) demonstrated a type B dissection with a compromised true lumen with the dissecting flap involving the left renal artery and progressing distally to involve the left common iliac artery. A renal duplex ultrasound performed demonstrated elevated systolic and diastolic velocities consistent with 80% stenosis of the left renal artery. An aortogram performed demonstrated an infrarenal dissection with the true lumen supplying the celiac trunk, superior mesenteric artery, and the right renal artery and the left renal artery supplied by the false lumen in a retrograde manner from a distal reentry site at the proximal left iliac artery. The left lumen flow was compromised by a dissecting septum causing stenosis of the artery resulting in compromised flow and potential cause of the uncontrolled hypertension.

## Endovascular procedure

The patient was brought to the operating room and after general anesthesia was achieved, percutaneous retrograde access of the left common femoral artery was performed with an 18-G needle and a 0.035-in. soft-tip angled glide wire was exchanged for a 9-F (French) short sheath. Heparin was given to achieve an activated clotting time of greater than 200 seconds. The 0.035-in. glide wire was advanced into the

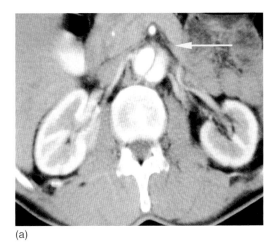

(a)

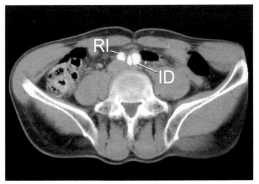

(b)

**Figure 1** (a) A CT scan demonstrating a type B dissection with a compromised true lumen. Flow to the left renal artery is diminished by a dissecting flap and is false lumen dependent. (b) A CT scan demonstrating a dissection involving the left common iliac artery ID with the right common iliac artery supplied by a nondissected true lumen. RI, right iliac artery; ID, internal diameter.

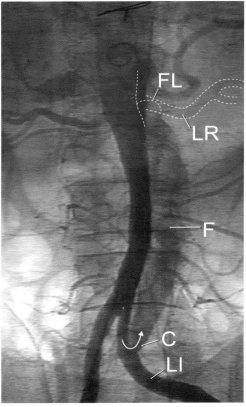

**Figure 2** An angiogram demonstrating a dissecting flap (FL) obstructing the ostium of the left renal artery (LR) perfused from the false lumen (F) with a distal reentry point at the level of the left common iliac artery (LI).

true lumen and a 5-F pigtail angiographic catheter was advanced over it for a true lumen angiogram. The angiogram demonstrated an infrarenal dissection with the true lumen supplying the celiac trunk, superior mesenteric artery, and the right renal artery with the left renal artery supplied by the false lumen in a retrograde manner from a distal reentry site at the proximal left iliac artery. The left renal lumen flow was compromised by a dissecting septum causing stenosis of the artery resulting in compromised flow and potential cause of the uncontrolled hypertension (Figure 2). The pigtail catheter was exchanged for a 5-F Bentson catheter and cannu-

lation of the distal communication at the level of the left iliac artery was performed to access the false lumen channel for determination of a pressure gradient. A 5-F Bentson catheter was advanced into the false lumen for determination of a gradient and a false lumen angiogram. A false lumen angiogram performed demonstrated a double-density shadow of the left renal artery compatible with a dissecting flap (Figure 3). The left renal artery was easily cannulated from the false channel and a Marshal balloon (Boston Scientific, Natick, MA) 5 mm × 2 cm was used to balloon angioplasty the origin of the left renal artery resulting in a break of the dissecting septum. There was resolution of the double-density image on completion angiogram with brisk flow to the left renal artery with resolution of the pressure gradient (Figure 4). A repeat duplex

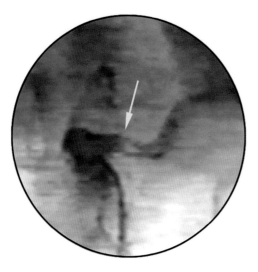

**Figure 3** False lumen angiogram demonstrating a compromised flow to the left renal artery with a dissecting flap (arrow) resulting in a double-density pattern on angiogram.

ultrasound performed the following day demonstrated normal renal artery velocities. The patient continued to do well with resolution of his hypertension and restoration of his renal function to normal.

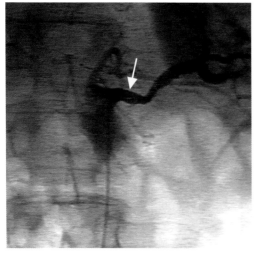

**Figure 4** A completion angiogram demonstrating brisk flow to the left renal artery with resolution of the double-density pattern on angiogram (white arrow).

## Discussion

Percutaneous endovascular techniques including deployment of endoluminal grafts, fenestration techniques, and deployment of stents are sometimes necessary to treat malperfusion syndromes. The understanding of the pathophysiologic mechanisms of aortic dissection needs to be thoroughly understood for successful management of the patient with aortic dissection and malperfusion syndrome. Percutaneous angioplasty and stent deployment have proven to be reliable methods of treating ischemic complications of aortic dissections [2–4]. The identification of the true and false lumen as well as the behavior of the true lumen is crucial for the endovascular management of aortic dissection. Treatment of malperfusion syndromes must be directed at the dissection flap in the thoracic aorta. Coverage of the entry tear by means of an endograft restores true lumen flow with partial collapse or thrombosis of the false lumen in dynamic obstruction where as techniques of fenestration, balloon angioplasty, and stent deployment may reestablishes flow across a flap into the compromised true lumen in cases of static obstruction.

In conclusion, the understanding of the pathoanatomy of branch vessel occlusion is important to determine the appropriate pecutaneous intervention techniques applicable for the management of branch vessel compromise.

## References

1 Williams DM, Lee DY, Hamilton B *et al*. The dissected aorta. Part III: Anatomy and radiologic diagnostics of branch-vessel compromise. *Radiology* 1997; **203**: 37–44.

2 Chavan A, Hausmann D, Dresler C *et al*. Intravascular ultrasound-guided percutaneous fenestration of the intimal flap in the dissected aorta. *Circulation* 1997; **96**: 2124–2127.

3 Slonim SM, Nyman U, Semba CP, Miller DC, Mitchell RS, Dake MD. Aortic dissection: percutaneous management of ischemic complications with endovascular stentsand balloon fenestration. *J Vasc Surg* 1996; **23**: 241–253.

4 Williams DM, Lee DY, Hamilton BH *et al*. The dissected aorta: percutaneous treatment of ischemic complications—principles and results. *J Vasc Interv Radiol* 1997; **8**(4): 605–625.

# Endovascular management of a chronic type B dissection complicated with a new dissection and left renal artery compromise

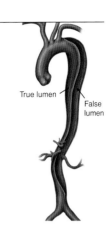

True lumen

False lumen

## Introduction

Aortic dissection is defined as the separation of the aortic media with presence of extraluminal blood within the layers of the aortic wall. The two mechanisms regarding the initial event in aortic dissection are primary intimal tear and initial delamination of the tunica media produced by the formation of an intramural hemorrhage and the second mechanism arises from bleeding of the vasa vasorum of the media. Aortic vascular bed compromise including ischemia of the lower limbs, mesenteric, and renal vessels arising from critical branch vessel occlusion may complicate aortic dissection in up to 31% of patients [1–4]. The mechanism by which malperfusion results from a dissection is a twofold dynamic obstruction in 80% of cases [5] and static obstruction. Identifying the mechanisms of branch compromise is critical to formulating effective treatment modalities. In dynamic obstruction, the compressed true lumen is unable to provide adequate flow volume or the dissection flap may prolapse into the vessel ostium, which remains anatomically intact. The severity of true lumen collapse and the degree of the aortic level ostial vessel occlusion is determined by the circumference of the aorta dissected, the blood pressure, heart rate, and peripheral resistance of the outflow vessel.

In static obstruction results from two mechanisms. In the first mechanism intra-arterial

dissection results in exposure of the thrombogenic false lumen with thrombus formation which may occur in the blind end of the dissection column. If the blind end or the propagating end of the dissection column enters and constricts the ostia of a branch vessel, organ injury can occur by thrombosis or hypoperfusion of the involved vessel.

In the second mechanism the dissecting process extends into the branch vessel proper, narrowing it to a variable degree—the so-called static obstruction [5]. This mechanism is unlikely to resolve with restoration of aortic true lumen flow alone, and some manipulation of the vessel itself either by fenestration, using a stent, balloon angioplasty, or by bypass graft will typically be required. A thorough familiarity with the mechanism of malperfusion [6] as well as a wide array of endovascular techniques must be available to the cardiovascular specialist who treats patients with aortic dissection.

## Case scenario

A 63-year-old male with history of hypertension was found to have lung nodule on routine chest X-ray. As part of his work-up, a CT scan of the chest and abdomen (Figure 1a and 1b) was performed that demonstrated a type B dissection with aneurysmal dilatation of the thoracic aorta to 6.0-cm in diameter with dissection beginning in the proximal descending thoracic aorta and extending into the left

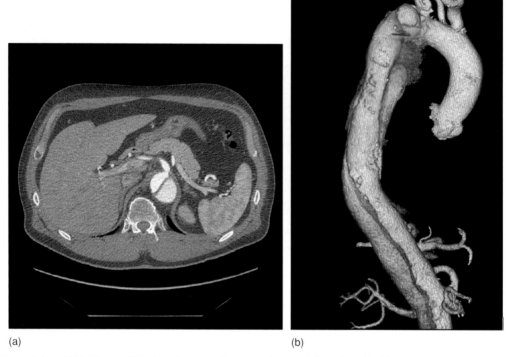

(a)                                    (b)

**Figure 1** (a and b) A CT scan of the chest demonstrating a complex type B dissection with false lumen aneurysmal expansion.

common iliac artery. The visceral and renal arteries arose from the true lumen and were well perfused. The abdominal component of the dissection was also aneurysmal with a diameter of 4.3-cm below the renal arteries. Due to concerns of thoracic aortic rupture, he was considered a candidate for endoluminal graft therapy of the aneurysmal segment of the thoracic aorta.

## Endovascular procedure 1

Under general anesthesia open retrograde cannulation of the right common femoral artery was performed with an 18-G needle and a 0.035-in. soft-tip angled glide wire (Medi-tech/Boston Scientific, Natick, MA) was advanced into the proximal thoracic aorta and exchanged to a 9-F (French) sheath under fluoroscopic visualization. Percutaneous access of the left common femoral artery was similarly performed and a 6-F sheath introduced. Five thousand units of heparin were given to keep the activated clotted time greater than 200 seconds.

A 5-F pigtail catheter was advanced through the left groin sheath into the thoracic aorta. The fluoroscopic C-arm was positioned in a left anterior oblique angle and an oblique thoracic arch aortogram was performed to visualize the orifices of the arch vessels and the dissecting thoracic aneurysm (Figure 2). Intravascular ultrasound (IVUS) was performed using an 8.2-F probe (Volcano Therapeutics, Inc., Rancho Cordova, CA) to further delineate the characteristics of the true and false lumen. The IVUS catheter was advanced through the right groin sheath and demonstrated a compressed true lumen with a thickened dissecting flap; the proximal neck diameter was measured to be 28 mm × 31 mm in diameter; the visceral and renal vessels were originating from the compressed true lumen as confirmed by CT scan (Figure 1a and 1b). A 34 mm × 15 cm Gore TAG stent graft (W.L. Gore & Associates, Flagstaff, AZ) was chosen firstly to expand the true lumen and secondly to exclude the aneurysmal false lumen to prevent aortic rupture. On completion of IVUS, the IVUS catheter was

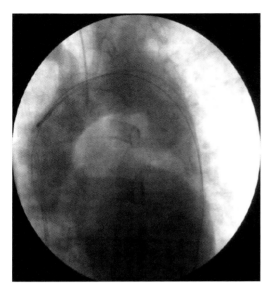

**Figure 2** An angiogram demonstrating a dissecting thoracic aortic aneurysm.

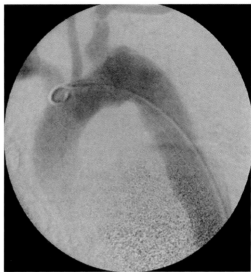

**Figure 3** A completion angiogram with exclusion of dissecting thoracic aortic aneurysm with absence of endoleak.

exchanged for an extra-stiff 260-cm Lunderquist wire (Cook Inc., Bloomington, IN). The right 9-F sheath was exchanged for a 22-F Gore sheath and a 34 mm × 15 cm TAG stent-graft device was advanced through the Gore sheath and subsequently deployed over an extra-stiff wire after marking the exact proximal and distal landing zones on our road map angiogram. A Gore trilobe balloon was used to perform postdeployment balloon angioplasty to the proximal and distal segments of the graft for good fixation. A completion angiogram (Figure 3) demonstrated exclusion of the aneurysm with a retrograde late filling of the false lumen possibly from a distal reentry point. Postdeployment IVUS confirmed reexpansion of the true lumen with a collapsed false lumen. All wires and sheaths were removed; the right common femoral artery was closed in a transverse fashion with restoration of flow. An 8-F angioseal closure device was deployed to the left common femoral artery. Patient had bilateral palpable pulses at the end of the procedure was extubated and transferred to recovery room. Patient was discharged on the second postoperative day in satisfactory condition with a CT scan of the chest (Figure 4a and 4b) performed on prior to discharge demonstrating exclusion of the dissecting aneurysm.

Patient returned 3 weeks after deployment of endoluminal graft for a dissecting aneurysm complaining of worsening left flank pain. On physical examination he was noted to be hypertensive with reproducible left flank tenderness with a moderately impaired renal function. A CT scan performed (Figure 5) demonstrated compromised flow to the left renal artery resulting from a possible progression of the dissection in a spiral fashion with a static obstruction. Patient was therefore scheduled for an angiogram, IVUS, and possible intervention.

## Endovascular procedure 2

Percutaneous retrograde access of the right common femoral artery was performed with an 8-F sheath. Five thousand units of heparin were given to the patient to achieve an activated clotted time greater than 200 seconds. An 0.035-in. soft-tip angled glide wire was advanced through the true lumen into the distal thoracic aorta. A C2 Cobra catheter was then used to selectively cannulate the left renal artery. A left renal angiogram demonstrated a dissecting flap with a false and true lumen with a reentry site (Figure 6). A multipurpose glide catheter was advanced through the C2 Cobra catheter and an 0.018-in. Platinum Plus wire was advanced into the true lumen of the left renal artery. An IVUS 5-F probe (Volcano Therapeutics, Inc., Rancho Cordova, CA) was advanced over the

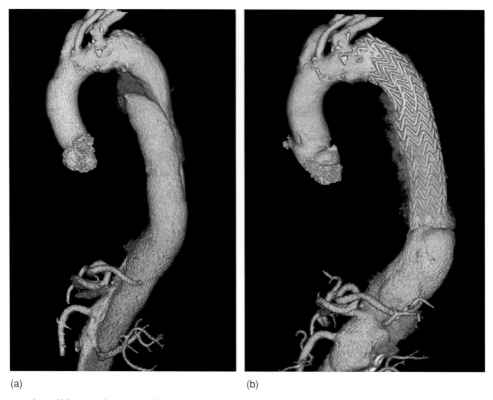

(a)                                    (b)

**Figure 4** (a and b) Pre- and postoperative CT scan with true lumen expansion and exclusion of 6-cm dissecting false aneurysm.

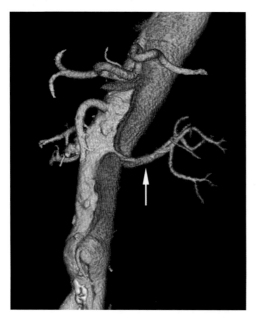

**Figure 5** A 64-slice CT scan demonstrating compromised flow to the left renal artery with a dissecting septum with most of the left renal artery flow false lumen dependent (arrow).

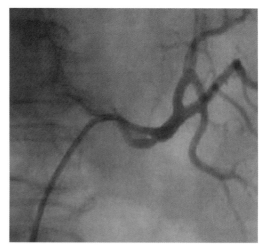

**Figure 6** Renal angiogram demonstrating a compressed true lumen ostium with a dissecting flap separating both lumens.

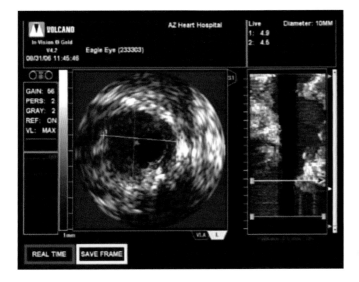

**Figure 7** IVUS demonstrating a compressed left renal artery true lumen.

0.018-in wire to confirm a collapsed true lumen with a dissecting flap at the ostium of the vessel as well as a entry and reentry point communicating with the false lumen (Figure 7). The left renal artery diameter was measured at 6 mm with length of dissection measured at 3 cm. Since we did not want to jeopardize the branched vessels, an uncovered stent 7 mm × 9 mm × 30 mm with enough radial force was chosen and deployed with postdeployment balloon angioplasty with a 7 mm × 2 cm OPTA Pro balloon. A repeat IVUS demonstrated marked true luminal gain (Figure 8). A repeat angiogram demonstrated flow in the false lumen believed to be from

accessory branches of the left renal artery feeding the false lumen as well as from distal retrograde flow from a reentry point identified from the left common iliac artery. The presence of false lumen flow to the left renal artery increased the risk of a false lumen aneurysm with a potential risk of rupture. Selective false lumen cannulation with coil embolization of the feeding vessels was therefore contemplated.

Percutaneous retrograde access of the left common femoral artery was performed with a 6-F sheath and a 0.035-in. glide wire was used to cannulate the distal reentry point at the level of the left common iliac artery with the help of a RIM

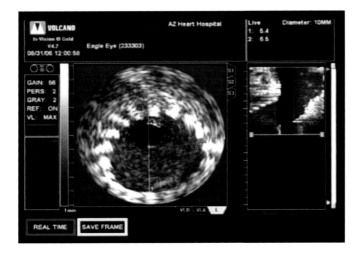

**Figure 8** IVUS poststent deployment with expanded true lumen.

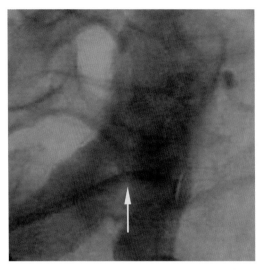

**Figure 9** An angiogram demonstrating cannulation of the false lumen entry point at the level of the left common iliac artery with a RIM catheter (arrow).

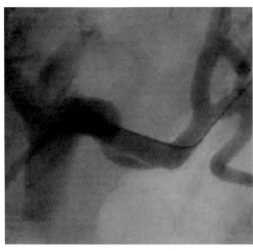

**Figure 10** An angiogram poststent deployment demonstrating an expanded true lumen with brisk flow to the left renal artery branches.

catheter to cannulate the false channel (Figure 9). A multipurpose catheter was advanced into the false lumen and a contrast injection demonstrated filling of the false lumen of the dissected left renal artery from a selective accessory branch of the left renal artery. Since none of the visceral branches depended on the false lumen flow, a decision was made to coil embolize the vessels supplying flow to the false lumen of the dissected left renal artery. Six 5 mm × 10 mm embolization coils and two 8 mm × 10 mm embolization coils were deployed in the false lumen sac at the level of the left renal artery. Selective false lumen angiogram through the multipurpose catheter demonstrated marked decrease flow to the false lumen of the renal artery; however, we could identify a few lumbar arteries feeding the false lumen distally and a decision was made not to coil embolize those for the fear of thrombosing those lumbar vessels with potential compromise to spinal cord flow. Selective true lumen left renal artery angiogram from the C2 Cobra catheter demonstrated brisk flow to the left renal artery with true lumen expansion (Figure 10). Once satisfied with the angiographic picture, all wires and sheaths were removed and an angioseal closure device was deployed in the left groin. Postoperatively, patient had a complete resolution of the left flank pain and a CT scan of the chest and abdomen (Figure 11) demonstrated

satisfactory flow to the left renal artery. His renal function improved and remained stable at 6 months follow-up with no symptoms.

## Discussion

Malperfusion syndromes may complicate the initial presentation of acute aortic dissection in 25–40% of patients. Operative mortality for open repair has been reported to be greater than 20% in most contemporary series [7]. In the initial arteriographic evaluation of the patient with an acute aortic dissection complicated by malperfusion, true and false lumen access must be obtained. The confirmation of position within the true or false lumen is facilitated by IVUS scans and fluoroscopy. Angiography should be performed in the proximal, undissected aorta to fully appreciate intimal flap mobility and any dynamic aortic obstruction, and may be assured by brachial artery cannulation in most cases.

Morbid events related to the entry tear itself are uncommon, with patients heretofore been managed with directed peripheral vascular intervention (either surgical or endovascular), a "complication-specific" approach. Stent-graft repair at the aortic entry tear site has become an additional "revascularization" modality likely to be effective in most patients with dynamic aortic obstruction

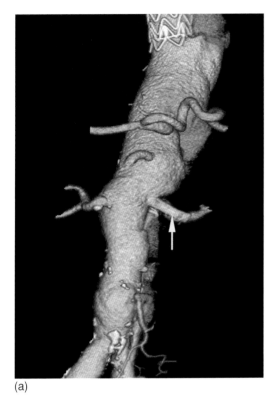

(a)

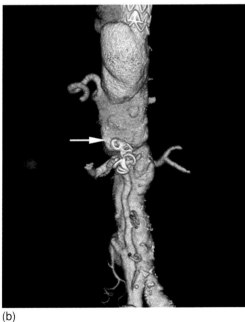

(b)

**Figure 11** (a) Postoperative CT scan demonstrating stent in the left renal artery (arrow) with increased luminal gain. (b) Postoperative CT scan demonstrating embolization coils deployed in the false lumen with false lumen thrombosis.

mechanisms. More complex is the treatment algorithm in patients with type A dissections complicated by malperfusion syndromes. Involvement of the mesenteric circulation constitutes one of the exceptions to prompt central aortic repair for type A dissection. Deeb *et al.* [8] found that the likelihood of death was 33 times greater in patients with acute type A dissections associated with malperfusion syndrome who first underwent immediate ascending aortic surgery as opposed to endovascular peripheral revascularization.

The goal of fenestration of the dissected intima is decompression of the false lumen, allowing for unrestricted flow in both the true and false lumens. The inexistence of a reentry tear in the distal aorta or its branches may jeopardize perfusion through the true lumen to such an extent that the true lumen collapses from the pressure of the thrombosis of the false channel. If compromise of any aortic branch vessel is identified by the dissection, wire access into the distal true lumen of the vessel should be secured. In general, placement of self-expanding stents in a potentially compromised aortic branch should precede aortic fenestration, as the latter may unpredictably alter aortic flow and make it extremely difficult to regain endovascular access to compromised vessels [9]. Fenestration is most commonly performed from the smaller (usually true lumen) to the larger false lumen. One technique uses an endovascular puncture needle to access the false lumen. After contrast injection confirms placement in the opposite lumen, an angioplasty balloon of at least 12–15 mm in diameter and 20–40 mm in length is used to create a fenestration tear.

The largest reported series of percutaneous balloon fenestration and endovascular stenting for peripheral ischemic complications in the setting of acute aortic dissection was reported by Dake *et al.* [7]. In their series of 40 patients with malperfusion syndromes, 14 patients underwent combined stenting and balloon fenestration, 24 underwent stenting alone, and 2 fenestration alone. Overall, flow was restored to the ischemic territories in 37 (93%) of 40 patients. Thirty-day mortality was 25% (10 of 40). The variables found to be significant predictors of death on multivariate analysis were ischemia of three vascular beds, which carries a nearly fourfold increase in risk, and advanced age.

The role of stent-graft therapy in the treatment of acute distal dissection with malperfusion syndrome or aortic rupture was also studied by Greenberg [10]. The indication for treatment in their series of 31 patients was malperfusion syndrome (77%) or aortic rupture (23%). Of the 31 patients, 29 were treated by stent-graft therapy alone and 2 by fenestrations when definitive true lumen access could not be established. When true lumen compression resulted in visceral vessel malperfusion, the authors established definitive true lumen access to a minimum of at least two visceral vessels (typically the superior mesenteric artery and a renal artery). Early mortality was 29% in these critically ill patients, compared with a historically documented mortality in the 80% range [1]. Four of the deaths occurred immediately after stent grafting because of massive reperfusion injuries with hyperkalemic cardiac arrest. Overall, mesenteric infarction accounted for 44% of the early deaths. The authors concluded that morbidity and mortality associated with a stent-graft approach to acute distal aortic dissection with end organ ischemia may be lower than conventional surgical approaches but still carries a significant risk [10].

The effect of fenestration on long-term outcome of false lumen expansion in patients with distal dissections remains to be determined since the false lumen remains pressurized and at risk for continued progression to aneurysm. Available data from series of patients treated with open surgical fenestration suggest that the incidence of aortic intervention at the site of previous open surgical fenestration is low and that (0 of 9 patients at 33 months follow-up) the presumed risk of late aneurysm formation may be overestimated [11].

# References

1 DeBakey ME, Henly WS, Cooley DA, Morris GC, Crawford ES. Dissection and dissecting aneurysms of the aorta (twenty-year follow-up of five hundred twenty seven patients treated surgically). *Surgery* 1982; **92**: 1118–1134.

2 Fann JI, Smith JA, Miller DC *et al.* Surgical management of aortic dissection during a 30-year period. *Circulation* 1995; **92**(Suppl II): 113–121.

3 Bernard Y, Zimmermann H, Chocron S *et al.* False lumen patency as a predictor of late outcome in aortic dissection. *Am J Cardiol* 2001; **87**: 1378–1382.

4 Pacifico L, Spodick D. ILEAD-ischemia of the lower extremities due to aortic dissection: the isolated presentation. *Clin Cardiol* 1999; **22**: 353–356.

5 Cambria RP. Surgical treatment of complicated distal aortic dissection. *Semin Vasc Surg* 2002; **15**: 97–107.

6 Nienaber CA, Eagle KA. Aortic dissection: new frontiers in diagnosis and management. Part II: Therapeutic management and follow-up. *Circulation* 2003; **108**: 772–778.

7 Dake MD, Kato N, Mitchell RS *et al.* Endovascular stent-graft placement for the treatment of acute aortic dissection. *N Engl J Med* 1999; **340**: 1546–1552.

8 Deeb GM, Williams DM, Bolling SF *et al.* Surgical delay for acute type A dissection with malperfusion. *Ann Thorac Surg* 1997; **64**: 1669–1675.

9 Hansen CJ, Bui H, Donayre CE *et al.* Complications of endovascular repair of high-risk and emergent descending thoracic aortic aneurysms and dissections. *J Vasc Surg* 2004; **40**: 228–234.

10 Greenberg R. Treatment of aortic dissections with endovascular stent grafts. *Semin Vasc Surg* 2002; **15**: 122–127.

11 Atkins MD, Jr, Black JH, III. Cambria RP. Aortic dissection: perspectives in the era of stent-graft repair. *J Vasc Surg* 2006; **43**(2): A30–A43.

# Hybrid management of a retrograde type B dissection after endoluminal stent grafting

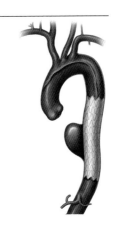

## Introduction

Thoracic endografting has recently been approved by the Food and Drug Administration in the United States for the treatment of descending thoracic aortic aneurysms. The first thoracic stent graft for the treatment of thoracic aortic aneurysm (TAA) was reported by Dake *et al.* [1]. Kato *et al.* [2] described the use of stent graft to treat dissecting aneurysms at about the same time. Stanford type B dissections are managed conservatively with meticulous control of blood pressure and pain medication for uncomplicated cases. As many as 43% of medically treated acute type B dissections will progress to aortic enlargement. Approximately 30% of the patients are dilated to 6 cm or greater within a mean of 59 months [3]. Surgical treatment of acute type B dissections is reserved for patients with a complicated course, such as frank or impending rupture, branch vessel occlusion with visceral and/or leg ischemia, refractory hypertension or pain. Despite significant improvement in anesthesia, surgical and postoperative techniques, the mortality rate in emergent surgical repair of type B aortic dissections can range between 29 and 50% [4, 5]. Frequent complications are respiratory failure 51% [6], renal failure 17% [7], or paraplegia 7–24% [6, 7]. Other notable complications include severe bleeding, stroke, cardiac events, or sepsis. Closure of the entry tear of a type B dissection is essential to reduce aortic diameter and promote both depressurization and shrinkage of the false lumen. This can lead to thrombosis, fibrous transformation, and subsequent remodeling and stabilization of the aorta [8–10]. Retrograde type A dissection following stent-graft placement for the treatment of type B dissection is a rare but fatal complication associated with a high mortality [11–17]. Once an ascending aortic dissection occurs, emergent treatment should be performed as soon as possible [18]. Hybrid management of this potentially devastating complication of stent grafting can be performed with less surgical morbidity and mortality than conventional open surgical repair of the ascending aorta with arch replacement.

## Case scenario

A 53-year-old male with a past medical history significant for hypertension and coronary artery disease developed sudden, severe crushing chest pain associated with a hypertensive crisis. This was accompanied by monocular blindness and compromised renal function. Aggressive management of his pain and blood pressure was undertaken and a subsequent CT scan of his chest showed the presence of an acute type B dissection (Figure 1).

Medical management was instituted and maximized to control his blood pressure and pain. Even with the administration of intravenous antihypertensive medications, it became increasingly difficult to control both his pain and blood pressure. His renal function also continued to deteriorate and, at

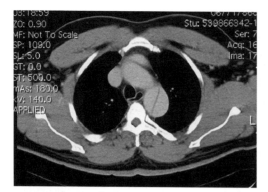

**Figure 1** A CT scan image demonstrating a type B dissection.

that time, he was referred to the surgical service for an endovascular repair of his dissection.

## Technical details of endoluminal graft deployment

Open retrograde cannulation of the right common femoral artery using an 18-G needle was performed and a 9-F (French) sheath was introduced over a 0.035-in. soft-tip angled glide wire. Percutaneous retrograde access of the left common femoral artery was similarly performed and a 5-F sheath was introduced. Heparin was given to achieve an activated clotted time of more than 200 seconds. An oblique thoracic aortogram was performed using a 5-F pigtail angiographic catheter advanced through the left groin sheath, which demonstrated a bovine arch with a collapsed true lumen and an intimal flap juxtadistal to the left subclavian artery (Figure 2a). An intravascular ultrasound was also performed through the 9-F sheath to identify the true lumen, the false lumen, and any entry points of the dissection. One entry point was identified approximately 2-cm distal to the left subclavian artery. A 9-F sheath in the right common femoral artery was exchanged to a 24-F Gore sheath. A 37 mm × 20 cm Gore TAG device (W.L. Gore & Associates, Flagstaff, AZ) was deployed at the level of the mid-descending thoracic aorta followed by a 40 mm × 20 cm Gore TAG device deployed distal to innominate artery stent to exclude the entry point. A completion angiogram showed that the deployed thoracic endografts collapsed the false lumen and expanded the true lumen with no visible sign of an endoleak (Figure 2b). Wires and sheaths were removed from the

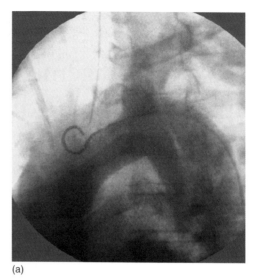

(a)

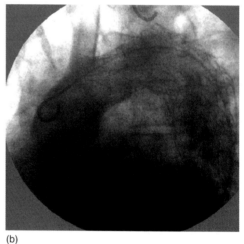

(b)

**Figure 2** (a) An angiogram demonstrating a type B dissection. (b) A completion angiogram demonstrating adequate deployment of endoluminal graft with no endoleak.

right common femoral artery with a primary repair done to close the incision site. A closure device was deployed to the left common femoral artery. A postoperative CT scan demonstrated complete thrombosis of the false lumen and exclusion of the principal entry tear.

## Postoperative surveillance (retrograde type A dissection)

The patient was discharged from the hospital in satisfactory condition and presented 1 month later to

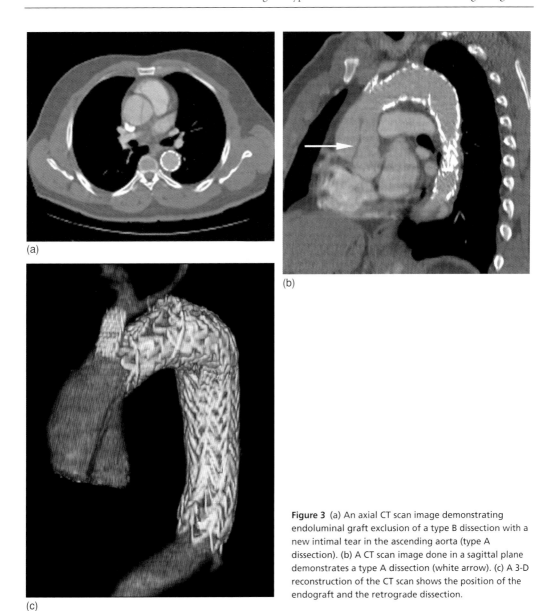

Figure 3 (a) An axial CT scan image demonstrating endoluminal graft exclusion of a type B dissection with a new intimal tear in the ascending aorta (type A dissection). (b) A CT scan image done in a sagittal plane demonstrates a type A dissection (white arrow). (c) A 3-D reconstruction of the CT scan shows the position of the endograft and the retrograde dissection.

the emergency room with an acute episode of chest pain. He was taken to the catheterization laboratory and angiogram revealed a retrograde type B dissection. CT scan showed a retrograde type A dissection (Figure 3a–3c). He was taken to the operating room where replacement of the ascending aorta was done with a 32-mm Hemashield Dacron graft (Boston Scientific, Natick, MA) (Figure 4). He was subsequently discharged from the hospital in satisfactory condition.

## Discussion

Acute, retrograde type A dissection after endovascular stent-graft repair is a fatal complication following stent-graft treatment of thoracic aortic pathologies. The incidence tends to be more common in the use of stent-graft deployment to treat Stanford type B dissection. Dissections that originate in the descending aorta and extend in a retrograde direction into the ascending aorta may lead to aortic

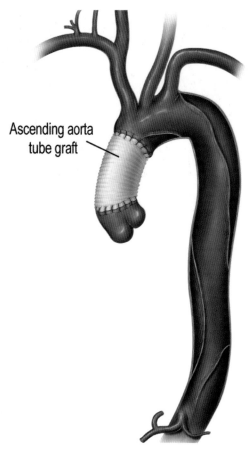

Ascending aorta
tube graft

**Figure 4** Replacement of the ascending aorta with a 32-mm Hemashield graft.

valve regurgitation, cerebrovascular ischemia, pericardial tamponade, and obstruction of the coronary artery. Open surgery is the treatment of choice in an effort to avert these life-threatening complications. Possible etiologies for this rare but fatal complication can be classified as procedure-related, device-related, and natural progression of disease.

Formation of a new intimal tear leading to a dissection or a pseudoaneurysm may occur at the margin of a stent graft [19, 20]. The time between stent-graft implantation and identification of a complicating intimal tear or dissection can vary from immediately postoperative deployment of stent graft to months after the procedure [21, 22]. In a report by Won *et al.*, retrograde type A dissection was diagnosed at 1–5 months post-procedure (mean 3.2 mo).

Procedure-related complications of retrograde type A dissection following stent-graft placement arise from wires and sheath manipulation in the aortic arch during the endovascular procedure that may cause localized intimal tears in the extremely fragile and easily injured intimal flap and aortic wall. Wire and sheath handling or balloon dilatation during the endovascular procedure may cause intimal injuries during the endovascular procedure and extend in a retrograde manner during the following days, weeks, or months.

Device-related complications arise from semi-rigid designed grafts not able to conform perfectly in an aortic curve that is significantly angulated. Multiple balloon dilations are done in an attempt to help the deivce conform to the aorta which may be intimal tears that may progress to a frank dissection. Stent grafts with bare springs used for anchoring at their proximal ends can create new intimal tears especially in a fragile, dissected aorta. In addition, routine stent-graft oversizing may contribute to intimal injuries despite exact measurements Oversizing of stent grafts more than 10% results in a higher radial force against the aortic wall, with potential intimal injury and tears occurring if oversizing is more than 20% of instructions for use (IFU) recommendations.

Progression of the aortic disease could result in the formation of new intimal injuries and dissections at sites unrelated to the stent-graft procedure. Congenital weakness of the aortic wall must also be considered in patients who have no obvious cause of dissection. Stent-graft implantation in such patients must be performed very cautiously. We suspect that the fragility of the aortic wall caused by this pathology finally results in a retrograde type A dissection, which is triggered by the stent-graft procedure. We recommend that the use of stent graft in patients with Marfan should be discouraged because of the fragility of the aortic wall.

Persistent blood flow into the false lumen at the end of the procedure might also be a positive predictor for retrograde type A dissection. The influence of the different stent grafts on intimal injury is questionable. Retrograde type A dissection has been reported in patients who were treated with a

**Table 1** Patients who developed a retrograde type A dissection at our institution following stent-graft therapy for various thoracic aortic pathologies.

| Age (year) | Sex | Etiology | Time to discovery | Result |
|---|---|---|---|---|
| 73 | F | Aneurysm | POD 1 | Death |
| 83 | F | Dissection | POD 1 | Death |
| 78 | F | Dissection | POD 10 | Death |
| 53 | M | Dissection | 1 mo | Ascending aorta repair—tube graft |
| 78 | F | PAU | 7 mo | Ascending aorta repair—tube graft |
| 67 | M | Dissection | 19 mo | Ascending aorta repair—tube graft |
| 60 | M | Dissection | 21 mo | Ascending aorta repair—death 2 wk postoperative |
| 74 | F | Dissection rupture | 30 mo | Pt. declined open repair—death |

POD, postoperative day; PAU, penetrating atherosclerotic ulcer, Pt, patient.

Talent endoprosthesis with a free flow design on the proximal cage, resulting in death. The cause may be related to the limited flexibility of the currently available devices that produce forced wall stress at the outer curvature leading to intimal injuries [23–25]. Although forced and repeated balloon dilation is an important factor that contributed to intimal injuries, careful balloon dilation is recommended since the self-expanding action of the stent grafts also results in continuous expansion of the true lumen over time.

Despite the minimal invasive nature of stent-graft implantation, sometimes fatal complications may arise from its deployment with retrograde ascending aortic dissection, one of the most severe one. Between 1998 and 2007 we have treated a total of 512 patients with a thoracic aortic stent graft for various aortic pathologies. The Gore TAG excluder device was used in 400 patients with 8 patients developing a retrograde type A dissection (2.0%); there were 3 males and 5 females with the diagnosis made at a median of 116 days. Fifty percent of patients were identified during the perioperative period. Retrograde type A dissection was diagnosed within the perioperative period in 3 patients with 100% mortality. Of the 8 patients who developed a retrograde type A dissection, 1 patient was previously treated for a TAA, 1 patient for a penetrating aortic ulcer, and 6 patients for a type B dissection (75%) (Table 1). There were 97 patients treated for type B dissection during that time period resulting in a 6/97 (6.2%) incidence of a retrograde type dissection in

that group category. The mortality rate for a retrograde type A dissection was 5/8 (62.5%) mostly as a result of complications with 3 deaths within the perioperative period (Table 1). The 3 surviving patients were diagnosed at 1 month, 7 months, and 19 months, respectively, and all had an ascending aorta replacement with a tube graft. Possible etiologies for retrograde type A dissection that we knew of were possibly related to oversizing more than 20% the indication for use. The larger the stent graft, the greater the radial force it gives to the aortic wall, resulting in good apposition to the aortic wall. Occasionally oversizing has resulted in intimal injuries especially in fragile aortas. In the treatment of 2 patients oversizing of the aorta was responsible for retrograde type A dissection with 1 patient receiving an endograft that had been oversized by 27.4%. Incomplete seal of the entry tear of a type B dissection occurred in 1 patient with progression of disease of the aorta responsible in 1 patient diagnosed at 19 months previously stent-graft placement for a type B dissection. Other possible etiologies could have been related to balloon dilatation of endografts to achieve good wall apposition resulting in aortic intimal injury and the tips of the guide wire and the delivery system could cause damage to the aortic intima. In our report we did not use any stent grafts with uncovered struts which have been known to cause intimal injuries at the proximal and distal fixation points.

Retrograde type A dissection, a potentially lethal complication following endovascular stent-graft repair of thoracic aortic pathologies may have an acute or delayed presentation. Better patient selection, precise stent-graft deployment, careful wire and sheath manipulation in the arch of the aorta, coverage of a large part of the descending aorta in the straight portion as opposed to the angled or curved part of the aorta, and avoidance of aggressive ballooning of stent grafts in the treatment of type B dissection can reduce the incidence of retrograde type A dissection. The inflexibility of stent grafts and pulsatile forces of the aorta have as much adverse effects as acutely dissected intima. The development of stent grafts with smoother edges, flexible bodies, and avoidance of stents with barbs at proximal ends that could create new intimal tears could further help decrease this fatal complication of endoluminal stent-graft use especially in the treatment of type B dissections.

# References

1 Dake MD, Miller DC, Semba CP *et al.* Transluminal placement of endovascular stent-grafts for the treatment of descending thoracic aortic aneurysms. *N Engl J Med* 1994; **331**: 1729–1734.

2 Kato N, Hirano T, Takeda K *et al.* Treatment of aortic dissections with a percutaneous intravascular endoprosthesis: comparison of covered and bare stents. *J Vasc Interv Radiol* 1994; **5**: 805–812.

3 Marui A, Mochizuki T, Mitsui N *et al.* Toward the best treatment for uncomplicated patients with type B acute aortic dissection: a consideration for sound surgical indication. *Circulation* 1999; **100**: II275–II280.

4 Miller DC, Mitchell RS, Oyer PE *et al.* Independent determinants of operative mortality for patients with aortic dissections. *Circulation* 1984; **70**: I153–I164.

5 Cambria RP, Brewster DC, Gertler J *et al.* Vascular complications associated with spontaneous aortic dissection. *J Vasc Surg* 1988; **7**: 199–209.

6 Crawford ES, Hess KR, Cohen ES *et al.* Ruptured aneurysm of the descending thoracic and thoracoabdominal aorta: analysis according to size and treatment. *Ann Surg* 1991; **213**: 417–426.

7 Velazquez OC, Bavaria JE, Pochettino A *et al.* Emergency repair of thoracoabdominal aortic aneurysms with immediate presentation. *J Vasc Surg* 1999; **30**: 996–1003.

8 Nienaber CA, Fattori R, Lund G *et al.* Nonsurgical reconstruction of thoracic aortic dissection by stent-graft placement. *N Engl J Med* 1999; **340**: 1539–1545.

9 Czermak BV, Waldenberger P, Fraedrich G *et al.* Treatment of Stanford type B aortic dissection with stent-grafts: preliminary results. *Radiology* 2000; **217**: 544–550.

10 Czermak BV, Mallouhi A, Perkmann R *et al.* Serial CT volume and thrombus length measurements after endovascular repair of Stanford type B aortic dissection. *J Endovasc Ther* 2004; **11**: 1–12.

11 Totaro M, Miraldi F, Fanelli F *et al.* Emergency surgery for retrograde extension of type B dissection after endovascular stent graft repair. *Eur J Cardiothorac Surg* 2001; **20**: 1057–1058.

12 Fanelli F, Salvatori FM, Marcelli G *et al.* Type A aortic dissection developing during endovascular repair of an acute type B dissection. *J Endovasc Ther* 2003; **10**: 254–259.

13 Nienaber CA, Eagle KA. Aortic dissection: new frontiers in diagnosis and management. Part II: Therapeutic management and follow-up. *Circulation* 2003; **108**: 772–778.

14 Pasic M, Bergs P, Knollmann F *et al.* Delayed retrograde aortic dissection after endovascular stenting of the descending thoracic aorta. *J Vasc Surg* 2002; **36**: 184–186.

15 Grabenwoger M, Fleck T, Ehrlich M *et al.* Secondary surgical interventions after endovascular stent-grafting of the thoracic aorta. *Eur J Cardiothorac Surg* 2004; **26**: 608–613.

16 Bethuyne N, Bove T, Van den Brande P *et al.* Acute retrograde aortic dissection during endovascular repair of a thoracic aortic aneurysm. *Ann Thorac Surg* 2003; **75**: 1967–1969.

17 Misfeld M, Notzold A, Geist V *et al.* Retrograde type A dissection after endovascular stent grafting of type B dissection [in German]. *Z Kardiol* 2002; **91**: 274–277.

18 Totaro M, Miraldi F, Fanelli F, Mazzesi G. Emergency surgery for retrograde extension of type B dissection after endovascular stent graft repair. *Eur J Cardiothorac Surg* 2001; **20**: 1057–1058.

19 Kato N, Hirano T, Kawaguchi T *et al.* Aneurysmal degeneration of the aorta after stent graft repair of acute aortic dissection. *J Vasc Surg* **34**: 513–518.

20 Pamler RS, Kotsis T, Gorich J, Kapfer X, Orend KH, Plassmann LS. Complications after endovascular repair of type B aortic dissection. *J Endovasc Ther* **9**: 822–828.

21 Totaro M, Miraldi F, Fanelli F *et al.* Emergency surgery for retrograde extension of type B dissection after endovascular stent graft repair. *Eur J Cardiothorac Surg* 2001; **20**: 1057–1058.

22 Fanelli F, Salvatori FM, Marcelli G *et al.* Type A aortic dissection developing during endovascular repair of an acute type B dissection. *J Endovasc Ther* 2003; **10**: 254–259.

23 Duebener LF, Lorenzen P, Richardt G *et al.* Emergency endovascular stent-grafting for life-threatening acute type B aortic dissections. *Ann Thorac Surg* 2004; **78**: 1261–1267.

24 Fattori R, Napoli G, Lovato L *et al.* Descending thoracic aortic diseases: stent-graft repair. *Radiology* 2003; **229**: 176–183.

25 Totaro M, Miraldi F, Fanelli F, Mazzesi G. Emergency surgery for retrograde extension of type B dissection after endovascular stent graft repair. *Eur J Cardiothorac Surg* 2001; **20**: 1057–1058.

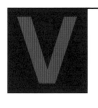

# SECTION V
# Thoracic aortic pseudoaneurysms

# Endovascular management of thoracic aortic pseudoaneurysms

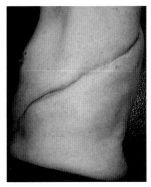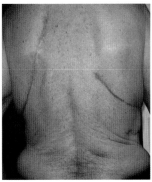

*The scars of others should teach us caution.*

–St. Jerome

## Introduction

Pseudoaneurysms of the thoracic aorta result from transmural disruption of the aortic wall, with the leak contained by surrounding mediastinal structures. Pseudoaneurysms commonly occur from previous cardiovascular operations [1], trauma [2], and infection [3]. Pseudoaneurysms are located at previous anastomotic sites, aortototomy sites, cannulation sites, cardioplegia and venting sites as well as proximal vein graft anastomotic sites [4]. Pseudoaneurysms affect the ascending aorta in 70%, ascending aorta and arch in 15%, descending aorta in 10%, and arch alone in 5% of cases [5]. Open surgical repair of such pseudoaneurysms can be challenging and are associated with a high morbidity and mortality in less experienced centers. The use of endovascular and hybrid techniques can be applied safely to treat patients with pseudoaneurysms. We describe the endovascular management of a patient with a thoracic pseudoaneurysm with three previous thoracic and aortic surgical repairs.

## Case scenario

A 72-year-old male with significant coronary artery disease with congestive heart failure, history of atrial fibrillation, hypertension, and three previous abdominal and thoracic aortic surgeries which consisted of an open infrarenal abdominal aneurysm repair followed 10 years later with a thoracoabdominal aneurysm repair and 3 years later a redo operation for a thoracoabdominal pseudoaneurysm presented to an outside facility with chest pain. As part of his work-up a diagnostic cardiac catheterization and angiogram performed (Figure 1) demonstrated severe ventricular dysfunction with an ejection fraction of 30%, normal coronary arteries were noted and a large thoracic aortic saccular aneurysm measuring 7.9 cm in diameter. Due to the extreme high risk with a reoperation, he underwent an intravascular ultrasound (IVUS) and angiogram with plans for exclusion of the thoracic aortic pseudoaneurysm with an endoluminal graft.

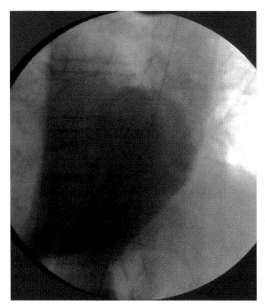

**Figure 1** Thoracic aortogram demonstrating a thoracic pseudoaneurysm measuring 7.9 cm in diameter.

## Endovascular procedure

Under general anesthesia open retrograde cannulation of the right common femoral artery was performed with an 18-G needle and a 0.035-in. soft-tip angled glide wire (Medi-tech/Boston Scientific, Natick, MA) was passed into the distal thoracic aorta and exchanged to a 9-F (French) sheath under fluoroscopic visualization. Percutaneous access of the left common femoral artery was similarly performed and a 5-F sheath introduced. Five thousand units of heparin were given to keep the activated clotted time greater than 200 seconds. A 5-F pigtail catheter was advanced through the left groin sheath into the thoracic aorta. The fluoroscopic C-arm was positioned in a left anterior oblique angle and an oblique thoracic arch aortogram was performed to visualize the orifices of the arch vessels and the descending thoracic aortic aneurysm. An IVUS was performed using an IVUS 8.2-F probe (Volcano Therapeutics, Inc., Rancho Cordova, CA) to determine the proximal and distal neck diameter, characteristic of saccular aneurysm, length of proximal and distal landing zones, and amount of thoracic aorta to be covered. IVUS measured the proximal neck diameter to be 35 mm

× 34 mm and the distal neck diameter to be 34 mm × 34 mm, the proximal neck length of the aneurysm from the left subclavian artery was 11 cm and the total length of aorta to be covered 15 cm. Based on the measurements a 40 mm × 15 cm TAG stent graft was chosen. The IVUS catheter was exchanged for an extra-stiff 260-cm Lunderquist wire (Cook Inc., Bloomington, IN). The right 9-F sheath was exchanged for a 24-F Gore sheath and a 40 mm × 15 cm Gore TAG stent-graft device was advanced through the Gore sheath and subsequently deployed over an extra-stiff wire after marking the exact proximal and distal landing zones on our road map angiogram. A Gore trilobe balloon was used to perform postdeployment balloon angioplasty to the proximal and distal segments of the graft for good fixation. A completion angiogram (Figure 2) demonstrated exclusion of the aneurysm with no endoleak. All wires and sheaths were removed; the right common femoral artery was closed in a transverse fashion with restoration of flow. An 8-F angioseal vascular closure device (St. Jude Medical, Inc., St. Paul, MN) was deployed to the left common femoral artery. Patient had

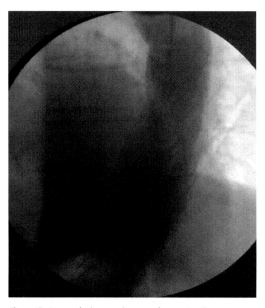

**Figure 2** A completion angiogram demonstrating satisfactory exclusion of the thoracic aortic aneurysm with no endoleak.

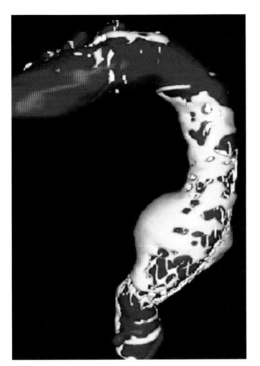

**Figure 3** Reconstructed CT scan of the chest demonstrating exclusion of thoracic aortic aneurysm with no endoleak.

bilateral palpable pulses at the end of the procedure was extubated and transferred to recovery room. Patient was discharged on postoperative day (POD) 2 in satisfactory condition. A CT scan of the chest performed on POD 1 showed exclusion of the 7.9-cm thoracic aortic aneurysm with no identifiable endoleak (Figure 3). At 1-year follow-up (Figure 4a and 4b) there is regression of thoracic aortic aneurysm sac volume.

## Discussion

Open surgical management of aortic pseudoaneurysms depends on the etiology and location of pseudoaneurysm. Hypothermic low-flow cardiopulmonary bypass or deep hypothermic circulatory arrest is sometimes required for surgical management of psueudoaneurysms. Majority of pseudoaneurysms involve the ascending aorta and are related to previous cardiac surgery operations. Trauma and infection are the commonest cause of pseudoaneuryms of the descending thoracic aorta. Redo operations are often very complex and hazardous to the patient with an increased risk of paraplegia. Endovascular management with a thoracic endograft provides a less invasive alternative. The principle of management is to use the shortest piece of graft to exclude the pseudoaneurysm. Although controversy still remains about using an endoluminal graft to treat mycotic aneurysms, we have reported success with this treatment with total regression of the aneurysm sac at mid-term follow-up [6].

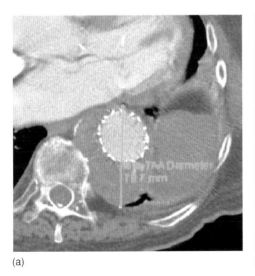

(a)

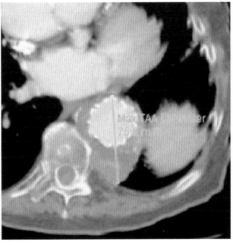

(b)

**Figure 4** (a) An axial CT scan demonstrating exclusion of thoracic aortic aneurysm with no endoleak. (b) At 1-year follow-up there is regression of thoracic aortic aneurysm sac.

In summary, endoluminal graft therapy is a less invasive approach used to treat pseudoaneurysms of the thoracic aorta in patients considered high risk for open surgical repair.

## References

1 Fleischaker RJ, Mazur JH, Baisch BF. Surgical treatment of acute traumatic rupture of the thoracic aorta. *J Thorac Cardiovasc Surg* 1964; **47**: 289–297.

2 Aebert H, Birnbaum DE. Tuberculous pseudoaneurysms of the aortic arch. *J Thorac Cardiovasc Surg* 2003; **125**: 411–412.

3 Sullivan KL, Steiner RM, Smullens SN, Griska L, Meister SG. Pseudoaneurysm of the ascending aorta following cardiac surgery. *Chest* 1988; **93**: 138–143.

4 Stassano P, De Amicis V, Gagliardi C, Di Lello F, Spampinato N. False aneurysm from the aortic vent site. *J Cardiovasc Surg (Torino)* 1982; **23**: 401–402.

5 Atik FA, Navia JL, Svensson LG *et al.* Surgical treatment of pseudoaneurysm of the thoracic aorta. *J Thorac Cardiovasc Surg* 2006; **132**(2): 379–385.

6 Kpodonu J, Williams JP, Ramaiah VG, Diethrich EB. Endovascular management of a descending thoracic aortic mycotic aneurysm: mid-term follow-up. *Eur J Cardiothorac Surg* 2007; **32**(1): 178–179.

# CASE 24

# Endovascular management of thoracic mycotic aneurysms

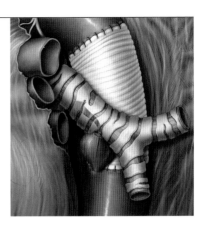

## Introduction

Mycotic aneurysms of the thoracic aorta are a rare but life-threatening events. They are characterized by an endarteritis of an infectious origin generally followed by the formation of an aneurysm. The physiopathology of mycotic aneurysm includes (i) secondary aneurysm with the embolism of the vasa vasorum by the germ in question, (ii) arterial infection of the intima injured at the time of a bacteremia, (iii) traumatism of the arterial wall with direct contamination, and (iv) infection of the vascular wall by extension of a contiguous infectious site [1]. Risk factors for mycotic aneurysms include male sex, age, tobacco use, hypertension, diabetes mellitus, dyslipidemia [2–4], and congenital anomalies such as coarctation of the aorta or ductus arteriosus [5]. Patients with atherosclerosis and a depressed immunity system are also at an increased risk for developing a mycotic aneurysm. The most common offending microorganisms are gram-positive cocci which occur in 60% of cases, among them including *Staphylococcus aureus* (30–50%), *Streptococcus*, and *Enteroccus* [6–8]. Gram-negative bacilli comprise between 20 and 40% of cases among them include *Salmonellas* which is the most prevalent and the less common *Campylobacter fetus* [9–12], *Listeria monocytogenes* [13], *Clostridium septicum* [14], and *Haemophilus influenza* [15]. Clinical signs are not specific but a strong correlation of fever is present (70%) shoulder, dorsal, or thoracic pains (60%). Compressive signs in the event of large aneurysms include dysphagia, dyspnea, cough, voice alterations by compression of the recurrent laryngeal nerve. Aortobronchial and aortoesophageal fistulas can arise in the event of fistulization or rupture leading to massive hemoptysis or gastrointestinal bleeding [16, 17]. Diagnosis consists of blood cultures which may be positive in 50–90% of cases; CT scan with contrast is the most useful to determine precise location of aneurysm. Thinning of the aortic wall, air in the aortic wall, or periaortic fluid collections are indicators of an infectious etiology. Leukocytosis with polynuclear neutrophils higher than 10,000/mm$^3$ may be found in 65–83% of the cases [2, 5]. The principal contributing factor to patient mortality is delayed diagnosis. Medical treatment is associated with 100% mortality from aortic rupture. Treatment consists of open surgical resection of the infected thoracic aorta with surrounding tissue, followed by revascularization via in situ or extra-anatomic grafting in combination with long-term bactericidal antibiotics [18]. The high mortality and morbidity rates associated with conventional open, surgical treatment of mycotic aneurysms have been reported to be as high as 40% [19, 20] directs surgeons to explore alternative less invasive options.

## Case scenario 1

A 70-year-old man presented with several comorbidities and a past surgical history notable for extensive debridement of a thoracic vertebrae perispinal abscess cavity with stabilization of the spine with metal plates. The procedure was performed 3 years ago and a left thoracotomy with decortication for left pleural space empyema within the same year

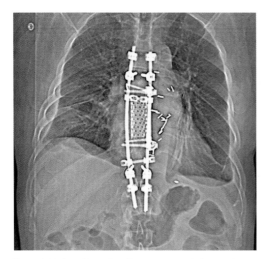

**Figure 1** A chest X-ray showing extensive plating and screws from the treatment of a paraspinal abscess.

at which time the aorta had been noted to be normal developed severe back pain, hemoptysis, and fevers. Blood and urine cultures were positive for *Enterobacter* species growth and a sputum culture grew methicillin-resistant *Staphylococcus aureus* (MRSA). A chest X-ray demonstrated stabilization of the spine with metal plating (Figure 1). A CT scan of the chest revealed a 10 cm × 12 cm aneurysm (Figure 2a and 2b). The patient was diagnosed with a mycotic aneurysm and immediately started on intravenous antibiotics consisting of Vancomycin and Primaxin. He was transferred to our facility for endoluminal graft therapy after been refusing open surgical repair. Upon arrival, the patient underwent another battery of bacterial tests that showed no culture growth. Due to the size of the aneurysm and stable infectious disease status, the patient was referred to the vascular surgeons for endovascular therapy.

### Endovascular procedure

Under general anesthesia, open retrograde cannulation of the right common femoral artery was performed with an 18-G needle with a 0.035-in. soft-tip angled glide wire (Medi-tech/Boston Scientific, Natick, MA) passed into the thoracic aorta and exchanged to a 9-F (French) sheath under fluoroscopic visualization. Percutaneous access of the left common femoral artery was similarly performed and a 5-F sheath introduced. Five thousand units

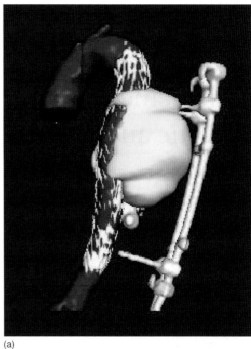

(a)

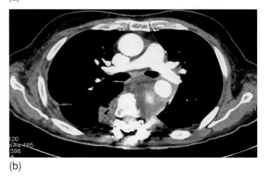

(b)

**Figure 2** (a and b) A CT scan demonstrating a 12 cm × 10 cm descending thoracic mycotic aneurysm with spinal rods used to stabilize spine.

of heparin were given to keep the activated clotted time greater than 200 seconds. A 5-F pigtail catheter was advanced through the left groin sheath into the thoracic aorta. The fluoroscopic C-arm was positioned in a left anterior oblique angle and an oblique thoracic arch aortogram was performed to visualize the orifices of the arch vessels and the descending thoracic mycotic aneurysm (Figure 3a). The intravascular ultrasound (IVUS) catheter was advanced through the right groin sheath to confirm the size of the aneurysm, presence or absence

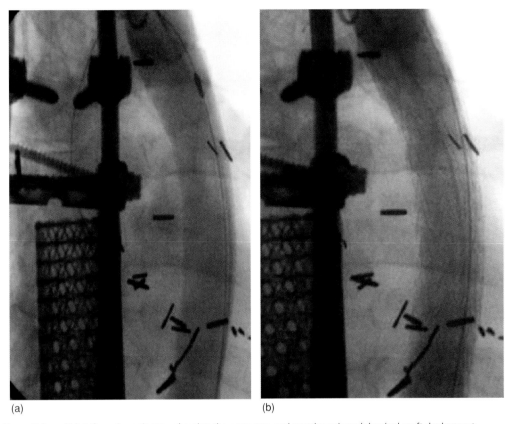

(a)                                    (b)

**Figure 3** (a and b) A thoracic angiogram showing the aorta pre- and postthoracic endoluminal graft deployment.

of thrombus, proximal neck diameter/length, and distal neck diameter/length. IVUS confirmed the measurements taken from the CT scan. Based on these measurements, a 34 mm × 20 cm Gore TAG stent graft (W.L. Gore & Associates, Flagstaff, AZ) was chosen. The IVUS catheter was exchanged for an extra-stiff 260-cm Lunderquist wire (Cook Inc., Bloomington, IN). The right 9-F sheath was exchanged for a 22-F Gore sheath and the 34 mm × 20 cm TAG stent-graft device was advanced through the Gore sheath. It was subsequently deployed after marking the exact proximal and distal landing zones on our "road map" angiogram. A Gore trilobe balloon was used to perform postdeployment balloon angioplasty to all fixation sites. A completion angiogram demonstrated exclusion of the aneurysm with no endoleak (Figure 3b). All wires and sheaths were removed and the right common femoral artery was closed in a transverse fashion with restoration of arterial flow. An 8-F angioseal vascular closure

device (St. Jude Medical, Inc., St. Paul, MN) was deployed to the left common femoral artery. The patient had bilateral palpable pulses at the end of the procedure; he was extubated and transferred to the recovery room. The patient was discharged home on postoperative day (POD) 2 in satisfactory condition. A CT scan of the chest performed on POD 1 demonstrated exclusion of the mycotic aneurysm with no endoleak (Figure 4a and 4b). The patient was subsequently placed on 6 weeks of intravenous antibiotics with recommendations of lifelong oral antibiotics. He remains asymptomatic at 36-month follow-up and exhibits a marked regression of the mycotic aneurysmal sac with remodeling of the thoracic aorta (Figure 5a and 5b).

## Case scenario 2

This is a 71-year-old male who developed fever, chills, and back pain and was diagnosed with a

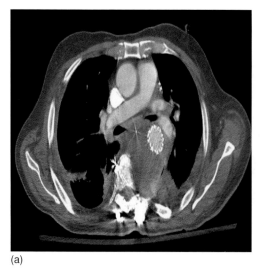

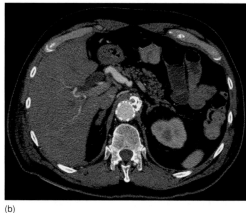

(a)  (b)

**Figure 4** (a and b) An axial CT scan image showing complete exclusion of the pseudoaneurysm.

discitis complicated by a paraspinal abscess. He underwent paraspinal abscess drainage with disc repair by a neurosurgeon. Cultures from the abscess cavity grew MRSA.

His hospitalization was complicated by MRSA septicemia. Upon discharge, he was started on antibiotic therapy consisting of Vancomycin and Clindamcin. Four months after his procedure, he complained of left flank pain. A CT scan of the chest was performed that demonstrated the resolution of the spinal abscess cavity but a 3.8 cm × 2.5 cm pseudoaneurysm involving the takeoff of the celiac

trunk was present (Figure 6). Suspicion of a mycotic aneurysm was entertained. With his previous surgery and complications from that procedure, the patient was brought to the endovascular suite for evaluation and treatment of his pseudoaneurysm by endovascular therapy.

### Angiogram and IVUS

Under local anesthesia, percutaneous access of the right common femoral artery was performed with an 18-G needle (Cook Inc., Bloomington, IN). A 0.035-in. soft-tip angled glide wire was advanced

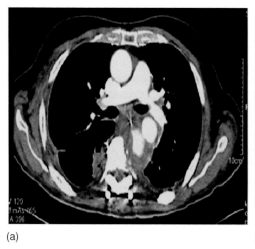

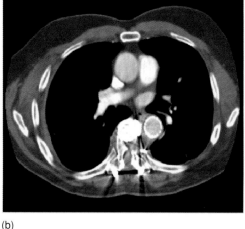

(a)  (b)

**Figure 5** A preprocedure CT scan image (a) with its counterpart done approximately 36 months after the procedure (b) demonstrating remodeling of the thoracic aorta.

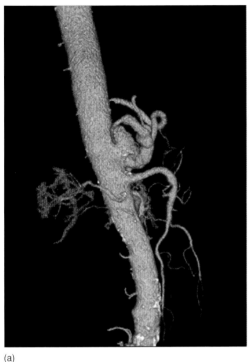

(a)

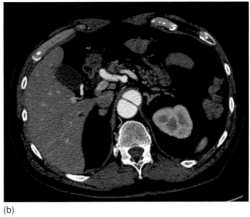

(b)

**Figure 6** (a and b) A CT scan of the chest demonstrating a 2.0-cm pseudoaneurysm of the thoracic aorta at the takeoff of the celiac trunk.

into the thoracic aorta under fluoroscopic guidance and exchanged to a 9-F sheath. Heparin was given to achieve an activated clotting time more than 200 seconds. A 5-F angiographic catheter was advanced into the thoracic aorta and an anterior–posterior plus a lateral angiogram demonstrated a pseudoaneurysm of the thoracic aorta at the level of the celiac trunk takeoff. A visceral angiogram demonstrated adequate collateralization between the celiac trunk and the superior mesenteric artery (SMA) from the gastroduodenal branch of the common hepatic artery. The angiographic catheter was exchanged for an IVUS 8.2-F probe. On IVUS, the area above the pseudoaneurysm was measured to be 24 mm with the area distal measuring 28 mm. The SMA was spared. The length of aorta to be covered was 5.0 cm. On completing the IVUS study, the wires and sheaths were removed and a closure device deployed to the right groin.

**Endovascular procedure**

Under general anesthesia open retrograde cannulation of the right common femoral artery was performed with an 18-G needle and a 0.035-in.

soft-tip angled glide wire (Medi-tech/Boston Scientific, Natick, MA) was passed into the distal thoracic aorta and exchanged to a 9-F sheath under fluoroscopic visualization. Percutaneous access of the left common femoral artery was similarly performed and a 9-F sheath introduced. Five thousand units of heparin were given to keep the activated clotted time greater than 200 seconds. A 5-F pigtail catheter was advanced through the left groin sheath into the thoracic aorta. An anteroposterior and a lateral thoracic aortogram were performed which confirmed the pseudoaneurysm (Figure 7) as well as collateralization of the celiac trunk and the SMA by the gastroduodenal artery. Using a 5-F internal mammary (LIMA) catheter cannulation of the SMA was performed and a 0.035-in. glide wire was positioned. Percutaneous retrograde cannulation of the left brachial artery was performed and with the help of a long (LIMA) catheter cannulation of the celiac trunk was achieved and left into position. A Power-link (Endologix) abdominal endoluminal graft cuff measuring 28 mm × 5.5 cm was then selected due to its short length and its ability to be delivered in a controlled fashion with incremental deployment.

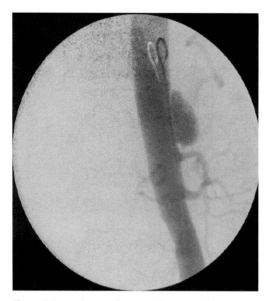

**Figure 7** An angiogram demonstrating a pseudoaneurysm of the thoracic aorta involving the celiac artery.

An exchange of the right groin 9-F sheath for the device sheath was performed. Under fluoroscopic visualization, the endoluminal graft was maneuvered and deployed in such a manner that its distal end was approximately 2 mm proximal to the ostium of the SMA. This was done in conjunction with a previously conducted road map that documented the takeoffs of each vessel in good fashion. Coil embolization of the celiac trunk was carried out through the existing LIMA catheter by deploying two 8 mm × 10 mm coils and six 5 mm × 8 mm coils to seal off the ostium of the celiac trunk in an attempt to prevent any endoleaks. A selective celiac angiogram was performed and showed satisfactory embolization of the celiac trunk. The device sheath was exchanged for a 12-F sheath and a 32-mm Coda balloon (Cook Inc., Bloomington, IN) was used to profile the endoluminal graft. The Endologix cuff was being used in an off-label fashion because it is not commercially approved for use in the thoracic aorta. With no studies on the migration of this device in the thoracic aorta, it was prudent to protect the SMA. With this in mind, a stent was to be placed in the SMA with the stent extending into the aorta. Should the Endologix cuff slip from its precarious position, the stent should protect the inflow. An angled glide wire positioned into the SMA was exchanged to a stiff 0.035-in. Amplatz wire (Cook Inc., Bloomington, IN) using an exchange catheter. A 7-F renal curved guiding catheter was positioned at the ostium of the SMA and an 6 mm × 17 mm Express LD stent (Boston Scientific, Natick, MA) was deployed accordingly. In keeping with the surgical plan, part of the stent was extending into the lumen of the aorta to prevent distal migration of the endoluminal graft. Satisfactory deployment of both the covered and uncovered stent were assured by an angiogram (Figure 8). The angiogram showed satisfactory exclusion of the pseudoaneurysm and a patent SMA with collateralization of the common hepatic, splenic, and left gastric arteries from the gastrodudenal artery. Wire and sheaths were removed with repair of the right common femoral artery. Closure devices were deployed to the left common femoral and left brachial artery. The patient spent 2 days in the hospital with no perioperative complications. A CT scan (Figure 9) conducted prior to discharge confirmed satisfactory exclusion of pseudoaneurysm with demonstrable migration of the endoluminal graft. A year has passed since his surgery with no complication or additional hospitalizations. The annual imaging indicated the pseudoaneurysm to be stable in size with a well-placed endoluminal graft.

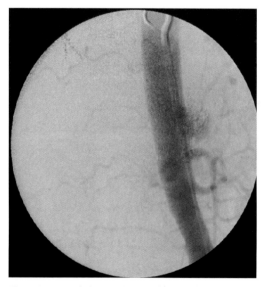

**Figure 8** A completion angiogram demonstrating exclusion of pseudoaneurysm with coil embolization of the celiac artery and stent placement in the SMA.

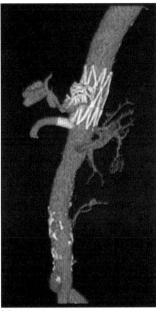

(a)

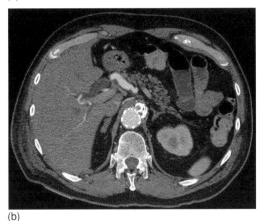

(b)

**Figure 9** (a and b) A postoperative CT scan of the chest demonstrating satisfactory exclusion of pseudoaneurysm with an abdominal Powerlink (Endologix) device. Coils are visualized in the celiac trunk and a stent placed in the SMA to prevent distal migration of endoluminal graft.

## Discussion

Mycotic aneurysms comprise less than 1% of aortic aneurysms and have a high risk of rupture, if not treated urgently. Endovascular therapy of thoracic aneurysms is associated with lower morbidity, mortality, and a lower risk of paraplegia compared to open surgical repair [21, 22]. Results of open surgical repair consist of intensive antibiotic administration, extensive excision/debridement of the infected field associated with extra-anatomic or in situ prosthetic bypass grafting are associated with mortality rates ranging from 5–75% [23, 24]. An endovascular approach to the treatment of mycotic aneurysms avoids the extensive excision and debridement of the infected field. The potential benefit of the endovascular approach is thus compared to the obvious risk of recurrence of the infection. The endovascular approach avoids full heparinization, aortic cross clamping, distal ischemia, and the possible use of shunts leading to less aggressive surgery with earlier extubation, better hemodynamics, less organ failure, and neurologic complications [25]. The few series reported in the literature managed by an endovascular approach to manage their mycotic aneurysms have shown encouraging results with patients alive as long as 62 months postendovascular therapy [26]. Despite the advantages with the endovascular approach, cases of perioperative rupture [26], stent migration [27], and malposition with a type I endoleak have been reported as well [26].

Stent grafts chosen should be selected for availability size and conform to the lesion to be covered. An extended zone proximal and distal to the aortic wall abnormality should be chosen because of the likelihood of more extended arterial lesions. Commercially available grafts can be presoaked in antibiotic solutions or the antibiotic solution can be injected perioperatively into the device delivery system. Reduction in aneurysm sac size, as shown in our patient, has been observed by other authors [28, 29]. The duration of antibiotic therapy remains debatable as some authors have not used antibiotics with others using as little as 6 weeks or as long as lifetime therapy [27–31]. Generally, antibiotic coverage should be tailored to the individual patient based on his or her general condition and results of serial blood cultures.

Due to the few reported series on the use of endoluminal grafts to treat mycotic aneurysms, it is difficult to formulate general guidelines. The creation of a registry could help answer lingering questions regarding the use of this technology in a high-risk patient pool. Only after collecting data on the length of antibiotic coverage, rate of endoleaks, types of endoleaks, residual aneurysm sac size, aortic rupture rates, bleeding, failed endovascular therapies, short-, mid-, and long-term follow-ups and deaths can we clarify the role of endoluminal graft therapy in such a specialized population. Until such data is available, the use of endovascular grafts to treat a thoracic mycotic aneurysm should be approached with caution and appraised on an individual basis. Patients considered ineligible for open surgery should be offered the endovascular approach to palliate rupture and death. Other patients with temporary contraindications could be offered the endovascular approach as a bridge to open surgical repair in the future. All patients should be on a life-long surveillance protocol to monitor for recurrent infection with annual CT scans.

# References

1 Jarrett F, Darling RC, Munth ED, Austen WCG. The management of infected atrial aneurysms. *J Cardiovasc Surg (Torino)* 1977; **18**: 361–366.

2 Miller DV, Oderich GS, Aubry MC, Panneton JM, Edwards WD. Surgical pathology of infected aneurysms of the descending thoracic and abdominal aorta: clinicopathological correlations in 29 cases (1976 to 1999). *Hum Pathol* 2004; **35**: 1112–1120.

3 Kearney RA, Eisen HJ, Wolf JE. Nonvalvular infections of the cardiovascular system. *Ann Intern Med* 1994; **121**: 219–230.

4 Gomes MN, Choyke PL, Wallace RB. Infected aortic aneurysms: a changing entity. *Ann Surg* 1992; **215**: 435–442.

5 Scheld W, Sande M. Endocarditis and intravascular infections. In: Mandell GL, Bennett JE, & Dolin R, eds. *Principles and Practice of Infectious Diseases*, 4th edn. Churchill Livingstone, New York, 1995: 740–783.

6 Maclennan AC, Doyle DL, Sacks SL. Infectious aortitis due to penicillin-resistant *Streptococcus pneumoniae. Ann Vasc Surg* 1997; **11**: 533–535.

7 Hoogendoorn EH, Oyen WJ, van Dijk AP, van der Meer JW. Pneumococcal aortitis, report of a case with emphasis on the contribution to diagnosis of positron emission tomography using fluorinated deoxyglucose. *Clin Microbiol Infect* 2003; **9**: 73–76.

8 Bronze MS, Shirwany A, and Corbett C, Schaberg DR. Infectious aortitis: an uncommon manifestation of infection with streptococcus pneumoniae. *Am J Med* 1999; **107**: 627–630.

9 Sebesta P, Klika T, Mach T *et al.* Bacterial aortitits. *Rozhl Chir* 2004; **83**: 209–216.

10 Fiessinger JN, Paul JF. Inflammatory and infectious artistes. *Rev Prat* 2002; **52**: 1094–1099.

11 Johansen K, Devin J. Mycotic aortic aneurysms: a reappraisal. *Arch Surg* 1983; **118**: 583–588.

12 Johnson JR, Ledgerwood AM, Lucas CE. Mycotic aneurysm: new concepts in therapy. *Arch Surg* 1983; **118**: 577–582.

13 Navarro-martinez A, Gomez-Merino E, Gomez-Garrido M, Fernandez-Funez A. *Listeria monocytogenes* aortitis. *Rev Clin Esp* 2001; **201**: 490.

14 Zenati MA, Bonanomi G, Kostov D, Lee R. Images in cardiovascular medicine: fulminant *Clostridium septicum* aortitis. *Circulation* 2002; **105**: 1871.

15 Byrne G, Barber P, Farrington M. Aortitis caused by beta lactamase producing *Haemophylus influenza* type B. *J Clin Pathol* 1989; **42**: 438–439.

16 Tozzi FL, da Silva ES, Campos F, Fagundes Neto HO, Lucon OM, Lupinacci RM. Primary aortoentric fistula related to septic aortitits. *Sao Paulo Med J* 2001; **119**: 150–153.

17 Barth H, Moosdorf R, Bauer J, Schranz D, Akinturk H. Mycotic pseudo aneurysm of the aorta in children. *Pediatr Cardiol* 2000; **21**: 263–266.

18 Pasic M. Mycotic aneurysm of the aorta: evolving surgical concept. *Ann Thorac Surg.* 1996; **61**: 1053–1054.

19 Muller BT, Wegener OR, Grabitz K, Pillny M, Thomas L, Sandmann W. Mycotic aneurysms of the thoracic and abdominal aorta and iliac arteries: experience with anatomic and extra-anatomic repair in 33 cases. *J Vasc Surg* 2001; **33**: 106–113.

20 Fillmore AJ, Valentine RJ. Surgical mortality in patients with infected aortic aneurysms. *J Am Coll Surg* 2003; **196**: 435–441.

21 Makaroun MS, Dillavou ED, Kes ST *et al.* Endovascular treatment of thoracic aortic aneurysms: results of the phase II multicenter trial of the Gore TAG thoracic endoprosthesis. *J Vasc Surg* 2005; **41**: 1–9.

22 Bavaria JE, Appoo JJ, Makaroun MS, Verter J, Zi-Fan Yu, Scott Mitchell RS. Endovascular stent grafting versus open surgical repair of descending thoracic aortic aneurysms in low-risk patients: a multicenter comparative trial. *J Thorac Cardiovasc Surg* 2007; **133**: 369–377.

23 Hsu RB, Tsay YG, Wang SS, Chu SH. Surgical treatment for primary infected aneurysm of the descending thoracic aorta, abdominal aorta and iliac arteries. *J Vasc Surg* 2002; **36**: 746–750.

24 Cina CS, Arena GO, Fiture AO, Clase CM, Doobay B. Ruptured mycotic thoracoabdominal aortic aneurysms: a report of three cases and a systematic review. *J Vasc Surg* 2001; **33**: 861–867.

25 Lepore V, Lonn L, Delle M *et al.* Endograft therapy for diseases of the descending thoracic aorta: results in 43 high-risk patients. *J Endovasc Ther* 2002; **9**: 829–837.

26 Jones KG, Bell RE, Sabharwal T, Aukett M, Reidy JF, Taylor PR. Treatment of mycotic aortic aneurysms with endoluminal grafts. *Eu J Vasc Endovasc Surg* 2005; **29**: 139–144.

27 Stanley M, Semmens JB, Lawrence Brown MM, Denton M, Grosser D. Endoluminal repair of mycotic aneurysms. *J Endovasc Ther* 2003; **10**: 29–32.

28 Bell RE, Taylor PR, Aukett M, Evans GH, Reidy JF. Sucessful endoluminal repair of an infected thoracic pseudoaneurysm caused by methicillin-resistant *Staphylococcus aureus*. *J Endovasc Ther* 2003; **10**: 29–32.

29 Nishimoto M, Hasegawa S, Asada K, Tsunemi K, Sasaki S. Stent graft placement for mycotic aneurysm of the thoracic aorta: report of a case. *Circ J* 2004; **68**: 88–90.

30 Ting AC, Cheng SW, Ho P, Poon JT. Endovascular repair for multiple *Salmonella* mycotic aneurysms of the thoracic aorta presenting with cardiovocal syndrome. *Eur J Cardiothorac Surg* 2004; **26**: 221–224.

31 Kotzampassakis N, Delanaye P, Masy F, Creemers E. Endovascular stent-graft for thoracic aorta aneurysm caused by *Salmonella*. *Eur J Cardiothorac Surg* 2004; **26**: 225–227.

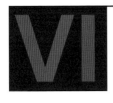

## SECTION VI

# Extending proximal landing zones

# Hybrid management of an arch aneurysm with a carotid–carotid bypass and deployment of an endoluminal graft

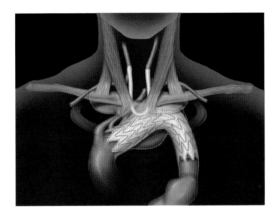

## Introduction

Thoracic aortic aneurysms (TAAs) are traditionally repaired with an open surgical replacement done with a synthetic tube graft [1]. The recent development of endograft technology for the treatment of TAAs has been associated with a lower morbidity and mortality [2]. Arch aneurysms have not been suitable for endovascular repair because of concerns about the supra-aortic vessels. Recently, there have been isolated reports of debranching techniques combined with the deployment thoracic endografts to treat both proximal and distal arch aneurysms [3, 4]. The hybrid technique avoids a median sternotomy, cardiopulmonary bypass, and circulatory arrest with a quicker postoperative recovery.

## Case scenario

An 88-year-old woman was found to have a widened mediastinum on a routine chest X-ray. A CT scan of the chest (Figure 1a and 1b) demonstrated an arch aneurysm measuring 5.7 cm with proximal neck diameter of 39 mm at the transverse aortic arch distal to the innominate artery takeoff. The location of the aneurysm did not allow for the conventional use of a thoracic endoluminal graft because coverage of the left carotid artery would be needed to attain proper seal of aneurysm (Figure 2a and 2b). The patient was not interested in an open repair due to her advanced age; she agreed to undergo the hybrid approach combining an arch vessel bypass with endograft technology.

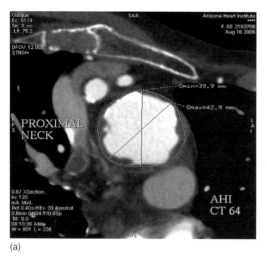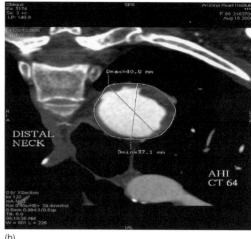

(a)　　　　　　　　　　　　　　　　　　(b)

**Figure 1** (a and b) An oblique CT scan image showing the proximal and distal neck diameters adjacent to the arch aneurysm.

## Surgical technique

Bilateral low-neck incisions were made parallel to the sternocleidomastoid muscle. Adequate mobilization of the common carotid artery was achieved so a low-lying bypass graft could be tunneled beneath the sternal notch for cosmetic reasons. An 8-mm Dacron Hemashield graft (Boston Scientific, Natick, MA) was tunneled beneath the sternal notch. Five thousand units of heparin were given to the patient followed by proximal and distal cross clamps to the right common carotid artery. Construction of an end-to-side anastomosis was accomplished using 5-0 polypropylene suture. Cross clamps were removed, the graft was clamped, and flow was reestablished to the right

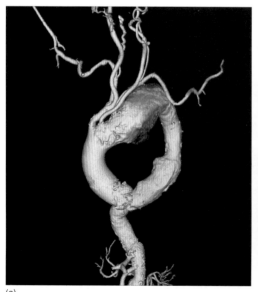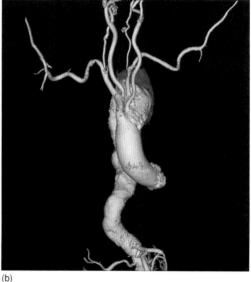

(a)　　　　　　　　　　　　　　　　　　(b)

**Figure 2** (a and b) A 3-D reconstruction of a 64-silce CT scan depicts the location of the arch aneurysm in relation to the arch vessels.

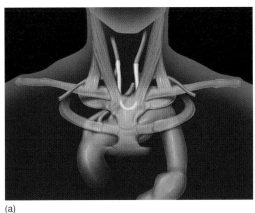 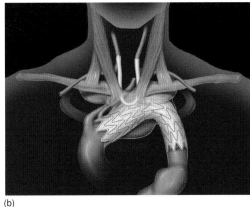

(a)                                    (b)

**Figure 3** (a and b) An illustration of a carotid–carotid bypass in conjunction with a thoracic endograft.

common carotid artery. The left common carotid artery was similarly mobilized up to its origin; proximal and distal cross clamp were applied; the artery was then transected close to the proximal clamp. The distal end of the left common carotid artery was anastomosed to an 8-mm Dacron Hemashield graft as an end-to-end anastomosis. The proximal left common carotid artery was oversewn with a 4-0 transfixing suture. The cross clamps were removed and flow was subsequently established to the left common carotid artery through the newly created carotid–carotid bypass (Figure 3a) with plan to exclude arch aneurysm with an endoluminal graft (Figure 3b).

## Deployment of endoluminl graft

Bilateral groin incisions were made to expose both common femoral arteries. Heparin was given to achieve an activated clotting time of greater than 200 seconds. Under fluoroscopic guidance, an 18-G needle (Cook Inc., Bloomington, IN) was used to access both common femoral arteries (CFAs). A 0.035-in. soft-tip angled glide wire was advanced to the arch of the aorta and 9-F (French) sheaths were placed in both groins. An oblique arch aortogram was performed using a 5-F pigtail angiographic catheter that was advanced through the left groin sheath. The aortogram demonstrated the arch aneurysm as well as the patent left to right carotid artery bypass (Figure 4a). After angiographic confirmation of the arch aneurysm and demarcating our proximal and distal landing zones, the 9-F sheath in

the right groin was exchanged to a 24-F Gore sheath. Under fluoroscopic surveillance, a 40 mm × 20 cm Gore TAG device (W.L. Gore & Associates, Flagstaff, AZ) was deployed over a stiff 260-cm Lunderquist wire (Cook Inc., Bloomington, IN) just distal to the takeoff of the innominate artery. A completion angiogram showed complete exclusion of the aneurysm with moderate flow to both common carotid arteries. A partial obstruction of the ostium of the innominate artery was caused by the flares of the endograft (Figure 4b). An 8 mm × 37 mm balloon expandable express stent (Boston Scientific, Natick, MA) was deployed to the ostium of the innominate artery with an improved, brisk flow to both carotid arteries. The sheaths and wires were removed; both CFAs were repaired and the patient extubated in the operating room with movement in all extremities. A CT scan performed prior to discharge showed adequate flow through the bypass graft, common carotid arteries, and with no endoleak identified with satisfactory position of the endograft (Figure 5). The patient continues to do well 9 months after the procedure.

## Discussion

Thoracic aneurysms with a diameter more than 5 cm are associated with a 2-year patient survival of less than 30% [5]. Most patients, if untreated, die from aneurysm rupture. The significant morbidity and mortality associated with open surgical repair of thoracic aneurysms has resulted in an increasing use of a less invasive and safer treatment

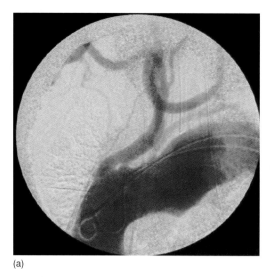

(a)

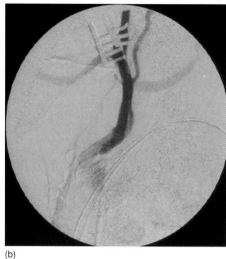

(b)

**Figure 4** (a) An angiogram demonstrating an arch aneurysm with a patent carotid–carotid artery bypass. (b) A completion angiogram showing total exclusion of the aneurysm with patent innominate artery and carotid bypass graft.

using endovascular therapy. Endovascular treatment of thoracic arch aneurysms is associated with fewer procedural-related complications, a shorter convalescence, and minimal neurological sequelae [6].

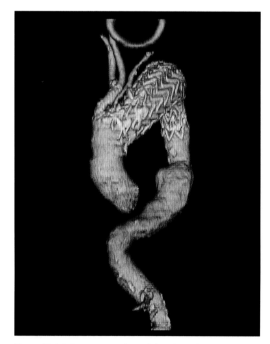

**Figure 5** A 3-D reconstruction of the chest showing an anterior view of the completed procedure.

Open graft replacement of arch aneurysms requires cardiopulmonary bypass, various degrees of hypothermia, and circulatory arrest, which increases the morbidity of the procedure. The use of a hybrid approach to treat aortic arch aneurysms can be satisfactorily performed with a lower morbidity and mortality than the traditional open surgical approach. This method gives high-risk patients another option for treatment should they be declined for open surgery due to significant comorbidities or they want a less invasive approach. Variations of reconstruction of common carotid and subclavian arteries can be performed to provide adequate landing zones for the treatment of TAA [7]. These variations in technique allow for a customized approach in terms of rerouting the arch vessels to achieve only the necessary length of healthy, normal aorta needed to seat an endoluminal graft properly.

The presternal approach as described in our report avoids the bypass graft from being visible and subject to injury as seen in the pretracheal approach. Secondly, it allows the possibility of the patient to undergo a tracheostomy in the near future. The disadvantage of this technique is that a sternotomy may be risky to perform if such a procedure was required in the future. Hybrid procedures using endografts with various combinations of supraaortic debranching procedures offer a less invasive approach to the management of arch pathologies.

However, long-term data is needed to validate the routine application of such a clinical practice.

## References

1 De Bakey ME, McCollum CH, Graham M. Surgical treatment of aneurysms of the descending thoracic aorta: long term results in 500 patients. *J Cardiovasc Surg (Torino)* 1978; **19**: 571–576.

2 Parodi J, Palmaz J, Barone H. Transfemoral intraluminal graft implantation for abdominal aortic aneurysm. *Ann Vasc Surg* 1991; **5**: 491–499.

3 Buth J, Penn O, Tielbeek A, Mersman M. Combined approach to stent-graft treatment of an aortic arch aneurysm. *J Endovasc Surg* 1998; **5**: 329–332.

4 Zhou W, Reardon ME, Peden EK, Lin PH, Bush RL, Lumsden AB. Endovascular repair of a proximal aortic arch aneurysm: a novel approach of supra-aortic debranching with antegrade endograft deployment via an anterior thoracotomy approach. *J Vasc Surg* 2006; **43**(5): 1045–1048.

5 Crawford ES, Denatale RW. Thoracoabdominal aortic aneurysm: observations regarding the natural course of the disease. *J Vasc Surg* 1986; **3**: 578–582.

6 Makaroun MS, Dillavou ED, Kee ST *et al.* Endovascular treatment of thoracic aortic aneurysms: results of phase II multicenter trial of the Gore TAG thoracic endoprosthesis. *J Vasc Surg* 2005; **41**: 1–9.

7 Criado FJ, Clark NS, Arnatan MF. Stent graft repair in the aortic arch and descending thoracic aorta: 4 year experience. *J Vasc Surg* 2002; **36**: 1121–1128.

# Endovascular management of transverse arch aneurysms

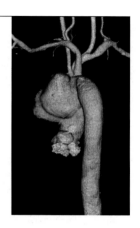

## Introduction

Transverse arch aneurysms comprise about 10% of thoracic aortic aneurysms. Etiologies include atherosclerosis, infection, trauma, Marfan's syndrome, and acute and chronic dissections. The majority of transverse arch aneurysms occur in association with an ascending, descending, or thoracoabdominal aneurysm. Patients may be asymptomatic and diagnosed by routine imaging performed for other conditions or they may present with compressive symptoms. Open surgical repair requires a median sternotomy, extracorporeal circulation deep hypothermic circulatory arrest (HCA) with various adjunct protective agents to protect the heart, brain, and spinal cord which results in an increased morbidity and mortality. Endovascular management of transverse arch aneurysms can be performed with a lower morbidity, mortality, and neurological sequelae and can sometimes require various types of debranching of the supra-aortic vessels to create an adequate proximal neck for fixation. We describe an endovascular approach to treat a transverse arch aneurysm.

## Case scenario

A 54-year-old male with a previous coronary artery bypass graft surgery for coronary artery disease and a history of hypertension developed a voice change with increasing shortness of breath. Significant past medical history was notable for a motor vehicle accident 15 years prior which did not result in any significant complications. His physical examination

was notable for a left vocal cord paralysis. A 64-slice CT scan of the chest was performed (Figure 1) showing a 7.6-cm saccular aneurysm involving the lesser arch with the (Figure 2) reconstruction depicting a bovine arch with left carotid artery and innominate artery originating from the same ostium. The saccular arch aneurysm is located at the isthmus of the aorta extending from the base of the left subclavian artery. A virtual angioscopic view demonstrating the arch of the aorta extibits the ostium of the arch vessels (Figure 3). Due to the previous median sternotomy with accompanying bypass graft involving the internal mammary artery, the patient was felt to be at high risk for a redo operation. He was offered a hybrid approach which would comprise a left carotid–left subclavian bypass to protect the internal mammary artery bypass graft and then followed by the deployment of a thoracic endoluminal graft to exclude the arch aneurysm.

## Technical details (left carotid–left subclavian bypass)

A left-sided supraclavicular incision was performed (Figure 4). The platysma was divided followed by the clavicular head of the sternocleidomastoid medially to reveal the carotid sheath. The carotid sheath was identified and incised to reveal the common carotid artery and the vagus nerve, which was protected. Next, we divided the omohyoid muscle and identified the scalene fat pad and mobilized it from lateral to medial to reveal the phrenic nerve overlying the scalenus anterior muscle. The phrenic nerve was preserved and the scalenus anterior muscle

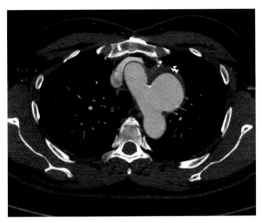

**Figure 1** A CT scan axial image demonstrating a saccular arch aneurysm measuring up to 7.6 cm in diameter.

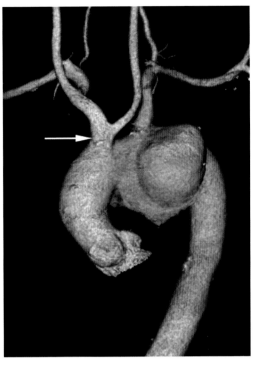

**Figure 2** A 3-D reconstruction clarifying the origin of all the arch vessels and the relative position of the arch aneurysm.

divided to reveal the aneurysmal ostium of the left subclavian artery. We then divided the left subclavian artery between clamps and oversewed the proximal subclavian artery with a 4-0 Prolene and sewed the distal end of the subclavian artery to an 8-mm Gore TAG graft (W.L. Gore & Associates, Flagstaff, AZ) in an end-to-end fashion after administering 5000 units of heparin. The graft was tunneled beneath the internal jugular vein and, after clamping,

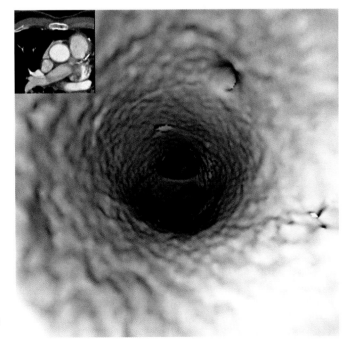

**Figure 3** A virtual angioscopic view of the arch of the aorta demonstrating the supra-aortic branch vessels.

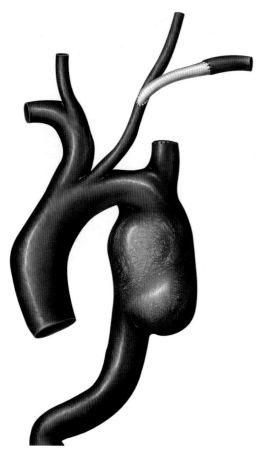

**Figure 4** Carotid left subclavian bypass.

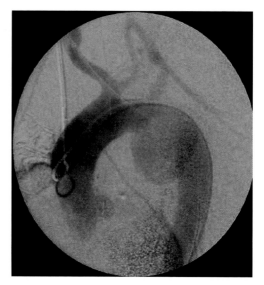

**Figure 5** Arch angiogram demonstrates arch secular aneurysm and a bovine arch.

oblique arch aortogram was performed using a 5-F pigtail angiographic catheter through the left groin which demonstrated a saccular arch aneurysm. Intravascular ultrasound probe was advance through the right groin sheath to determine the proximal neck and distal neck diameter (Figure 5). After angiographic confirmation and under fluoroscopic

the left common carotid artery proximally and distally the graft was sewn in an end-to-side fashion with 5-0 Prolene. De-airing maneuvers were performed prior to unclamping the artery to restore flow. The neck incision was closed and patient returned to the recovery room without any complications.

## Technical details (deployment of thoracic endograft)

Bilateral groin incisions were made to expose both common femoral arteries (CFAs). Heparin was given to achieve an activated clotting time of greater than 200 seconds. Under fluoroscopic guidance, an 18-G needle (Cook Inc., Bloomington, IN) was used to access both CFAs. A 0.035-in. soft-tip angled glide wire was advanced to the arch of the aorta and 9-F (French) sheaths were placed in both groins. An

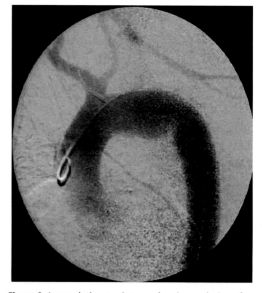

**Figure 6** A completion angiogram showing exclusion of aneurysm with endoluminal graft and no endoleak and patent left carotid to left subclavian bypass graft.

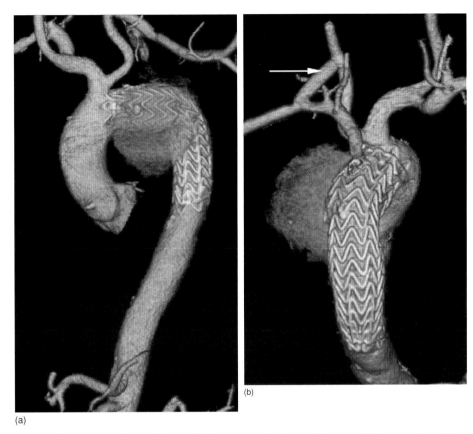

(a)

(b)

**Figure 7** (a and b) A CT scan performed prior to discharge showed adequate flow through the bypass graft (white arrow) and both common carotid arteries with no endoleak seen. There is satisfactory position of the endograft and exclusion of saccular ach aneurysm.

surveillance, the 9-F sheath was exchanged to a 24-F Gore sheath and a 40 mm × 20 cm Gore TAG device (W.L. Gore & Associates, Flagstaff, AZ) was deployed just distal to the takeoff of the innominate artery covering the ostium of the left subclavian artery. A completion angiogram showed complete exclusion of the saccular aneurysm with no endoleak (Figure 6). The sheaths and wires were removed, and both CFAs were repaired. The patient was extubated in the operating room and a neurological examination showed that movement to all the extremities was intact with no deficits. A postoperative CT scan showed successful exclusion of the arch aneurysm with no endoleak with a patent left carotid to left subclavian artery bypass (Figure 7a and 7b). A postprocedure virtual angioscopic view of the arch demonstrated patent arch vessels (Figure 8). The patient continues to do well at 5 months after the surgery.

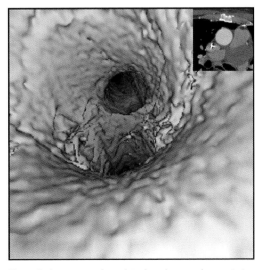

**Figure 8** A postprocedure virtual angioscopy demonstrates patent innominate artery.

## Discussion

Isolated transverse arch aneurysms are rare. Most aneurysms of the transverse arch occur in association with ascending, descending, or thoracoabdominal aneurysms. Surgical repair of such aneurysms present a surgical challenge as the heart, brain, and spinal cord must all be protected. A graft replacement of the ascending aorta, transverse arch, and descending aorta in a single operation is a lengthy procedure requiring multiple incisions, a number of complicated protective surgical adjuncts, longer clamp times, greater blood loss, HCA which can lead to an increased surgical morbidity and mortality.

The elephant trunk technique introduced in 1983 [1] permitted the surgeon to open the transverse arch and the descending thoracic aorta without dissecting the proximal native descending thoracic aorta thereby decreasing bleeding complications and overall mortality of this operation. Report of a documented cumulative mortality exceeding 20% has been reported with the elephant trunk technique which includes an in-house mortality for the two procedures as well as the risk of rupture between the two intervals [2, 3]. Surgery using the techniques of HCA for aortic arch surgery carries a risk of permanent stroke of 5–7% as well as a transient neurological deficit as high as 20% and a risk of neuropsychological deficit in the majority of patients [4–9]. The single largest operative determinant of neurological outcome in aortic arch surgery after HCA remains arrest duration. Arrest time of 25 minutes is associated with an increased risk of transient neurological deficit and times more than 40 minutes increases the risk of stroke with a sharp increase in mortality with arrest time more than 1 hour [10]. In a series of 150 aortic arch aneurysms reported by Spielvogel *et al.*, the etiologies of the arch aneurysms were atherosclerosis ($n = 48$, 32%), chronic dissections ($n = 56$, 37.3%), degenerative disease ($n = 29$, 19.3%), ruptured atherosclerotic ulcer ($n = 8$, 5.3%), Marfanic aneurysms ($n = 3$, 2.0%), trauma ($n = 2$, 1.3%), inflammatory aneurysms ($n = 2$, 1.3%), false aneurysms ($n = 1$, 0.7%), and other ($n = 1$, 0.7%). Isolated arch replacement was performed in 38 patients (25.3%) [11].

The frozen elephant trunk technique allows for a single stage repair of a combined aortic arch and the descending thoracic aorta using hybrid prosthesis with a stented and a nonstented end. With this procedure, the ascending and arch aorta are repaired using a conventional approach and, through the open-ended aortic arch; a stent graft is deployed using an antegrade approach. In a series of 39 patients treated with this modality, the indication was primarily acute type A dissection ($n = 11$, 28.2%), chronic type A dissection with aneurysmal expansion ($n = 3$, 7.7%), acute type B dissection ($n = 1$, 2.5%), and chronic type B dissection with aneurysmal expansion ($n = 3$, 7.7%). The second indication ($n = 18$, 46.2%) was an aneurysm proximal and distal to the left subclavian artery with a range in aneurysm diameter (49–73 mm) mean 59 $\pm$ 8 mm. The 30-day mortality was 12.8% with 2 deaths related to the procedure. Five patients developed neurological complications with full resolution in 2 patients. There were no cases of paraplegia [12]. The use of a hybrid approach to treat aortic arch aneurysms can be satisfactorily performed with a lower morbidity and mortality than traditional open surgical approach while providing high-risk patients the possibility of a less invasive repair. Variations of reconstruction techniques of common carotid and subclavian arteries can be performed to provide adequate landing zones for the treatment of transverse arch aneurysms.

## References

1 Borst HG, Walterbusch G, Schaps D. Extensive aortic replacement using "elephant trunk" prosthesis. *Thorac Cardiovasc Surg* 1983; **31**: 37–40.

2 Schepens MA, Dossche KM, Morshuis WJ, van den Barselaar PJ, Heijmen RH, Vermeulen FE. The elephant trunk technique: operative results in 100 consecutive patients. *Eur J Cardiothorac Surg* 2002; **21**: 276–281.

3 Estrera AL, Miller CC, III, Porat EE, Huynh TT, Winnerkvist A, Safi HJ. Staged repair of extensive aortic aneurysms. *Ann Thorac Surg* 2002; **74**: S1803–S1805.

4 Hagl C, Ergin M, Galla J *et al.* Neurologic outcome after ascending aorta-aortic arch operations: effect of brain protection technique in high-risk patients. *J Thorac Cardiovasc Surg* 2001; **121**: 1107–1121.

5 Immer F, Barmettler H, Berdat P *et al.* Effects of deep hypothermic circulatory arrest on outcome after resection of ascending aortic aneurysm. *Ann Thorac Surg* 2002; **74**: 422–425.

6 Czerny M, Fleck T, Zimpfer D *et al*. Risk factors of mortality and permanent neurologic injury in patients undergoing ascending aortic and arch repair. *J Thorac Cardiovasc Surg* 2003; **126**: 1296–1301.

7 Ehrlich M, Ergin M, McCullough J *et al*. Predictors of adverse outcome and transient neurological dysfunction after ascending aortic/hemiarch replacement. *Ann Thorac Surg* 2000; **69**: 1755–1763.

8 Harrington D, Bonser M, Moss A, Heafield M, Riddoch M, Bonser R. Neuropsychometric outcome following aortic arch surgery: a prospective randomised trial of retrograde cerebral perfusion. *J Thorac Cardiovasc Surg* 2003; **126**: 638–644.

9 Deborah KH, Fernanda F, Robert SB. Cerebral perfusion. *Ann Thorac Surg* 2007; **83**: S799–S804.

10 Svensson L, Crawford E, Hess K *et al*. Deep hypothermia with circulatory arrest: determinants of stroke and early mortality in 656 patients. *J Thorac Cardiovasc Surg* 1993; **106**: 19–31.

11 David S, Christian DE, Daniel S, Steven LL, Randall BG. Aortic arch replacement with a trifurcated graft. *Ann Thorac Surg* 2007; **83**: S791–S795.

12 Hassina B, Christian H, Narwid K *et al*. The frozen elephant trunk technique for treatment of thoracic aortic aneurysms. *Ann Thorac Surg* 2007; **83**: S819–S823.

# Hybrid endovascular management of an arch pseudoaneurysm using an antegrade deployment approach

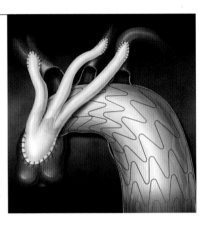

## Introduction

Open surgical replacement of the arch to treat arch aneurysms requires hypothermic circulatory arrest with extracorporeal circulation which increases morbidity and mortality. Endovascular management of arch aneurysms requires an adequate landing zone to achieve proximal seal. Due to the configuration of the arch combined with semirigid stent-graft designs longer than normal landing zones may be necessary requiring coverage of the left subclavian artery and sometimes more cephalad deployment of endograft. Supra-aortic vessel debranching is necessary to restore flow to the head vessels when the arch has to be excluded with an endoluminal graft. The hybrid approach can be performed through a minimal median sternotomy without requiring extracorporeal circulation and circulatory arrest.

## Case scenario

A 68-year-old lady with past medical history of hypertension and osteoarthritis developed pancreatitis and acute renal failure after replacement of a 10.0 cm × 13.0 cm distal arch and descending thoracic aortic aneurysm 3 years ago with a 34-mm Hemashield graft. She developed an upper respiratory tract infection and a chest X-ray demonstrated a tortuous and dilated thoracic aorta. A CT scan of

the chest (Figure 1a and 1b) demonstrated a pseudoaneurysm at the proximal anastomosis of her previous repair measuring 6.6 cm × 5.5 cm at its largest diameter. Due to the high risk associated with a redo operation, she was managed with a hybrid approach consisting of rerouting of the supra-aortic vessels and exclusion of the arch pseudoaneurysm with an endoluminal graft.

## Procedural technique

A median sternotomy incision approximately 8 cm long was made (Figure 2a) for exposure of the ascending aorta and arch vessels. The ascending aorta, origins of the innominate, and left common carotid arteries were mobilized. Mobilization of the left subclavian artery is performed only if transposition is indicated. A woven Dacron or polytetrafluoroethylene bifurcated graft was selected based upon the diameter of the ascending aorta and the branch arteries to be bypassed; in this case an 18 mm × 9 mm Hemashield Dacron bifurcated graft was used. A 10-mm straight graft was cut obliquely (60°) and anastomosed to the heel of the bifurcated graft using 5-0 Prolene suture. This conduit will be used to deliver the endoluminal graft antegrade across the aortic arch. After 5000 units of heparin were administered to the patient a partially occluding clamp was applied to the lateral curve of the ascending aorta, and the bifurcated conduit graft anastomosed with

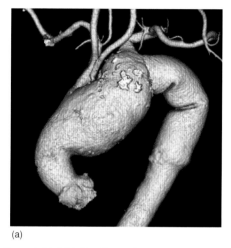
(a)

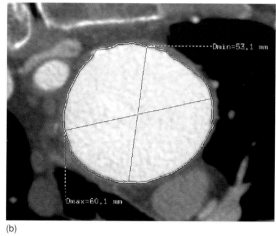
(b)

**Figure 1** (a) A 64-slice CT scan demonstrating an arch pseudoaneurysm measuring 6.6 cm × 5.5 cm. (b) A CT scan with an axial cut demonstrating a cross sectional area of arch aneurysm.

4-0 Prolene suture as an end-to-side anastomosis; the left common carotid artery was clamped proximally and distally, transected at the arch, and sutured proximally. The lateral limb of the graft was anastomosed in an end-to-end configuration. The innominate artery was similarly addressed. After each anastomosis the graft was flushed to eliminate any thrombus or air. All clamps were removed and the integrity of the suture line confirmed (Figure 2b). The left subclavian artery was to be excluded using an endoluminal graft.

Retrograde percutaneous access of both common femoral arteries was achieved with a 9-F (French) sheath. A 9-F sheath was secured in the 10-mm conduit, and a 250-cm angled hydrophilic guide wire passed to the desired right iliac artery, captured with a snare, and exteriorized through the right femoral sheath. The conduit was clamped, and the stent-graft delivery sheath was substituted for the 24-F sheath. A marker (opaque string, clips, or a sternal wire) was placed at a proximal portion on the conduit, which is important to assure that the stent graft's deployment was just beyond the limb origins of the bifurcated graft. The conduit was introduced across the aortic arch as tension was placed on the conduit–femoral artery wire. Once in the desired position, the 40 mm × 20 cm Gore TAG endoprosthesis (W.L. Gore & Associates, Flagstaff, AZ) was introduced and positioned at the marker as the sheath is withdrawn into the conduit. A final

angiogram of the ascending aortic arch was performed (Figure 2c) through a 5-F pigtail angiographic catheter that had been introduced through the left groin sheath which demonstrated patent debranched arch vessels, satisfactory placement of the endoluminal graft, and a type II endoleak from the left subclavian artery. A decision was made to reverse the heparin at this time and manage the endoleak conservatively. The delivery sheath was removed, and the conduit transected and oversewn. The sternal incision was closed, with one mediastinal drainage tube in place. Patient made an uneventful recovery and the postoperative CT scan (Figures 3 and 4) performed demonstrated patent debranched arch vessels with exclusion of the pseudoaneurysm with a demonstrable type II endoleak from the left subclavian artery. A decision was made to manage the endoleak conservatively with routine CT surveillance over the next few weeks.

## Discussion

Pseudoaneurysms of the arch regardless of their etiology are traditionally managed by open surgical techniques requiring a total arch replacement. Total arch replacement for this cohort group of patients requires hypothermic extracorporeal circulation which despite improvement in surgical techniques is associated with high morbidity and mortality.

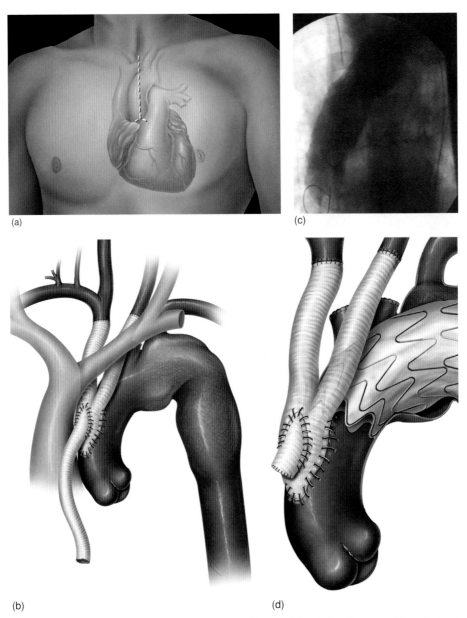

(a)

(c)

(b)

(d)

**Figure 2** (a) A median sternotomy incision. (b) Anastomosis of the bifurcated 9-mm limbs to the left common carotid artery and the innominate artery in an end-to-end fashion. (c) A completion angiogram demonstrating satisfactory exclusion of arch aneurysm with an endoluminal graft, patent debranched arch vessels, and a significant type II endoleak from the ostium of the left subclavian artery. (d) Deployment of endoluminal graft to exclude arch pseudoaneurysm with transection of the 10-mm side limb conduit.

Endoluminal grafting has recently been approved by Food and Drug Administration, United States, for the treatment of thoracic aortic aneurysms. The endoluminal approach has been associated with a decrease in morbidity, mortality, and paraplegia [1, 2]. The application of endoluminal graft therapy under investigational device exemption has been extended in our institution to treat acute dissecting aneurysms, chronic dissecting aneurysm with aortic expansion, penetrating aortic ulcer, adult

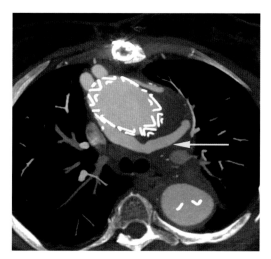

**Figure 3** Postoperative CT scan demonstrating a type II endoleak (arrow).

coarctation, pseudoaneurysms associated with previous repair acute traumatic transection aortobronchial and aortoesophageal fistulas, and the shaggy aorta [3]. Management of patients with arch aneurysms using endovascular stent grafts sometimes requires longer landing zones to achieve seal due to the relative rigidity of stent grafts in the arch [4]. Coverage of the left subclavian artery as a means

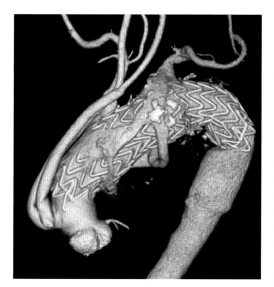

**Figure 4** A 64-slice CT scan demonstrating a type II endoleak from the subclavian artery.

to prolong the landing zone may not be adequate to achieve a satisfactory hemostatic seal requiring stent grafts to be deployed further cephalad with risk of covering the left carotid artery or the innominate artery. The hybrid approach to treating arch aneurysms [5–7] offers a benefit to patients who are at a higher risk for a more demanding operation. The hybrid approach as described can be performed off cardiopulmonary bypass using a partial occluding clamp without any hypothermia and circulatory arrest. Neurological sequelae are few due to a short partial aortic cross-clamp time and if present are more likely due to manipulation of wires in the arch during deployment of endograft. Bergeron *et al.* [6] treated aneurysms and dissections involving the aortic arch in 29 high-risk patients, deploying a variety of commercial stent grafts using preliminary arch vessel transposition in 26. They reported 1 (3.5%) major stroke and 2 (7.7%) deaths, the latter owing to catheterization-related complications (iliac rupture and left ventricle perforation) after endovascular exclusion. One (3.8%) patient had a delayed minor stroke. Schumacher *et al.* [7] encountered no neurological complications.

Retrograde arch deployment of endoluminal grafts is often complicated due to difficult arch configurations and specific deployment characteristics of these devices. The antegrade technique of deployment of endograft allows precise delivery of the endoluminal graft at the proximal aortic arch, thus avoiding problems with retrograde delivery. Threading the wire through the delivery conduit to the femoral artery facilitates the advancement of both the sheath and the endoluminal graft across the aortic arch and permits precise deployment of the stent graft within the tube graft on the ascending aorta.

Other applications of this technique include patients who previously had type A dissections repaired with a tube-graft replacement of the ascending aorta and later developed complications related to the aortic arch or proximal descending thoracic aorta and patients with a retrograde type A dissection involving the arch of the aorta.

The hybrid approach offers a less invasive approach to managing aortic arch pathology. The development of branched stent grafts may replace conventional open surgery of the aortic arch.

# References

1 Makaroun MS, Dillavou ED, Kee ST *et al*. Endovascular treatment of thoracic aortic aneurysms: results of the phase II multicenter trial of the Gore TAG thoracic prosthesis. *J Vasc Surg* 2005; **41**: 1–9.

2 Criado FJ, Clark NS, Barnatan MF. Stent graft repair in the aortic arch and descending thoracic aorta: a 4-year experience. *J Vasc Surg* 2002; **36**: 1121–1128.

3 Wheatley GH, Gurbuz AT, Rodriguez-Lopez JA *et al*. Midterm outcome in 158 consecutive Gore TAG thoracic endoprostheses: a single-center experience. *Ann Thorac Surg* 2006; **81**(5): 1570–1577; discussion 1577.

4 Tse LW, MacKenzie KS, Montreuil B, Obrand DI, Steinmetz OK. The proximal landing zone in endovascular repair of the thoracic aorta. *Ann Vasc Surg* 2004; **18**(2): 178–185.

5 Kato N, Shimono T, Hirano T *et al*. Aortic arch aneurysms: treatment with extraanatomical bypass and endovascular stent-grafting. *Cardiovasc Intervent Radiol* 2002; **25**: 419–422.

6 Bergeron P, Coulon P, De Chaumaray T *et al*. Great vessels transposition and aortic arch exclusion. *J Cardiovasc Surg (Torino)* 2005; **46**: 141–147.

7 Schumacher H, Böckler D, Bardenheuer H *et al*. Endovascular aortic arch reconstruction with supra-aortic transposition for symptomatic contained rupture and dissection: early experience in 8 high-risk patients. *J Endovasc Ther* 2003; **10**: 1066–1074.

# CASE 28

# Hybrid management of a retrograde type B dissection

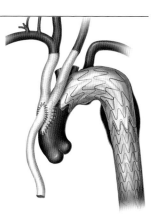

## Introduction

Retrograde type B dissection into the arch with the entry point in the descending thoracic aorta is associated with a high morbidity and mortality. Hybrid operations combining open surgical repair with endovascular stent grafting could potentially be associated with a lower morbidity and mortality. This approach allows surgeons to treat arch pathologies with endoluminal graft technology that would normally be prohibitive in nature. Hybrid procedures can be done without the use of cardiopulmonary bypass and circulatory arrest.

## Case scenario

A 51-year-old gentleman with a long history of hypertension and multiple medical problems was admitted to a local emergency room with severe chest pain. A chest X-ray showed a widened mediastinum, which in turn led to a contrast-enhanced CT scan of the chest where a type B dissection with proximal entry point, believed to be at the level of the left subclavian artery, was identified (Figure 1a and 1b). He was initially managed medically with intravenous antihypertensive and pain medication in the intensive care unit. Due to persistence of chest pain, he was taken to the operating room for an aortogram and an intravascular ultrasound to further assess his condition. The aortogram demonstrated a type B dissection with a compressed true and enlarged false lumen (Figure 2). The intravascular ultrasound confirmed a type B dissection with a retrograde progression of the dissecting flap from the level of the

subclavian artery to the innominate artery. Due to the concerns of increased surgical morbidity associated with aortic arch replacement using the open elephant trunk technique, an alternative hybrid approach composed of thoracic debranching of the arch vessels with an endoluminal graft deployed to the thoracic dissection was used to treat the patient with a remarkable recovery.

## Technical details

A median sternotomy was performed to expose the ascending aorta and the arch vessels. A bifurcated Dacron Hemashield graft (Boston Scientific, Natick, MA) 18 mm × 9 mm was the brought onto the field. A 10-mm arm was attached to the conduit to be used as possible access for an antegrade deployment of the endograft. A side-biting clamp was placed on the aorta and the 18-mm bifurcated limb was sewn to the ascending aorta. Heparinization was performed to keep the activated clotting time around 400 seconds. Cross clamps were placed on the innominate artery. Division of the innominate artery was performed close to the arch with the distal end of the innominate artery sewn to the 9-mm limb of the bifurcated graft in an end-to-end fashion. The proximal end of the inomminate artery was oversewn. Cross clamps were removed after various de-airing and flushing maneuvers. The same procedure was done to anastamose the other 9-mm limb to the left carotid artery with oversewing of the stump of the left common carotid artery. The cross clamp was removed from the left common carotid artery as well as the partial clamp on the

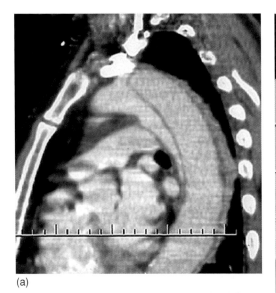

(a)

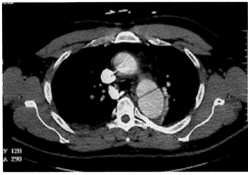

(b)

**Figure 1** (a and b) An axial and sagittal view of a CT scan show the extent of the dissection in the thoracic arch.

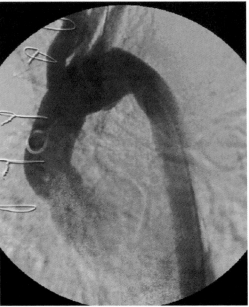

**Figure 2** An angiogram demonstrating a dissection with a true and false lumen.

aorta again after de-airing and flushing maneuvers to restore flow to the innominate artery and the left carotid artery (Figure 3).

## Endovascular approach

The second part of the procedure involved open retrograde access of the left common femoral artery with a 9-F (French) sheath; percutaneous retrograde access of the right common femoral artery was performed with 5-F sheath. Heparin was administered to keep the activated clotted time above 200 seconds. An oblique aortogram was performed through a 5-F pigtail angiographic catheter introduced through the 9-F sheath attached to the 10-mm conduit limb. Aortogram demonstrated the

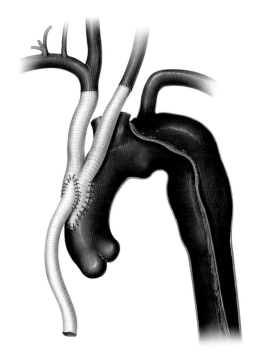

**Figure 3** Illustration of the debranching of the innominate and left carotid artery with a birfurcated graft. A 10-mm conduit is sewn to the graft for possible delivery of the endograft.

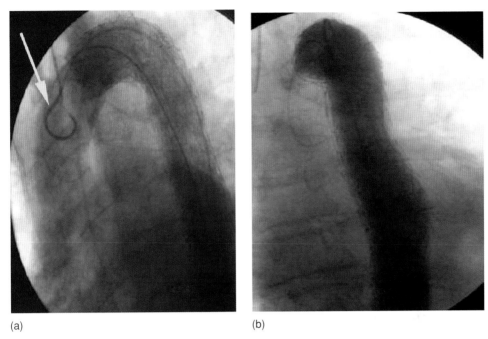

(a)                                          (b)

**Figure 4** (a and b) A completion angiogram demonstrates true lumen expansion with collapse of false lumen with flow seen through the debranched bifurcated graft to the supra-aortic vessels (arrow).

dissecting flap in the arch as well as the true lumen, which was compressed by an enlarged false lumen with the dissection progressing all the way to the aortic bifurcation. Care was taken to make sure we introduced our glide wires in both groins into the true lumen. Intravascular ultrasound was used to confirm that both wires were in the true lumen. A stiff 0.035-in. Lunderquist wire (Cook Inc., Bloomington, IN) was advanced to the arch and based on our measurements of the arch by aortogram, intravascular ultrasound and CT scan of the chest a 40-mm Gore TAG device (W.L. Gore & Associates, Flagstaff, AZ) was selected. Due to adequate iliac sizes the left 9-F common femoral sheath was then exchanged to a 24-F Gore sheath and a 40 mm × 20 cm Gore thoracic endograft was deployed via the left groin under fluoroscopic guidance to the arch excluding the entry point of the dissection in the arch at the level of the innominate artery that was debranched with coverage of the left subclavian artery. Completion angiogram did not demonstrate any endoleak with exclusion of the dissection flap in the arch and collapse of the false lumen (Figure 4a and 4b). The proximal stump of the 10-mm conduit was oversewn (Figure 5). Wires and sheaths

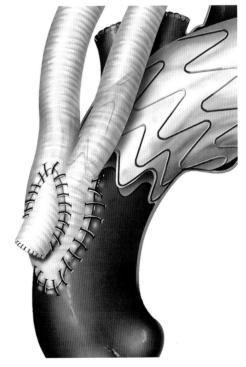

**Figure 5** An illustration of hybrid debranching of the arch vessels with deployment of endoluminal graft and oversewing of 10-mm conduit limb.

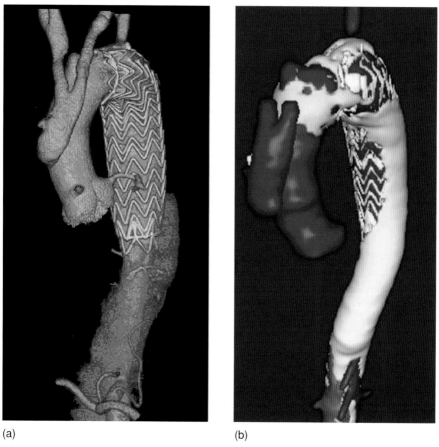

(a)                                    (b)

**Figure 6** (a and b) Reformatted images demonstrating a thoracic debranching for a retrograde type B dissection extending into the innominate artery with exclusion of the entry point with an endoluminal graft.

were taken out and the left common femoral artery was repaired and the groin closed. A closure device was used on the right groin. Postoperative CT scan (Figure 6a and 6b) demonstrates exclusion of entry point of dissection in arch with an endoluminal graft with debranched arch vessels and no endoleak. Patient continues to do well at 32-month follow-up with remodeling of the thoracic aorta and no demonstrated endoleak seen on 32-month follow-up axial images of the CT scan of the chest (Figure 7a and 7b).

## Discussion

The reported incidence of retrograde type B dissections with an entry tear in the descending aorta that has propagated up to the arch or to the ascending aorta varies from 10 to 27% [1]. Excision of the entry tear with replacement of both the ascending aorta and the arch is associated with a significant morbidity and mortality with reports of a 27% mortality rate according to the International Registry for Aortic Dissection (IRAD) [2]. The standard surgical approach of such patients involves the replacement of the ascending aorta; however, controversy does exist as to the management strategy when the predominant aortic lesion seems to be in the descending aorta. Von Segesser *et al.* [3] proposed that the replacement of the arch with a varying portion of ascending aorta via a median sternotomy be recommended in patients with enlarged aortic diameter, pericardial effusion, and/or aortic insufficiency while distal dissections with dilated descending thoracic aorta and or

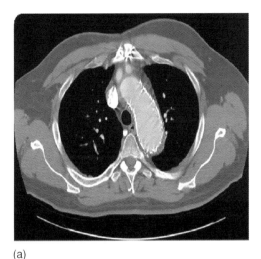 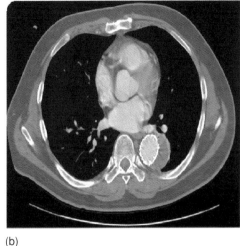

(a)  (b)

**Figure 7** (a and b) Axial CT scan images demonstrating thrombosis of false lumen with marked regression of the false lumen and remodeling of the thoracic aorta. The images are approximately 32 months apart.

distal complications best be approached via a lateral thoracotomy.

This type of hybrid approach [4–13] allows for endovascular treatment of complex arch pathology by excluding the entry point and providing a solution for the management of the supra-aortic vessels while avoiding the risk associated with the use of cardiopulmonary bypass and circulatory arrest, with ultimately a reduction in the morbidity, and mortality of the procedure. As demonstrated in the illustrations, once the arch vessels are debranched deployment of the thoracic endoluminal graft can be performed in an antegrade fashion through a 10-mm conduit sewn to the bifurcated graft for cases of small, tortuous, or calcified vessels or in a retrograde manner through the common femoral artery or through a retroperitoneal conduit. Proximal thrombosis of the false lumen by excluding the entry point of the dissection supports repositioning of the dissection lamella, progressive caudal thrombosis, and finally fibrosis of the false lumen, resulting in stent-induced aortic remodeling as demonstrated in our patient at 32 months.

In conclusion, hybrid surgical treatment of retrograde type B dissections is a promising option for those patients not suitable for conventional surgical repair. Long-term durability of this approach is uncertain and results of these less invasive procedures remain to be determined. Nevertheless, this approach may add as an alternative treatment adjunct especially in old and frail patients with multiple comorbidities and high surgical risk. Broader application of this technique will reveal its safety and efficacy, especially with regard to long-term outcome.

## References

1 Trimachi S, Nienaber CA, Rampoldi V *et al.* Role and results of surgery in acute type B aortic dissection: insights from the International Registry of Acute Aortic Dissection. *Circulation* 2006; **114**(Suppl 1): I357–I364.

2 Ehrlich MP, Schillinger M, Grabenwoger M *et al.* Predictors of adverse outcome and transient neurological dysfunction following surgical treatment of acute type A dissections. *Circulation* 2003; **108**(Suppl 1): II312–II317.

3 Von Segesser LK, Killer I, Ziswiler M *et al.* Dissection of the thoracic aorta extending into the ascending aorta: a therapeutic challenge. *J Thorac Cardiovasc Surg* 1994; **108**: 755–761.

4 Schumacher H, Böckler D, Bardenheuer H *et al.* Endovascular aortic arch reconstruction with supra-aortic transposition for symptomatic contained rupture and dissection: early experience in 8 high-risk patients. *J Endovasc Ther* 2003; **10**: 1066–1074.

5 Naganuma J, Ninomiya M, Miyairi T *et al.* Total aortic arch aneurysm repair using a stent graft without cardiac or cerebral ischemia. *Jpn J Thorac Cardiovasc Surg* 2002; **50**: 298–301.

6 Nathanson DR, Rodriguez-Lopez JA, Ramaiah VG *et al.* Endoluminal stent-graft stabilization for thoracic aortic dissection. *J Endovasc Ther* 2005; **12**: 354–359.

7 Carrel TP, Berdat PA, Baumgartner I *et al.* Combined surgical and endovascular approach to treat a complex aortic coarctation without extracorporeal circulation. *Ann Thorac Surg* 2004; **78**: 1462–1465.

8 Svensson LG. Progress in ascending and aortic arch surgery: minimally invasive surgery, blood conservation, and neurological deficit prevention. *Ann Thorac Surg* 2002; **74**: S1786–S1788.

9 Diethrich EB, Ghazoul M, Wheatley GH *et al.* Great vessel transposition for antegrade delivery of the TAG endoprosthesis in the proximal aortic arch. *J Endovasc Ther* 2005; **12**: 583–587.

10 Greenberg RK, Haddad F, Svensson L *et al.* Hybrid approaches to thoracic aortic aneurysms: the role of endovascular elephant trunk completion. *Circulation* 2005; **112**: 2619–2626.

11 Diethrich EB, Ghazoul M, Wheatley GH, III *et al.* Surgical correction of ascending type A thoracic aortic dissection: simultaneous endoluminal exclusion of the arch and distal aorta. *J Endovasc Ther* 2005; **12**: 660–666.

12 Zhou W, Reardon M, Peden EK, Lin PH, Lumsden AB. Hybrid approach to complex thoracic aortic aneurysms in high risk patients: surgical challenges and clinical outcomes. *J Vasc Surg* 2006; **44**(4): 688–693.

13 Criado FJ, Clark NS, Barnatan MF. Stent graft repair in the aortic arch and descending thoracic aorta: a 4-year experience. *J Vasc Surg* 2002; **36**: 1121–1128.

# Hybrid management of a chronic type B dissecting aneurysm with ascending aortic aneurysm

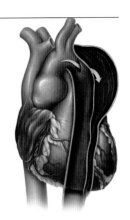

## Introduction

Management of the ascending aortic pathology requires open surgical replacement of the diseased aorta. Pathology extending into the arch requires hemireplacement or total replacement of the arch aorta which consists of hypothermic circulatory arrest and extracorporeal circulation. Dissection of the aortic arch is present in 30% of patients who develop a type A dissection [1, 2]. Twenty to thirty percent of patients with an arch dissection, irrespective of intimal flap resection, require some form of distal aortic operation [3]. Mortality associated with arch replacement in centers of excellence has been reported ranging from 15 to 35% [4]. Hybrid revascularization uses a technique of supra-aortic debranching of the head vessels on a partial clamp without the use of circulatory arrest and profound hypothermia. The hybrid approach provides a less invasive approach of managing arch pathologies like dissection or arch aneurysms.

## Case scenario

A 67-year-old female with a history of hypertension developed a Stanford type B dissection requiring a left to right femoral–femoral artery bypass for right lower extremity ischemia. Aggressive medical therapy was instituted with antihypertensive medication to manage the sequelae of the dissection. She had done well over the ensuing years until she developed new onset back pain and was found to have a dissecting thoracic aneurysm measuring 6.5 cm by CT scan (Figure 1a). Her physical examination was notable for hypertension and a patent left to right femoral–femoral artery bypass. A chest X-ray was performed with a widened mediastinum noted. Transesophageal echocardiogram demonstrated an ascending aortic aneurysm measuring 5.2 cm with moderate aortic insufficiency and a preserved left ventricular function. Closer examination of the CT scan indicated the presence of an aberrant right subclavian artery in a retropharyngeal position (Figure 1b and 1c). This, combined with both the ascending and descending aneurysm, required a catheterization to determine the location of the intimal flap and her candidacy for conventional endoluminal graft repair. Intravascular ultrasound performed during the catheterization demonstrated a thoracic aortic neck diameter of 44 mm. In addition, the intimal tear was identified in the proximal portion of the bovine arch and the right subclavian takeoff was distal to the one for the left subclavian artery (Figure 2). Due to the complexity of her aortic disease, she was felt to require both treatment of her ascending aorta and the descending thoracic aorta complete with dissection exclusion. Conventional surgery with the replacement of the ascending aorta, the arch aorta with elephant trunk technique, and the descending thoracic aortic is associated with high morbidity and mortality. A hybrid approach with the replacement of the ascending aorta combined with the debranching of the arch vessels and deployment of a thoracic endoluminal graft would allow

193

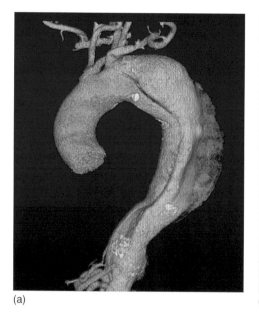

(a)

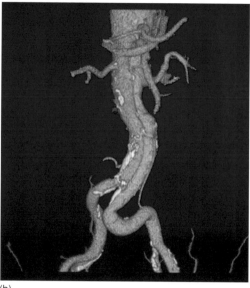

(b)

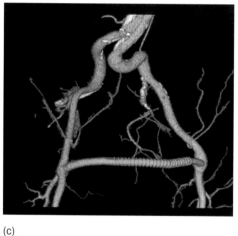

(c)

**Figure 1** (a–c) A 3-D model from a 64-slice CT scan shows the aberrant arch vessels and the extent of the dissection into the arch. The dissection continues to the iliac arteries with a patent femoral–femoral artery bypass graft.

for a one-stage treatment of such a complex aortic pathology.

## Hybrid debranching with deployment of endoluminal graft

A median sternotomy incision was created, the pericardium was opened with suspension, and dissection of the great vessels was undertaken. The patient was systemically heparinized. Cannulation of the arch, right atrium, and coronary sinus was done once the patient was placed on cardiopulmonary bypass. The aorta was cross clamped. Cardiac protection was achieved with antegrade and retrograde cardioplegia with prompt diastolic arrest of the heart and cooling of the heart. The ascending aorta was resected and a 34 mm × 30 mm Hemashield Dacron graft (Boston Scientific, Natick, MA) was then interposed without difficulty (Figure 3). The patient was weaned off cardiopulmonary bypass and arterial and venous decannulation was done after partial reversal of heparin. An 18-mm graft with a 10-mm side arm attachment was sewn in an end-to-side fashion with a partial clamp to the

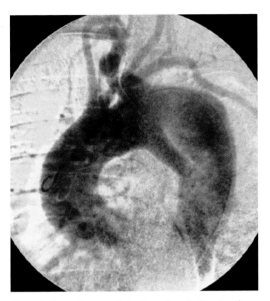

**Figure 2** An angiogram of the thoracic arch showing the great vessel takeoffs and the intimal flap.

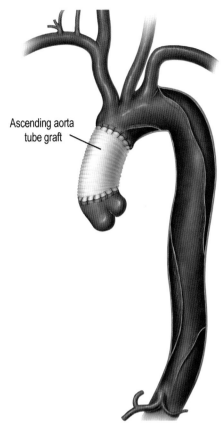

Ascending aorta
tube graft

**Figure 3** The replacement of 5.5-cm ascending aortic aneurysm with a 34-mm Hemashield graft (Boston Scientific, Natick, MA).

previously placed 34-mm interposition graft in the ascending aorta. Separate 10-mm grafts were then sewn to the common takeoff of the left carotid and innominate artery. After retrograde and antegrade flushing, the clamps were removed. An 8-mm graft was then taken off; the body of the 10-mm graft was then sewn end-to-end to the left subclavian artery. The left subclavian ostium was oversewn with 4-0 Prolene suture. The ostia of the left carotid and left innominate artery were also oversewn with 4-0 Prolene stitch. For antegrade delivery of an endoluminal graft, a 10-mm graft was sewn to the body of the 18-mm Hemashield graft. A radiopaque clip was positioned at the 18-mm inflow conduit for fluoroscopic identification of the inflow during endograft deployment. Using the 10-mm Hemashield graft that was sutured to the interposition graft, a 9-F (French) sheath was inserted. Through the 9-F sheath, under direct fluoroscopy, a 0.035-in. soft-tip angled glide wire was advanced through graft into the arch, as well as to the descending thoracic aorta. Open retrograde cannulation of the right limb of the femoral–femoral graft was performed with an 18-G needle and a 0.035-in. glide wire advanced into the true lumen. A snare was advanced and the antegrade-delivered 0.035-in. glide wire was snared and pulled through the right groin sheath. A 5-F

pigtail was advanced up the arch from the groin; the 9-F sheath through the 10-mm conduit was exchanged to a 24-F Gore sheath (Figure 4). Antegrade deployment of a 40 mm × 20 cm Gore TAG graft (W.L. Gore & Associates, Flagstaff, AZ) was deployed distally to exclude the dissecting aneurysm. Two additional TAG grafts measuring 40 × 20 and 40 × 10 were deployed cephalad to the first graft to exclude the arch dissection. Care was taken during the third graft deployment not to cover the inflow conduit which supplies blood to the supra-aortic vessels. The radiopaque band placed round the inflow graft served as a guide during fluoroscopic deployment of the endoluminal graft. Balloon angioplasty with a 40-mm Coda balloon (Cook Inc., Bloomington, IN) was performed for good apposition of the endograft to the aortic wall. A completion angiogram was performed and demonstrated

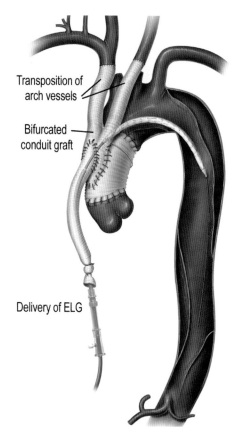

Transposition of arch vessels

Bifurcated conduit graft

Delivery of ELG

**Figure 4** An illustration of the inflow graft and the 10-mm conduit sutured to the tube graft used to reconstruct the ascending aorta with transposition of arch vessels and antegrade advancement of endoluminal graft for deployment.

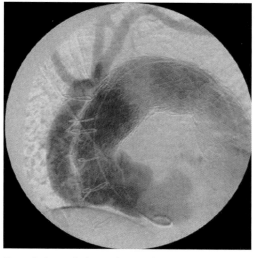

**Figure 5** A completion angiogram demonstrates patent-debranched arch vessels with satisfactory deployment of an endoluminal graft to exclude dissection flap with true lumen expansion.

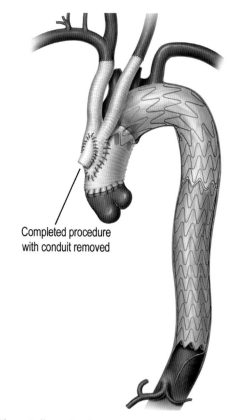

Completed procedure with conduit removed

**Figure 6** Illustration demonstrating retrograde deployment of endoluminal graft to exclude entry tears in the arch and reexpand of the compressed true lumen.

no endoleak with good visualization of supra-aortic vessels (Figure 5). The 9-F sheath was removed from the 10-mm conduit and the conduit was trimmed short and suture ligated to a short stump (Figure 6). Removal of sheaths and wires from groin was performed and the arteriotomy repaired and the groins closed. Hemostasis was achieved in the chest and after placement of drainage tubes. The sternum was rewired and the chest closed. A high-resolution 64-slice CT scan demonstrated obliteration of the false channel and no proximal endoleak. The ascending tube grafts to the brachiocephalic and left common carotid arteries were patent, as well as the endoluminal grafts in the descending thoracic artery (Figure 7a and 7b). In the distal abdominal aorta, the persistent dissection and a patent femoral–femoral bypass graft were documented.

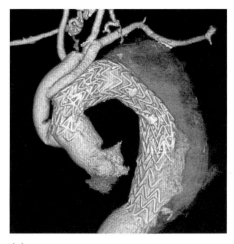

(a)

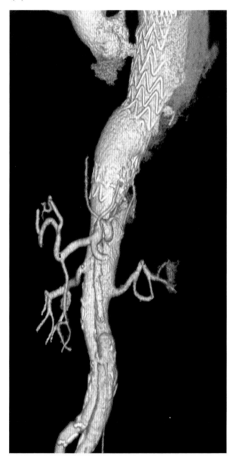

(b)

**Figure 7** (a and b) A discharge 64-slice CT scan examination showing exclusion of the dissection in the thoracic arch and the dissection continuing down to the abdominal aorta.

## Discussion

The management of a patient with both an ascending and a descending thoracic aneurysm as a result of the sequelae of a chronic type B dissection remains complex. Surgical replacement of the ascending aorta is performed for ascending aortic aneurysms diameter greater than 4.5–5.0 cm in the Marfan population [5] and 5.5–6.0 cm in the non-Marfan population. Similarly, prosthetic graft replacement of the aorta is carried out at aneurysm diameters of 6.0 cm. Twenty-five percent of aneurysm formation in the thoracic aorta and the thoracoabdominal aorta result from sequelae of a chronic type B dissection [6]. Predictors of aortic enlargement in the patient with a chronic type B dissection include the existence of a patent false lumen and a patent entry site in the thoracic aorta [7]. An initial aortic diameter greater than 40 mm is a predictor for aortic enlargement of greater than 60 mm and potential rupture [8]. The management of type B dissection within 6 months of acute event with an endoluminal graft may result in full or partial false lumen thrombosis in 85–100% of patients even in the setting of chronic and retrograde type A dissections preventing aneurysmal expansion [8].

Open surgical management of tears propagating into the arch of the aorta remains controversial. Resection of intimal tears may require partial or total arch replacement with elephant trunk technique if the entry tears propagate distally in the descending thoracic aorta. Complications associated with the open surgical approach include strokes, paraplegia, renal failure, visceral ischemia, and pulmonary failure. Money *et al.* reported a 21% respiratory failure following thoracic aortic repair with a mortality of 42% [9]. The morbidity and mortality for this type of surgery remains high even in centers of excellence despite improvement in surgical techniques. The hybrid operation provides a less invasive approach for management of the supra-aortic vessels. Debranching of the supra-aortic vessels is achieved without the need for extracorporeal circulation and hypothermic circulatory arrest. The hybrid operation can be applied to complex pathologies of the aorta with good outcomes.

In conclusion, the hybrid approach to the treatment of complex aortic pathologies provides a new treatment paradigm to provide patients with a less invasive therapeutic alternative that may concomitantly achieve gains in survival.

## References

1 Ergin MA, O'Connor J, Guinto R *et al*. Experience with profound hypothermia and circulatory arrest in the treatment of aneurysms of the aortic arch: aortic arch replacement for acute aortic arch dissections. *J Thorac Cardiovasc Surg* 1982; **84**: 649–655.

2 Nguyen B, Mueller M, Kipfer B *et al*. Different techniques of distal aortic repair in acute type A dissection: impact on late aortic morphology and reoperation. *Eur J Cardiothorac Surg* 1999; **15**: 496–500.

3 Schor JS, Yerlioglu ME, Galla JD *et al*. Selective management of acute type B dissection: long term follow-up. *Ann Thorac Surg* 1996; **61**: 1339–1341.

4 Kazui T, Washiyama N, Muhammad BA *et al*. Extended total arch replacement for acute type A aortic dissection: experience with 70 patients. *J Thorac Cardiovasc Surg* 2000; **119**: 558–565.

5 Finkbohner R, Johnston D, Crawford ES *et al*. Marfan syndrome. Long term survival and complications after aortic aneurysm repair. *Circulation* 1995; **91**: 728–733.

6 Safi HJ, Miller CC, Estrera AL *et al*. Chronic aortic dissection not a risk factor for neurologic deficit in thoracoabdominal aortic aneurysm repair. *Eur J Vasc Endovasc Surg* 2002; **23**: 244–250.

7 Akutsu K, Nejima J, Kiuchi K *et al*. Effect of the patient false lumen on the long term outcome of type B acute aortic dissections. *Eur J Cardiothorac Surg* 2004; **26**: 359–366.

8 Onitsuka S, Akashi H, Tayama K *et al*. Long term outcome and prognostic predictors of medically treated acute type B aortic dissections. *Ann Thorac Surg* 2004; **78**: 1268–1273.

9 Money SR, Rice K, Crokett D *et al*. Risk of respiratory failure after repair of thoracoabdominal aortic aneurysms. *Am J Surg* 1994; **168**: 152–155.

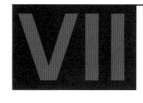

## SECTION VII
# Extending distal landing zones

# Hybrid repair of Extent II thoracoabdominal aneurysms

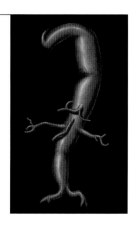

## Introduction

Crawford extent II thoracic aortic aneurysms involve all or most of the descending thoracic aorta and all or most of the abdominal aorta. Causes of thoracic aortic aneurysm can be attributed to various conditions including atherosclerotic medial degenerative disease (82%), type B dissections (17%) with various disorders representing the remainder [1]. Examples of these disorders are Marfan's syndrome, Ehlers-Danlos syndrome, and Takayasu's aortitis.

Due to the high risk of complications and mortality associated with open surgical repair, multiple centers of excellence are starting to offer a less invasive alternative. The hybrid approach combines components from both endovascular and open surgical approaches to create a procedure with a shorter clamp time. Short cross-clamp times have been correlated with diminished mortality and morbidity in the management of thracoabdominal aneurysms [2]. The hybrid approach in the management of extent II thoracoabdominal aneurysms avoids aortic cross clamping, thoracotomy, and is associated with limited ischemia time which constitutes the potential benefits of the hybrid approach.

## Case scenario

A 76-year-old female with a past medical history of hypertension, peripheral vascular disease, and a known thoracoabdominal aneurysm presented with severe back and chest pain to an outside facility. In the past, she had declined surgical management. A thorough cardiac work-up was performed to

exclude a myocardial infarction as a possible etiology from her symptoms. A repeat CT scan was done which measured the thoracoabdominal aneurysm at 9 cm but free of any aortic rupture (Figure 1a and 1b). Her symptoms combined with the large diameter of the aneurysm indicated that she was at high risk for aortic rupture. Options were again presented to the patient and she agreed to a hybrid approach which had elements of an open repair with the benefits of an endovascular procedure.

## Intravascular ultrasound (IVUS) and angiogram

The patient was taken to the operating room and the following measurements were collected using an IVUS probe. The proximal neck juxtadistal to the left subclavian artery measured at 32–34 mm with a length of 3 cm. The ostiums of the visceral and renal arteries were identified and documented. The distal landing zone at the distal infrarenal aorta was measured at 24 mm × 39 mm with a satisfactory neck length of 3 cm. There was no thrombus identified in either landing zones. The left common iliac artery was measured at 10.5 mm × 11 mm in diameter. Angiogram performed demonstrated the 9.0-cm thoracoabdominal aneurysm.

## Open surgical portion

A midline laparotomy incision was made. The retroperitoneum over the infrarenal abdominal aorta was incised. The infrarenal aorta was aneurysmal up to the bifurcation of the aorta sparing both

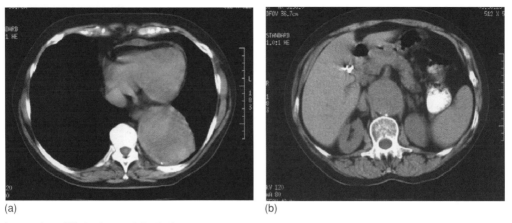

(a)                                                          (b)

**Figure 1** (a and b) The thoracoabdominal aneurysm as seen on a CT scan.

common iliac arteries. The right common iliac artery was moderately calcified and diseased compared to the left common iliac artery. The choice was made to use the left common iliac artery as the inflow source for the revascularization of the renal arteries, the superior mesenteric artery, and the celiac trunk. Mobilization of the visceral and the renal vessels were performed. Adequate heparinization was obtained as verified by activated clotting time. Using a trifurcated Dacron graft, we sewed the inflow to the left common iliac artery with a 4-0 Prolene suture after a partial cross clamp had been applied to the left common iliac artery. We then anastomosed a limb to the right and left renal arteries in an end-to-end fashion, making sure to ligate the ostium prior to removal of cross clamps (Figure 2a). The third limb was sewn in a side-to-side fashion in a lazy C format to the superior mesenteric artery and the end of the graft sewn to the celiac trunk in an end-to-end fashion after making sure the limb was passed retropancreatic (Figure 2b). The ostium of the celiac and superior mesenteric arteries was

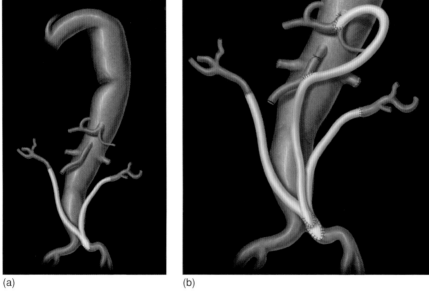

(a)                                                          (b)

**Figure 2** (a and b) An artist's illustration showing the various phases of the debranching process.

ligated. Completion angiogram showed all the four vessels were adequately revascularized (Figure 3). We placed a clip at the inflow to serve as a marker to prevent covering the inflow to aid in the future deployment of an endoluminal graft. We achieved hemostasis and closed the retroperitoneum over the trifurcated graft. The abdomen was closed with an intention to bring the patient back for the endovascular portion of the operation in a week's time.

## Endovascular portion

Open retrograde cannulation of the left common femoral artery was performed with an 18-G Cook needle and 0.035-in. soft-tip angled glide wire was passed in the aorta. This was exchanged to a 9-F (French) sheath after 5000 units of heparin were given.

Percutaneous access of the right common femoral artery was particularly difficult. A retrograde iliac angiogram was obtained and showed the presence of severe calcification with a tight stenosis in the colon iliac (Figure 4). Percutaneous balloon angioplasty of the stenosis was then performed using an OPTA Pro (Cordis) 6 mm × 4 cm balloon. Arch

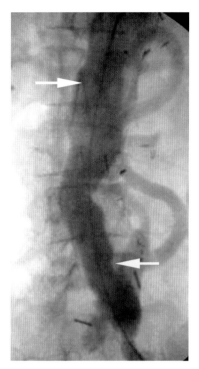

**Figure 3** A thoracoabdominal aortogram demonstrating the aneurysm (white arrow) with total visceral and renal artery debranching from the left common iliac artery inflow conduit (yellow arrow).

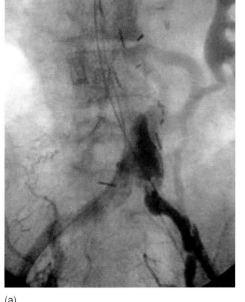

(a)

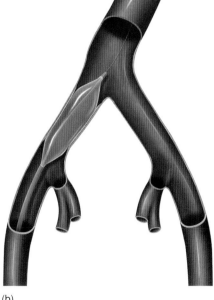

(b)

**Figure 4** (a) Retrograde iliac angiogram demonstrating a diseased right common iliac artery with a focal area of stenosis amenable to balloon angioplasty. (b) An artist's depiction of the procedure.

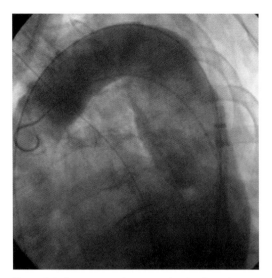

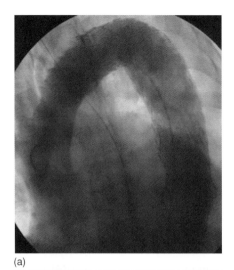

(a)

**Figure 5** Arch aortogram demonstrating the thoracic component of the thoracoabdominal aortic aneurysm.

aortogram was performed through the right sheath via a pigtail catheter to delineate the arch and the descending thoracoabdominal aneurysm (Figure 5). IVUS was performed using an 8.2-F probe to verify measurements obtained from the part of the procedure. These measurements indicated that a 40 mm × 20 cm Gore TAG graft would be needed to exclude the aneurysm.

The left 9-F sheath was exchanged for a 24-F sheath and the 40 mm × 20 cm Gore TAG device (W.L. Gore & Associates, Flagstaff, AZ) was advanced through the Gore sheath. It was subsequently deployed over an extra-stiff wire after verifying the exact position of the radiopaque marker, which marked the inflow conduit. A second and a third Gore TAG graft (40 mm × 20 cm and 40 mm × 15 cm) was subsequently deployed proximal to the first endograft to cover the rest of the aneurysm up to the level of the left subclavian artery. A Gore trilobe balloon was used to perform postdeployment balloon angioplasty to the proximal, the interdevice junctions, and the distal segments of the repair area to verify apposition to the aortic wall. A completion angiogram showed exclusion of the aneurysm with no endoleak and good visualization of all the bypassed visceral and renal vessels (Figure 6a and 6b). An Express 7 mm × 37 mm uncovered stent (Boston Scientific, Natick, MA) was deployed at the area of stenosis in right common

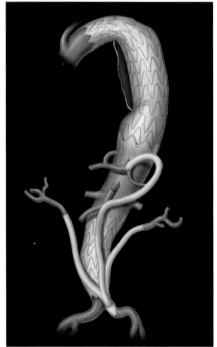

(b)

**Figure 6** (a and b) A completion angiogram with an illustration demonstrating the exclusion of the extent II thoracoabdominal aneurysm with no demonstrable endoleak.

iliac artery (Figure 7a and 7b). All wires and sheaths were removed; the left common femoral artery was closed in a transverse fashion with restoration of flow. An 8-F angioseal closure device was deployed to the right common femoral artery. The patient

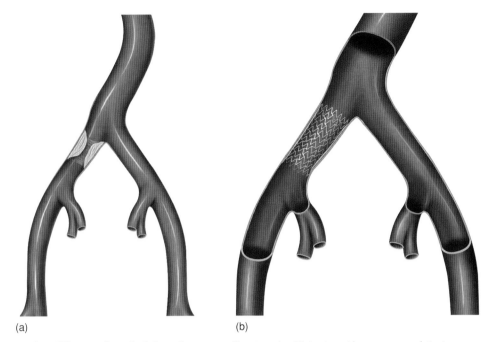

(a)                                          (b)

**Figure 7** (a and b) Pre- and postdepictions of a common iliac stenosis with treatment by an uncovered stent.

underwent a series of assessments prior to being extubated and transferred to the recovery room. A postoperative CT scan demonstrated patent bypass grafts with no endoleak and satisfactory exclusion of the extent II thoracoabdominal aneurysm (Figure 8a and 8b).

## Discussion

The 5-year survival for patients with nonoperated dissecting aneurysms was 7% compared to 19.2% for nondissecting aneurysms with rupture as the major cause of death [3]. Patients with atherosclerotic medial degenerative disease are more often older with multiple comorbidities including renal insufficiency and coronary artery disease, and have a higher incidence of adverse outcomes. Potential adverse outcomes include renal failure, paraplegia, myocardial infarction, and a higher mortality compared to those with dissecting aneurysms.

Pulmonary complications continue to remain the most common source of morbidity associated with thoracoabdominal aneurysm repair. The cause of respiratory failure is multifactorial and includes the extensive incision required, paralysis of the left hemidiaphragm during division of the diaphragm to access the aneurysm, high transfusion requirements, the high frequency of preoperative lung disease, and surgical trauma to the left lung. Svensson *et al.* [4] reported a 45% incidence of pulmonary complication in his series for the open surgical repair of Crawford extent II aneurysms. The perioperative mortality in this cohort was 9.7%; multivariate analysis showed that increasing age and preoperative renal, cardiac, and pulmonary diseases, as well as prolonged aortic cross-clamp time, were associated with an increased risk of mortality.

Paraplegia and paraparesis continues to remain a significant cause of morbidity after extent II thoracoabdominal aneurysm repair and often contribute to early mortality. Despite the use of several different adjuncts, paraplegia continues to occur from 7–32% in reported series from centers of excellence (Table 1) [5–13]. Recent advances—especially cerebrospinal fluid drainage and left heart bypass, hypothermia, and reattachment of intercostals arteries—have led to improved spinal cord protection and a reduction in the incidence of paraplegia.

Despite the use of various adjunctive techniques to protect the kidney, renal insufficiency continues to be a significant and lethal complication of type

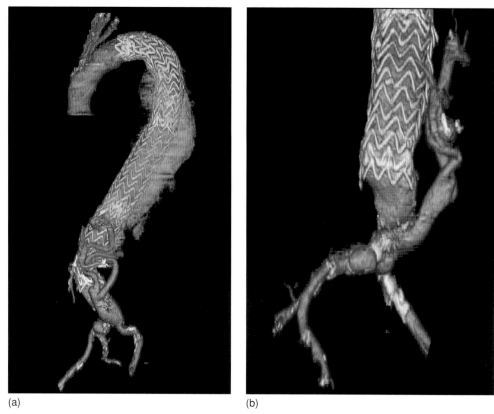

(a)                                                    (b)

**Figure 8**  (a and b) Postoperative CT scan demonstrating thrombosis of the aneurysm sac with debranched visceral and renal vessels with adequate placement of endoluminal grafts.

II thoracoabdominal aneurysm repair. Various adjunctive techniques currently employed to reduce renal failure include intraoperative administration

**Table 1** Paraplegia and paraparesis in contemporary series of extent II thoracoabdominal aortic aneurysm repairs.

| Author, year | Extent type II, n | Paraplegia/paraparesis, n (%) |
|---|---|---|
| Frank et al., 1994 [5] | 12 | 0 |
| Gilling-Smith et al., 1995 [6] | 19 | 6 (32%) |
| Kouchoukos et al., 1995 [7] | 13 | 0 |
| Bavaria et al., 1995 [8] | 18 | 4 (22%) |
| Mauney et al., 1996 [9] | 14 | 1 (7%) |
| Acher et al., 1998 [10] | 66 | 13 (20%) |
| Safi and Miller, 1999 [11] | 131 | 20 (15%) |
| Cambria et al., 2000 [12] | 30 | 4 (13%) |
| Cosseli et al., 2002 [13] | 439 | 33 (8%) |

of diuretics, minimization of ischemic times, renal hypothermia, and renal artery perfusion with oxygenated blood. However, despite the use of adjuvant techniques, the incidence of kidney failure after extent type II thoracoabdominal aneurysm repair still ranges from 16 to 26% (Table 2) [8, 9, 14–16].

Hybrid debranching provides a less invasive approach with a potentially less risk of paraplegia due to the avoidance of cross clamping, less risk of pulmonary failure due to avoidance of a painful thoracotomy incision, the lack of division of the diaphragm, and a lesser risk of renal failure due to decreased renal ischemic time associated with the renal debranching techniques. Long-term data, however, is lacking at this time to recommend this technique as the standard of care. The development of fenestrated and branched endograft [17, 18] will further reduce the invasiveness of treating patients

**Table 2** Postoperative renal failure in contemporary series of extent type II thoracoabdominal aortic aneurysm repair.

| Author, year | Extent type II, n | Renal failure, n (%) | Definition of renal failure |
|---|---|---|---|
| Bavaria et al., 1995 [8] | 18 | 4 (22%) | ↑Cr to 2 mg/dL above preoperative value or postoperative HD |
| Mauney et al., 1996 [9] | 14 | 3 (21%) | Postoperative HD |
| Safi et al., 1996 [14] | 99 | 26 (26%) | ↑Cr to 1 mg/dL above preoperative value for 2 consecutive days or postoperative HD |
| Schepens et al., 1995 [15] | 23 | 4 (17%) | Postoperative HD |
| Grabitz et al., 1996 [16] | 81 | 13 (16%) | Postoperative HD |

Cr, serum creatinine level; HD, hemodialysis; excludes 8 patients receiving preoperative hemodialysis.

with thoracoabdominal aneurysms in the near future.

# References

1 Panneton JM, Hollier LH. Non-dissecting thoracoabdominal aortic aneurysms: Part 1. *Ann Vasc Surg* 1995; **9**: 503–514.

2 Sarac TP, Clair DG, Hertzer NR *et al.* Contemporary results of juxta renal aneurysm repair. *J Vasc Surg* 2002; **36**: 1104–1111.

3 Bikerstaff LK, Paireloro PC, Hollier LH *et al.* Thoracic aortic aneurysms: a population based study. *Surgery* 1982; **92**: 1103–1108.

4 Svensson LG, Crawford ES, Hess KR *et al.* Experience with 1509 patients undergoing thoracoabdominal aortic operations. *J Vasc Surg* 1993; **17**: 357–370.

5 Frank SM, Parker SD, Rock P *et al.* Moderate hypothermia, with partial bypass and segmental sequential repair for thoracoabdominal aortic aneurysm. *J Vasc Surg* 1994; **19**: 687–697.

6 Gilling-Smith GL, Worswick L, Knight PF, Wolfe JHN, Mansfield AO. Surgical repair of thoracoabdominal aortic aneurysm: 10 years' experience. *Br J Surg* 1995; **82**: 624–629.

7 Kouchoukos NT, Daily BB, Rokkas CK, Murphy SF, Bauer S, Abboud N. Hypothermic bypass and circulatory arrest for operations on the descending thoracic and thoracoabdominal aorta. *Ann Thorac Surg* 1995; **60**: 67–77.

8 Bavaria JE, Woo YJ, Hall RA, Carpenter JP, Gardner TJ. Retrograde cerebral and distal aortic perfusion during ascending and thoracoabdominal aortic operations. *Ann Thorac Surg* 1995; **60**: 345–353.

9 Mauney MC, Tribble CG, Cope JT, Luctong A, Spotnitz WD, Kron IL. Is clamp and sew still viable for thoracic aortic resection? *Ann Surg* 1996; **223**: 534–543.

10 Acher CW, Wynn MM, Hoch JR, Kranner PW. Cardiac function is a risk factor for paralysis in thoracoabdominal aortic replacement. *J Vasc Surg* 1998; **27**: 821–830.

11 Safi HJ, Miller CC, III. Spinal cord protection in descending thoracic and thoracoabdominal aortic repair. *Ann Thorac Surg* 1999; **67**: 1937–1939.

12 Cambria RP, Davison JK, Carter C *et al.* Epidural cooling for spinal cord protection during thoracoabdominal aneurysm repair: a five year experience. *J Vasc Surg* 2000; **31**: 1093–1102.

13 Joseph SC, Scott AL, Lori DC, Cüneyt K, Zachary CS. Morbidity and mortality after extent II thoracoabdominal aortic aneurysm repair. *Ann Thorac Surg* 2002; **73**: 1107–1116.

14 Safi HJ, Harlin SA, Miller CC *et al.* Predictive factors for acute renal failure in thoracic and thoracoabdominal aortic aneurysm surgery. *J Vasc Surg* 1996; **24**: 338–345.

15 Schepens MA, Defauw JJ, Hamerlijnck RP, Vermeulen FE. Use of left heart bypass in the surgical repair of thoracoabdominal aortic aneurysms. *Ann Vasc Surg* 1995; **9**: 327–338.

16 Grabitz K, Sandmann W, Stuhmeier K *et al.* The risk of ischemic spinal cord injury in patients undergoing graft replacement for thoracoabdominal aneurysms. *J Vasc Surg* 1996; **23**: 230–240.

17 Anderson JL, Adam DJ, Berce M, Harley DE. Repair of thoracoabdominal aneurysms with fenestrated and ranched endovascular stent grafts. *J Vasc Surg* 2005; **42**: 600–607.

18 Stanley BM, Semmens JB, Lawrence-Brown MMD, Goodman MA, Hartley DE. Fenestration in endovascular grafts for aortic aneurysm repair (new horizons for preserving blood flow in branch vessels). *J Endovasc Ther* 2001; **8**: 16–24.

# Hybrid repair of an extent V thoracoabdominal aneurysm

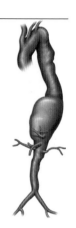

## Introduction

Extent V thoracoabdominal aneurysms involve the distal half of the descending thoracic aorta with varying segments of the abdominal aorta. Open surgical repair is associated with an increased morbidity and mortality from pulmonary, renal, cardiac, and neurology causes. Endovascular techniques have been used successfully to treat a variety of lesions in the thoracic aorta, including aneurysms, dissecting aneurysms, penetrating ulcers, aortobronchial fistulas, acute transections, and complications of previous aortic repair [1, 2]. Results of endoluminal grafting have been favorable, with reduced blood loss, fewer spinal cord complications, shorter operating times and hospital stays, and less convalescence after surgery.

Despite the advantages of endovascular interventions, the complexity of certain thoracic aortic pathologies frequently demands that techniques be modified to include more than one type of approach. Hybrid procedures that combine both open and endovascular procedures are often necessary to correct complex aortic pathologies [3, 4]. The hybrid approach to repair an extent V thoracoabdominal aneurysm with antegrade deployment of the endoluminal graft through a side limb of the bifurcated inflow conduit permits the deployment of an endoluminal graft in patients with tortuous, calcified, and small iliac arteries while at the same time avoiding a thoracotomy, left heart bypass, hypothermia, and aortic cross clamping.

## Case scenario

A 71-year-old female with complaints of back pain was found to have a type III thoracoabdominal aneurysm measuring 5.3 cm × 6.1 cm extending from the descending thoracic aorta up to the level of the renal arteries. A routine CT scan of the chest and abdomen was done to evaluate the anatomy for repair (Figure 1a, 1b and 1c). Due to her significant coronary artery disease and chronic obstructive lung disease, she was not considered a suitable candidate for a conventional repair. A hybrid approach consisting of total abdominal debranching with exclusion of the aneurysm using an endoluminal graft was chosen as a better option.

## Surgical techniques

A midline laparotomy incision was performed. The renal, celiac, and superior mesenteric arteries were exposed in a standard manner. Retrograde access of the right common femoral artery was performed and a 9-F (French) right groin sheath was inserted. An angiogram was performed to demonstrate a thoracocabdominal aneurysm (Figure 2). Using an intravascular probe, measurements were taken at both proposed landing zones (Figure 3). The total length to be covered was determined by placing the intravascular ultrasound (IVUS) probe at the proximal landing zone and pulling it back until it had reached the distal landing zone. The amount of wire that was pulled back was then measured

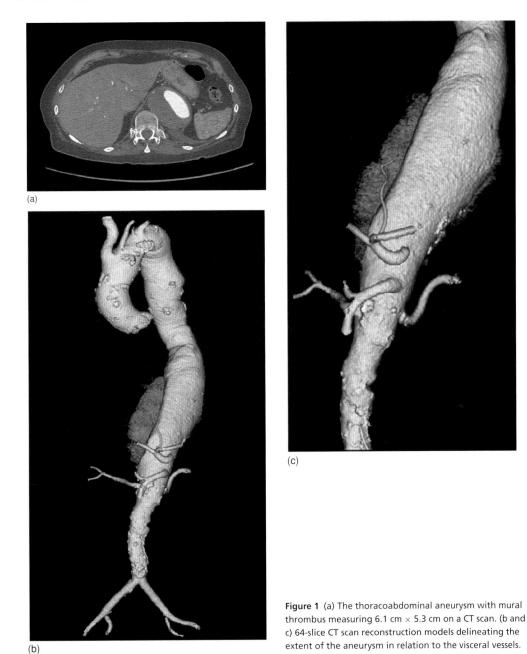

**Figure 1** (a) The thoracoabdominal aneurysm with mural thrombus measuring 6.1 cm × 5.3 cm on a CT scan. (b and c) 64-slice CT scan reconstruction models delineating the extent of the aneurysm in relation to the visceral vessels.

using a ruler. The IVUS probe was then removed and 5000 units of heparin were given. Once the activated clotting time was above 200 seconds, a partial clamp was placed on the distal aorta. A 6-mm Dacron Hemashield (Boston Scientific, Natick, MA) limb was sewn to a bifurcated 12-mm Hemashield Dacron graft as an end-to-side anastomosis (Figure 4a). The 12-mm bifurcated Dacron Hemashield graft was anastomosed to the distal abdominal aorta with a 4-0 Prolene suture to serve as the inflow blood source. The side limb of the bifurcated graft would be used for antegrade delivery of

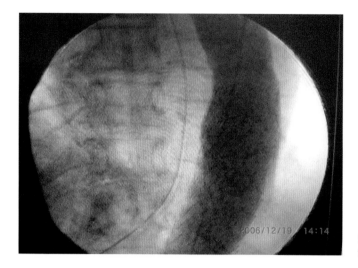

**Figure 2** An angiogram demonstrating the thoracoabdominal aneurysm.

the endoluminal graft. The attached 6-mm Dacron limb was then sewn as an end-to-end anastomosis to the celiac artery after ligating the ostium (Figure 4b). Subsequently, two 6-mm and an 8-mm Dacron graft were anastomosed as end-to-side anastomosis to the 12-mm inflow limb. An end-to-end anastomosis to the celiac artery, right renal artery (6-mm graft), and the left renal artery (8-mm graft) was performed after ligating each of these vessels at their ostium (Figure 4c and 4d). A radiopaque marker was then placed around the inflow portion of the 12-mm Hemashield graft to aid in the deployment of the thoracic endoluminal graft under fluoroscopic guidance. Due to the small, heavily diseased iliac arteries, the end of the 12-mm inflow graft was to be used as a conduit to advance the

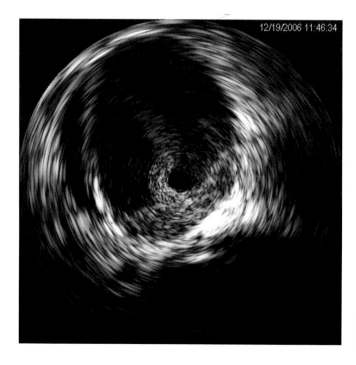

**Figure 3** An intravascular picture that shows the mural thrombus with the thoracoabdominal aneurysm.

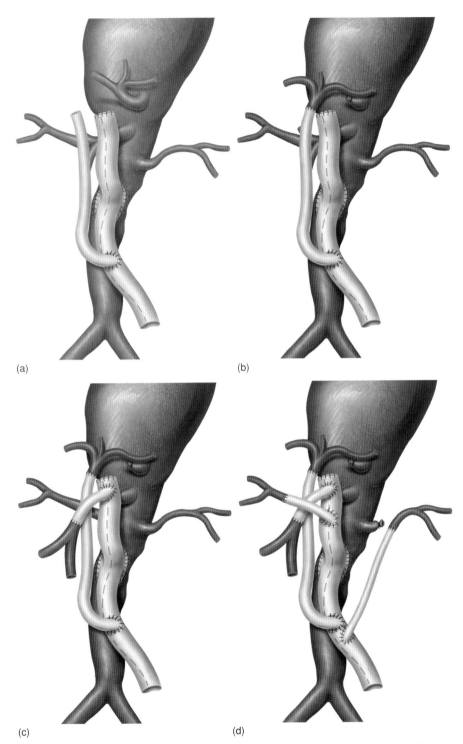

(a)

(b)

(c)

(d)

**Figure 4**  (a and b) A 12-mm bifurcated Dacron Hemashield graft anastomosed to the distal abdominal aorta with a side 6-mm limb anastomosed to celiac trunk. (c and d) Two 6-mm and an 8-mm Dacron grafts were anastomosed as end-to-side anastomosis to the 12-mm inflow limb and as end-to-end anastomosis to the superior mesenteric artery, right renal arteries (6-mm graft), and the left renal artery (8-mm graft) sequentially as end-to-end anastomosis.

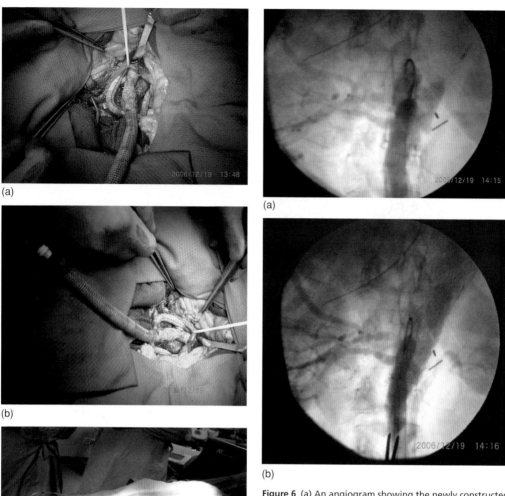

(a)

(b)

(c)

**Figure 5** (a) An operative view of debranched visceral and renal vessels with 12-mm limb to be used to deploy endoluminal graft. (b) The 9-F sheath inserted into the 12-mm conduit. (c) The 24-F Gore sheath inserted in the 12-mm conduit limb for delivery of endoluminal graft.

(a)

(b)

**Figure 6** (a) An angiogram showing the newly constructed visceral and renal bypasses. (b) A postdeployment angiogram showing exclusion of the aneurysm with no evidence of endoleak.

graft through the groin (Figure 5a). A 9-F sheath was secured to the side limb of the 12-mm bifurcated graft conduit (Figure 5b) and a 260-cm extra-stiff guide wire is passed through the conduit into the thoracic aorta. Contrast dye was injected to visualize all the bypass grafts as well as to mark the intended landing zone for the graft (Figure 6a). The conduit was clamped, and the TAG device's delivery sheath was substituted for the 9-F sheath (Figure 5c). A marker placed on the conduit assured that the stent graft was deployed just beyond the limb origins of the 12-mm Hemashield inflow graft. A Gore TAG (W.L. Gore & Associates, Flagstaff, AZ) endograft was positioned just proximal to the marker as the sheath was withdrawn from the conduit. The endograft was deployed successfully to exclude the aneurysm and completion angiography demonstrated adequate deployment of endoluminal graft.

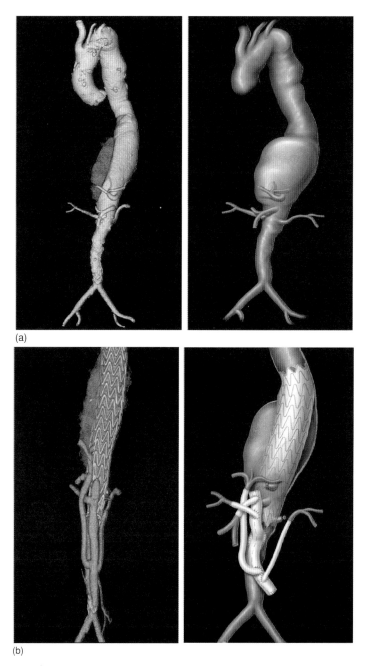

**Figure 7** (a) Illustrations of the thoracoabdominal aneurysm pre- and posthybrid repair. (b) A 3-D model from a 64-slice CT scan with an artist's depiction next to it.

Visualization of the visceral and renal debranched vessels was confirmed with no endoleak noted. The delivery sheath was removed, and the conduit transected and oversewn (Figure 6b). Upon reversing the Heparin, the abdominal incision was repaired.

The hospital stay after the operation was uneventful with a CT scan done prior to discharge. The CT scan verified the postprocedure angiogram showing no endoleak and intact flow to the viscera (Figure 7a and 7b).

## Discussion

The presence of significant calcification in iliac vessels that may be small in caliber or tortuous in nature can prove to be hazardous in advancing the sheaths necessary for endoluminal graft deployment. The use of temporary or permanent conduits to deliver the prosthesis can overcome these obstacles in the majority of patients. Direct deployment of an endoluminal graft through a side arm of an inflow conduit can technically avoid the numerous problems with access sometimes encountered during a retrograde femoral approach. The inflow conduit is marked with a radiopaque marker to prevent deploying the endoluminal graft across the arterial intake. Should the intake be occluded, both abdominal viscera and the kidneys would become ischemic and threaten the patient's life. Abdominal debranching of the viscerals and renal arteries is a formidable operation; however, this hybrid technique provides a unique opportunity for high-risk patients with thoracoabdominal aneurysms who would have no other option. The avoidance of a thoracotomy incision, possible left heart bypass, and aortic cross clamping may contribute to the decreased morbidity and mortality of the patient. We have performed this operation on 14 patients with Crawford type I ($n = 6$), type IV ($n = 6$), and type III ($n = 2$) thoracoabdominal aneurysm with a survival rate of 93%. There were no paraplegic events with 2 patients suffering from worsening renal failure, 2 patients with limb ischemia, and 1 patient with visceral ischemia who died within 30 days due to complications from the procedure.

This technique can be applied to the treatment of arch aneurysms with translocation of the great vessels and the delivery of the endoluminal graft by antegrade or retrograde delivery [5].

In conclusion, total visceral and renal debranching with the deployment of an endoluminal graft avoids the morbidity associated with cross clamping of the aorta, left heart bypass, and thoracotomy. Antegrade deployment of endoluminal graft via a side arm of a bifurcated graft is a novel technique to deploy an endoluminal graft in cases when the iliac arteries are not amenable to large-bore sheath advancement.

## References

1 Makaroun MS, Dillavou ED, Kee ST *et al.* Endovascular treatment of thoracic aortic aneurysms: results of the phase II multicenter trial of the GORE TAG thoracic prosthesis. *J Vasc Surg* 2005; **41**: 1–9.

2 Wheatley GH, Gurbuz AT, Rodriguez-Lopez JA *et al.* Midterm outcome in 158 consecutive Gore TAG thoracic endoprostheses: a single-center experience. *Ann Thorac Surg* 2006; **81**(5): 1570–1577.

3 Fulton JJ, Farber MA, Martson WA *et al.* Endovascular stent-graft repair of pararenal and type IV thoracoabdominal aneurysms with visceral reconstruction. *J Vasc Surg* 2005; **41**: 191–198.

4 Chiesa R, Melissano G, Civilini E *et al.* Two stage combined endovascular and surgical approach for recurrent thoracoabdominal aorticaneurysm. *J Endovasc Ther* 2004; **11**: 330–333.

5 Bergeron P, Coulon P, De Chaumaray T *et al.* Great vessels transposition and aortic arch exclusion. *J Cardiovasc Surg (Torino)* 2005; **46**: 141–147.

# Hybrid (combined open and endovascular) repair of thoracoabdominal aneurysms

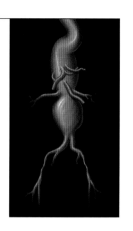

## Classification of thoracoabdominal aneurysm (TAAA)

Extent I TAAAs involve most of the descending thoracic aorta from the left subclavian artery down to vessels in the abdomen. Usually the renal arteries are not involved in extent I aneurysms. Extent II aneurysms begin at the left subclavian artery and reach the infrarenal abdominal aorta even as far as the inguinal area. Extent III aneurysms involve the distal half or less of the descending thoracic aorta and substantial segments of the abdominal aorta. Extent IV aneurysms are those that involve the upper abdominal aorta and all or none of the infrarenal aorta. Extent V aneurysms involve the distal half of the descending thoracic aorta and the abdominal aorta up to the level of the renal arteries.

## Introduction

Atherosclerotic medial degenerative disease (82%) and aortic dissection (17%) account for nearly all reported cases of TAAA [1]. The morbidity of TAAA repair remains significant with major complications, including spinal cord ischemia, as high as 15%, significant pulmonary problems in up to 40% of patients, and renal impairment in up to 30% [2–5]. Despite these daunting risks in patients with significant comorbidity, surgery remains an option because the mortality rate of conservative treatment at 2 years may be 76%; half of these deaths are due to aneurysm rupture [6]. There is a 30% 5-year risk of rupture when a thoracic aortic aneurysm (TAA) is greater than 6 cm, and thus the general recommendation of 6 cm as an appropriate size for repair seems warranted in acceptable-risk patients [7]. Pain and

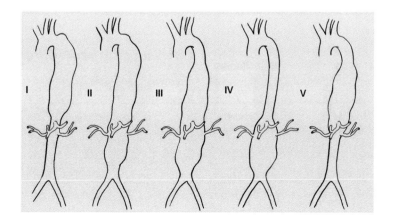

chronic obstructive disease have been found to be higher indicators for rupture. Open surgical repair of thoracoadominal aneurysms is associated with a 30-day mortality of 20 and 28% in an octogenarian population. An increase of 32 and 44% in octogenarian mortality at 1 year is mostly due to cardiovascular-related complications [8]. The application of stent-graft repair to the more complex TAAAs has been limited by the origin of the visceral vessels off the aneurysm itself. Randomization to open surgical repair of TAA was compared to endovascular stent graft in the recently presented phase II study [9]. Ninety-four patients who underwent TAA repair were compared to a similar cohort of 140 patients who underwent endovascular stent-graft repair [10]. The surgical technique for thoracic aortic replacement included extracorporeal support in 78% patients with spinal drainage not routinely used [11]. There was no significant difference in the mean age, aortic morphology, and past medical history between the endovascular and open TAA groups. The 30-day mortality was 11.7% in the open TAA "controls" versus 2.1% in the endovascular group. Paraplegia/paraparesis was encountered in 13.8% of the open TAA patients versus 3% of those undergoing endovascular repairs. Renal failure was noted in 12% and respiratory failure, defined as more than 24 hours mechanical ventilation or reintubation, in 20% of open TAA patients versus 1 and 4% in the endovascular group. This series represents perhaps the best assessment available of comparative real-world results of open TAA versus stent-graft repair in the nation.

Hybrid revascularization incorporates both open surgical repair and endovascular stent grafts to manage TAAA. It has recently provided a less invasive approach to the repair of TAAA [12–17] (H. Schumacher and J. Allenberg, personal communication). The hybrid procedure presents an attractive alternative to open repair because it avoids a thoracotomy and cross clamping of the aorta in the supraceliac region. This is accomplished by having a bypass sewn into the abdominal aorta provide vascularization through retrograde flow into the viscera. With vascularization protected, there is sufficient area for an endoluminal graft to be placed to exclude the thoracoabdominal aneurysm. In the hybrid repair, the placement of individual bypasses to the visceral branches and/or renal vessels are performed with ligation of the vessels at their origin to prevent type II endoleaks. Endoluminal grafts are deployed to exclude the thoracovisceral/thoracoviscerorenal aorta in either the same procedure or as part of a staged procedure that can occur days after the bypass part of the procedure. The endograft is inserted to cover the aneurysmal thoracovisceral aorta through a small incision in the groin. In endovascular exclusion, proper fixation zones and substantial overlap of endoprostheses are mandatory to withstand the substantial hemodynamic forces present. Clearly, long-term data regarding this very creative approach to extensive TAAAs are lacking, yet the complication rates particularly paraplegia, and paraparesis compare favorably with series detailing open TAAA repair [18–23].

## Case scenario

A 66-year-old female with a history of chronic obstructive pulmonary disease, osteoporosis, chronic back pain, and an active smoker presented with worsening back pain radiating to the flanks. A CT scan demonstrated a thoracoadominal aneurysm with the thoracic component measuring 8.0 cm with the abdominal component measuring at 6.8 cm at the infrarenal level (Figure 1a and 1b). There was a normal segment of aorta at the level of the renal arteries. She was managed using a hybrid approach which comprised an open surgical repair of the infrarenal abdominal aortic aneurysm combined with visceral and renal debranching followed by the deployment of an endoluminal graft to exclude the thoracic component of the aneurysm.

## Open surgical procedure

A midline laparotomy incision was performed. The retroperitoneum over the abdominal aorta was incised to reveal the large infrarenal component of a thoracoabdominal aneurysm (Figure 2a and 2b). There was heavy calcification of the bilateral common iliac arteries with the external iliac arteries too small to serve as an inflow conduit. The aorta at the level of the renal arteries was less aneurysmal

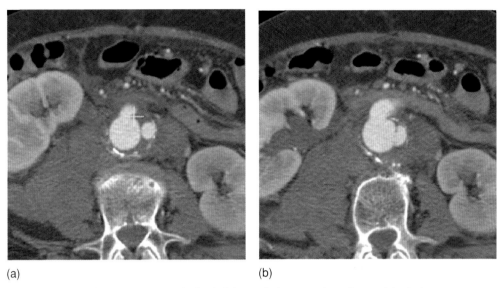

(a)                                         (b)

**Figure 1** (a and b) Axial CT scans images at the level of the renals demonstrating a thoracoabdominal aneurysm.

and was suitable for a proximal cross clamp. Mobilization of the renal arteries, superior mesenteric artery, and celiac artery was performed. Heparin was given to achieve an activated clotting time of over 200 seconds. A cross clamp was applied to the infrarenal aorta and the infrarenal portion of the thoracoabdominal aneurysm with replacement using a 22-mm Hemashield Dacron graft (Boston Scientific, Natick, MA) using 4-0 Prolene suture (Figure 3a and 3b). A partial cross clamp was applied to the distal abdominal aorta and a 14 mm × 7 mm bifurcated Hemashield graft was then sewn to the distal abdominal aorta to serve as an inflow conduit for the revascularization of both renal arteries and the visceral arteries. The 7-mm limbs of the bifurcated grafts were sewn end-to-end to both the right and left renal arteries using a 5-0 Prolene suture after cross clamping (Figure 4a and 4b). Ligation of the ostiums was then carried out prior to restoring blood flow. A side-biting clamp was applied to the left renal graft and the superior mesenteric artery with a side-to-side anastomosis constructed using a 5-0 Prolene suture. Ligation of the ostium of the superior mesenteric artery was then performed. A 7-mm graft was then anastomosed to the bifurcated graft and passed retropancreatic and anastomosed to the celiac trunk after a cross clamp had been applied (Figure 5a and 5b). Ligation of the celiac

trunk was performed prior to restoring flow. Due to the small calcified iliac arteries, a 10-mm graft was then sewn to the distal aorta with a 5-0 Prolene using partial cross clamp to serve as a left 10-mm aortofemoral conduit for delivery of the endoluminal graft. The conduit was then tunneled in a retroperitoneal fashion and then anastomosed to the left common femoral artery in an end-to-side fashion using 5-0 Prolene suture after proximal and distal cross clamps were applied (Figure 6). Usual flushing maneuvers were performed and the cross clamps were released. The inflow was marked with a clip to serve as a guide during the deployment of the endoluminal graft from the 10-mm conduit. The retroperitoneum was closed over the abdominal graft and bypass grafts and the laparotomy incision was closed.

Percutaneous access of the left 10-mm conduit was then performed with an 18-G needle and exchanged for a (9-French) sheath. An angled glide wire was then advanced in the aorta and exchanged to a 5-F pigtail. An aortogram demonstrated a type IV tortuous aorta with three curvatures of more than 60° angulation (Figure 7). The visceral branches and the renal arteries were well visualized with the inflow source from the distal aorta. An intravascular ultrasound (IVUS) probe was introduced and measurements were taken. The

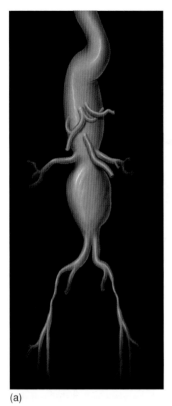

(a)

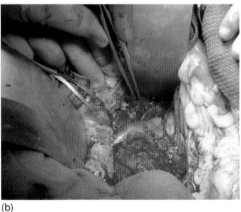

(b)

**Figure 2** (a and b) Comparative views of a thoracoabdominal aneurysm.

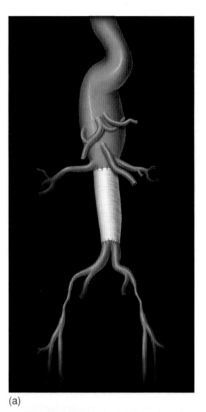

(a)

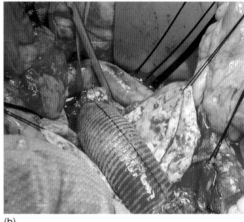

(b)

**Figure 3** (a and b) The replacement of the infrarenal aorta accomplished with a Dacron graft.

intended proximal landing zone measured 32–34 mm in width with a target length for full coverage measured at approximately 25 cm. A decision was made to end the procedure, and with the arteriotomy repaired, the patient was to be brought back to the operating room within the span of a week for the endoluminal graft.

## Endovascular procedure

Ten days after the visceral and renal debranching of an extent II thoracoabdominal aneurysm, the patient was brought back to the operating room and arterial access was obtained. A thoracoabdominal aortogram was performed to demonstrate the

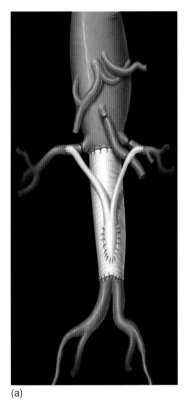

(a)

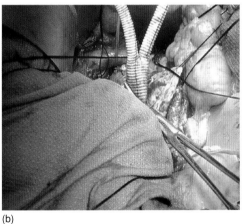

(b)

**Figure 4** (a and b) A bifurcated 14 mm × 7 mm Hemashield graft was sewn to the distal abdominal aorta with 7-mm limbs sewn to both renal arteries.

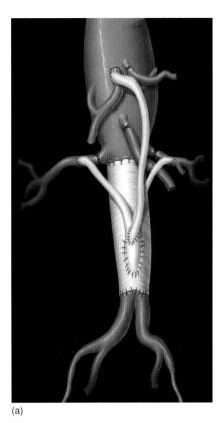

(a)

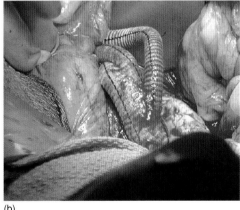

(b)

**Figure 5** (a and b) A 7-mm Dacron limb was anastomosed to celiac trunk and a sequential side-to-side anastomosis from renal limb to superior mesenteric artery was created.

thoracoabdominal aneurysm as well as continued patency of the visceral and renal bypass grafts. The IVUS probe was introduced again to identify the target landing area. An extra-stiff wire (Lunderquist) was advanced upon proper heparinization of the patient. The left 9-F sheath was exchanged for a

24-F Gore sheath. A 28 mm × 15 cm Gore TAG graft (W.L. Gore & Associates, Flagstaff, AZ) was deployed within the 24-mm Dacron graft. Proper position was ensured by placing the graft above the radiopaque clip that marked the inflow conduit

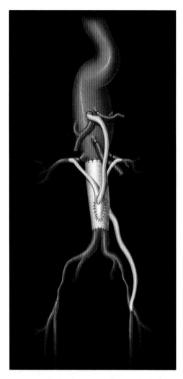

**Figure 6** A 10-mm Dacron limb conduit is sewn from distal abdominal graft to left common femoral artery for future delivery of endoluminal graft due to the condition of the iliac vessels.

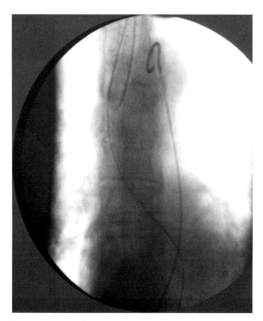

**Figure 7** An angiogram performed prior to the deployment of an endoluminal graft.

placed during the previous procedure. We then deployed a second endoluminal 37 mm × 20 cm Gore TAG graft into the smaller graft building proximally to exclude the thoracoabdominal aneurysm (Figure 7). Adequate overlap was ensured to prevent a type III endoleak. Postdeployment balloon angioplasty was conducted with a 40-mm Coda balloon (Cook Inc., Bloomington, IN). The proximal portion of the endoluminal graft, the interdevice junction, and the abdominal graft were profiled with the balloon. A completion angiogram did not demonstrate any endoleak with satisfactory exclusion of thoracoabdominal aneurysm and brisk flow to both the renal and visceral arteries. Wires and sheaths were removed, the arteriotomy in the conduit repaired, and the left groin incision closed. Manual pressure was applied after removal of right groin 5-F sheath to secure hemostasis. Figure 8 demonstrates an

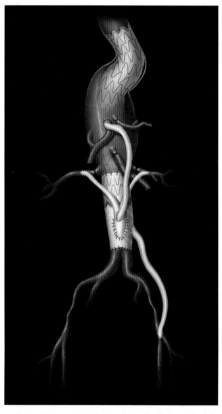

**Figure 8** An illustration of the abdominal visceral and renal arteries rerouting with deployment of thoracic endoluminal grafts for treatment of a thoracoabdominal aneurysm.

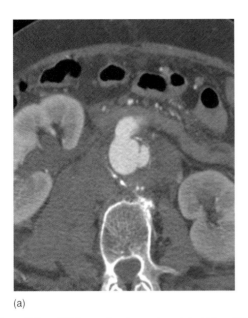 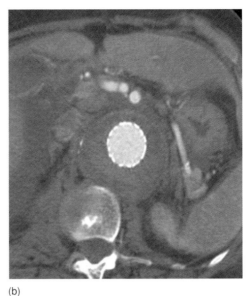

(a)                                          (b)

**Figure 9** (a and b) Pre- and postprocedure pictures showing exclusion of the aneurysm.

illustration of the abdominal visceral and renal arteries rerouting with deployment of thoracic endoluminal grafts for treatment of a TAAA. Pre- and postoperative CT scans performed on postoperative day 1 are illustrated in (Figure 9a and 9b). There was no endoleak with exclusion of the thoracoadominal aneurysm and patent visceral and renal vessels. The patient continues to do well with a 1-year follow-up CT scan demonstrating exclusion of thoracoabdominal aneurysm with no endoleak (Figure 10a and 10b).

## Discussion

The hybrid approach to manage thoracoabdominal aneurysms is a less invasive approach that combines open surgical repair, debranching of visceral and/or renal vessels with final aneurysm exclusion by endoluminal graft. The advantage of this technique is the lack of a thoracotomy incision associated with division of the diaphragm. This is thought to be the cause of an increased respiratory failure rate that is often associated with this surgery in combination with aortic cross clamping and risk of paraplegia.

Over a period of 22 months, March 2005 to January 2007, we have applied this procedure to 14 patients with varying degrees of thoracoabdominal aneurysms. There were 9 males and 5 females

with a mean age 69.2 years range (36–93). The extent of thoracoabdominal aneurysms included patients with Crawford extent I ($n = 6$), extent IV ($n = 6$), extent III ($n = 1$), and extent V ($n = 1$). The endografts were implanted through the usual means by either a Dacron graft or through common femoral access. Patients' medical histories were analyzed with the following comorbidities: hypertension (100%), peripheral vascular disease (100%), chronic obstructive pulmonary disease (78%), coronary artery disease (64%), renal insufficiency (29%), and obesity at 21%. Six of the fourteen patients had previous abdominal aortic surgery. A total of 38 graft bypasses were performed. Thirteen of fourteen patients (93%) survived with no paraplegia. Complications included transient left extremity weakness (1), renal insufficiency not requiring hemodialysis (1), lower limb ischemia (2), mesenteric ischemia (1), and respiratory failure (1). There was no perioperative myocardial infarction. The mean operating time was 4.25 hours with a mean blood loss of 1.1 L range (0.25–5.0 L). One patient died within 30 days from complications relating to surgery. There was one type I endoleak with no graft migration, graft collapse, aortic rupture, or open conversion. Various authors have reported their experience with the management of various extents of thoracoabdominal aneurysms with

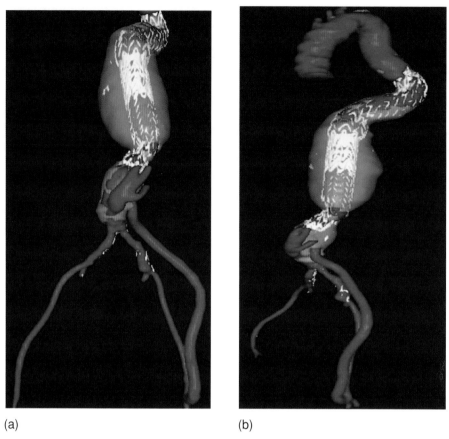

(a)                                                 (b)

**Figure 10** (a and b) 3-D models depicting the location of the endoluminal grafts and the presence of bypass grafts.

satisfactory results [24–26]. Despite extensive coverage of the thoracic and abdominal aorta in our experience and also in the series summarized in Table 1, there was no incidence of paraplegia.

Extent I and III endoleaks were the most common endoleaks encountered. Distal type I endoleaks are a more specific concern when the hybrid repair is performed because many of the patients have no

**Table 1** Results of hybrid thoracoabdominal aneurysm repair.

| Author, year | Patient (n) | Extent (n) | Follow-up (months) | 30-day mortality | Type I or III leak (%) | Complication (n) | Paraplegia (%) |
|---|---|---|---|---|---|---|---|
| Flye *et al.*, 2004 [24] | 3 | III, IV, patch | 11–21 | 0 | 33 (III) | TIA [1] | 0 |
| Fulton *et al.*, 2005 [25] | 10 | IV [2] | 0–13 | 0 | 10 (I) | CV (2); pulm (2) | 0 |
| | | JAAA (8) | | | | GI (1) | |
| Black *et al.*, 2005 (26) | 29 | I (3) | 2–28 | 15% | 23 (I) | CV (7); pulm (9) | 0 |
| | | II (18) | | | 4 (III) | Renal 4; GI (3) | |
| | | III (7) | | | | | |
| | | IV (1) | | | | | |

GI, gastrointestinal; CV, cardiovascular; pulm, pulmonary; JAAA, juxtarenal abdominal aortic aneurysm; TIA, transient ischemic attack.

adequate landing zone in the distal aorta. Distal type I endoleaks nevertheless can be successfully coiled and embolized. Pulmonary, renal, and gastrointestinal complications were the most common types encountered with the hybrid approach.

Patency rates for bypass grafts, as assessed by Kaplan-Maier life-table analysis, have been reported at 90–95% at 36 months in some series [27], which is encouraging. Furthermore, Kansal *et al.* [28] found no difference in patency between antegrade and retrograde grafts in this later series [27].

Branched and fenestrated stent grafts allow a total endovascular repair of thoracoabdominal aneurysms [29]. The approach has obvious advantages over a conventional open repair and hybrid open/endovascular techniques in that laparotomy or thoracotomy and aortic cross clamping are avoided. This procedure also minimizes cardiovascular instability, operative blood loss, and visceral ischemia. One potential disadvantage, however, is that this technique does not facilitate preservation of flow to the intercostal arteries which may be associated with an increased risk of spinal cord ischemia. Until branched and fenestrated grafts become more available, the hybrid procedure will be the least invasive approach to manage thoracoabdominal aneurysms.

As comparative studies of open TAA repair and stent-graft repair continue to emerge, endovascular repair will likely continue to demonstrate impressive reductions in overall perioperative morbidity and mortality. This type of procedure does come with an increased risk for secondary interventions. The risk is mitigated when one considers the target population that is composed of either high-risk or prohibitive surgical candidates. With the improvement in surgical techniques and endovascular technology, variations in open surgical techniques to maintain end-organ perfusion and achieve "hybrid" endovascular reconstruction of TAA and TAAA are more likely to become complementary.

# References

1 Panneton JM, Hollier LH. Non dissecting thoracoabdominal aortic aneurysms: Part 1. *Ann Vasc Surg* 1995; **9**: 503–514.

2 Cox GS, O'Hara PJ, Hertzer NR, Piedmonte MR, Krajewski LP, Beven EG. Thoracoabdominal aneurysm repair (a representative experience). *J Vasc Surg* 1992; **15**: 780–787.

3 Dardik A, Perler BA, Roseborough GS, Williams GM. Aneurysmal expansion of the visceral patch after thoracoabdominal aortic replacement (an argument for limiting patch size?). *J Vasc Surg* 2001; **34**: 405–409.

4 Vaccaro PS, Elkhammas E, Smead WL. Clinical observations and lessons learned in the treatment of patients with thoracoabdominal aortic aneurysms. *Surg Gynecol Obstet* 1988; **166**: 461–465.

5 Schepens MA, Defauw JJ, Hamerlijnck RP, De Geest R, Vermeulen FE. Surgical treatment of thoracoabdominal aortic aneurysms by simple cross clamping: risk factors and late results. *J Thorac Cardiovasc Surg* 1994; **107**: 134–142.

6 Crawford ES, DeNatale RW. Thoracoabdominal aortic aneurysm (observations regarding the natural course of the disease). *J Vasc Surg* 1986; **3**: 578–582.

7 Elefteriades JA. Natural history of thoracic aortic aneurysms (indications for surgery, and surgical versus nonsurgical risks). *Ann Thorac Surg* 2002; **74**: S1877–S1880; discussion S1892–S1898.

8 Rigberg DA, Zingmond D, Maggard M, Agustin M, Lawrence PF, Ko C. 30-day mortality statistics underestimate the risk of repair of thoracoabdominal aneurysms (TAA): a statewide experience. Presented at Society for Vascular Surgery Annual Meeting, Chicago, IL, 2005.

9 Bavaria JE, Appoo JJ, Makaroun MS, Verter J, Yu ZF, Mitchell SR. Endovascular stent-grafting versus open surgical repair of descending thoracic aortic aneurysms: a multi-center comparative trial. Presented at the American Association for Thoracic Surgery, San Francisco, CA, 2005.

10 Makaroun MS, Dillavou ED, Kee ST *et al*, for the GORE TAG Investigators. Endovascular treatment of thoracic aortic aneurysms (results of the phase II multicenter trial of the GOR TAG thoracic endoprosthesis). *J Vasc Surg* 2005; **41**: 1–9.

11 Cowan JA, Dimick JB, Henke PK, Huber TS, Stanley JC, Upchurch GR. Surgical treatment of intact thoracoabdominal aortic aneurysms in the United States (hospital and surgeon volume-related outcomes). *J Vasc Surg* 2003; **37**: 1169–1174

12 Kotsis T, Scharrer-Pamler R, Kapfer X *et al*. Treatment of thoracoabdominal aortic aneurysms with a combined endovascular and surgical approach. *Int Angiol* 2003; **22**: 125–133.

13 Watanabe Y, Ishimaru S, Kawaguchi S *et al*. Successful endografting with simultaneous visceral artery bypass grafting for severely calcified thoracoabdominal aortic aneurysm. *J Vasc Surg* 2002; **35**: 397–399.

14 Lundbom J, Hatlinghus S, Odegard A *et al.* Combined open and endovascular treatment of complex aortic disease. *Vascular* 2004; **12**: 93–98.

15 Chiesa R, Melissano G, Civilini E, Setacci F, Tshomba Y, Anzuini A. Two-stage combined endovascular and surgical approach for recurrent thoracoabdominal aortic aneurysm. *J Endovasc Ther* 2004; **11**: 330–333.

16 Quinones-Baldrich WJ, Panetta TF, Vescera CL, Kashyap VS. Repair of type IV thoracoabdominal aneurysm with a combined endovascular and surgical approach. *J Vasc Surg* 1999; **30**: 555–560.

17 Macierewicz JA, Jameel MM, Whitaker SC, Ludman CN, Davidson IR, Hopkinson BR. Endovascular repair of perisplanchnic abdominal aortic aneurysm with visceral vessel transposition. *J Endovasc Ther* 2000; **7**: 410–414.

18 Jacobs MJ, Meylaerts SA, de Haan P, de Mol BA, Kalkman CJ. Strategies to prevent neurologic deficit based on motor-evoked potentials in type I and II thoracoabdominal aortic aneurysm repair. *J Vasc Surg* 1999; **29**: 48–57; discussion 57–59.

19 Svensson LG, Crawford ES, Hess KR *et al.* Experience with 1509 patients undergoing thoracoabdominal aortic operations. *J Vasc Surg* 1993; **17**: 357–368; discussion 368–370.

20 Coselli JS, LeMaire SA, Conklin LD, Koksoy C, Schmittling ZC. Morbidity and mortality after extent II thoracoabdominal aortic aneurysm repair. *Ann Thorac Surg* 2002; 73: 1107–1115; discussion 1115–1116.

21 Coselli JS, LeMaire SA, Miller CC *et al.* Mortality and paraplegia after thoracoabdominal aortic aneurysm repair (a risk factor analysis). *Ann Thorac Surg* 2000; **69**: 409–414.

22 Safi HJ, Winnerkvist A, Miller CC *et al.* Effect of extended cross-clamp time during thoracoabdominal aortic aneurysm repair. *Ann Thorac Surg* 1998; **66**: 1204–1209.

23 Cambria RP, Giglia JS. Prevention of spinal cord ischaemic complications after thoracoabdominal aortic surgery. *Eur J Vasc Endovasc Surg* 1998; **15**: 96–109.

24 Flye MW, Choi ET, Sanchez LA *et al.* Retrograde visceral vessel revascularization followed by endovascular aneurysm exclusion as an alternative to open repair of thoracoabdominal aortic aneurysm. *J Vasc Surg* 2004; **39**: 454–458.

25 Fulton JJ, Farber MA, Marston WA, Mendes R, Mauro MA, Keagy BA. Endovascular stent-graft repair of pararenal and type IV thoracoabdominal aortic aneurysms with adjunctive visceral reconstruction. *J Vasc Surg* 2005; **41**: 191–198.

26 Black SA, Wolfe JHN, Clark M, Hamady M, Cheshire NJW, Jenkins MP. Complex thoracoabdominal aortic aneurysms: endovascular exclusion with visceral revascularization. Presented at Society for Vascular Surgery, Chicago, IL, 2005.

27 McMillan WD, McCarthy WJ, Bresticker MR Golan JF, *et al.* Mesenteric artery bypasses (objective patency determination). *J Vasc Surg* 1995; **21**: 729–740.

28 Kansal N, LoGerfo FW, Belfield AK *et al.* A comparison of antegrade and retrograde mesenteric bypass. *Ann Vasc Surg* 2002; **16**: 591–596.

29 McWilliams RG, Murphy M, Hartley D, Lawrence-Brouwn MM, Harris PL. In situ stent graft-fenestration to preserve the left subclavian artery. *J Endovasc Ther* 2004; **11**: 170–174.

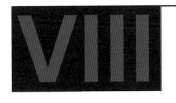

# SECTION VIII

# Thoracic aortic coarctations

## CASE 33

# Endovascular management of adult primary coarctation of the aorta

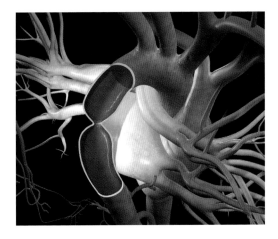

## Introduction

Primary coarctation of the aorta in an adult population usually presents with systemic hypertension and a differential blood pressure between the upper and lower extremities. A differential of more than 20 mm Hg warrants further investigation. Echocardiography can be performed to rule out associated cardiac lesions with a CT scan to check for anatomical variances including arterial collateralization. Once a significant coarctation is identified, there are two options for treatment. An open surgical repair involves a left thoracotomy with an end-to-end anastomosis [1], a subclavian flap angioplasty [2], an extended end-to-end anastomosis [3], or an end-to-side anastomosis [4]. An open repair has been considered the "gold standard" for this aortic defect. With the rapid growth of the endovascular field, there are preliminary reports of successful treatment at a limited number of sites. The advantage to an endovascular approach over an open surgical repair is that this less invasive approach is often associated with a shorter hospital stay and fewer complications.

## Case scenario

A 59-year-old gentleman with severe hypertension presented to the emergency room with chest pain. He was suspected to have coronary artery disease and was subsequently taken to the catheterization laboratory. Significant disease was found in two coronary artery vessels and a percutaneous coronary intervention was conducted with the placement of stents. Incidentally, an arch angiogram performed at that time revealed a severe native coarctation with a gradient of 65 mm Hg. He was referred for endovascular management of his coarctation. A CT scan of his chest approximates the area of coarctation to be 5 mm with the presence of a poststenotic dilatation (Figure 1a and 1b).

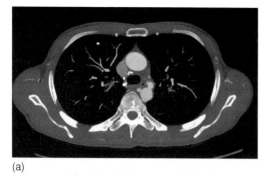

(a)

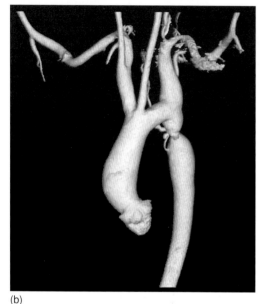

(b)

**Figure 1** (a) A CT scan image demonstrating the area of coarctation. (b) A 3-D reconstruction model further documents the extent of the disease (arrow).

## Endovascular therapy

Arterial lines were placed in both upper extremities. Under general anesthesia, open retrograde cannulation of the right common femoral artery was performed with an 18-G Cook needle (Cook Inc., Bloomington, IN) and a 0.035-in. soft-tip angled glide wire was passed in the thoracic aorta and exchanged to a 9-F (French) sheath. The patient was then heparinized. Percutaneous access of the left common femoral artery was similarly performed and a 5-F sheath was introduced. An angiogram of the thoracic aorta was conducted to document the extent of the disease and to identify the target area (Figure 2a). The measured gradient across the area

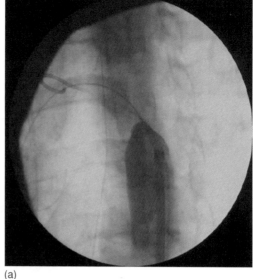

(a)

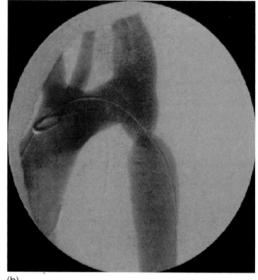

(b)

**Figure 2** (a and b) An angiographic depiction of a severe coarctation demonstrating the change after balloon angioplasty was carried out.

of coarctation was 65 mm Hg. Intravascular ultrasound (IVUS) was performed using an 8.2-F probe (Volcano Therapeutics, Inc., Rancho Cordova, CA) that was advanced through the right groin sheath (Figure 3a). A measurement of the coarctation was done (7 mm) with the lesion approximately 2-cm distal to the left subclavian artery. The landing zones were evaluated with the proximal aorta at

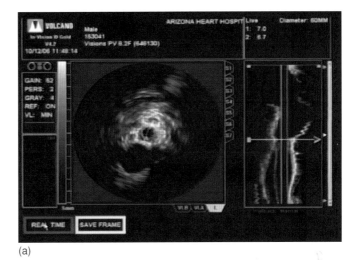

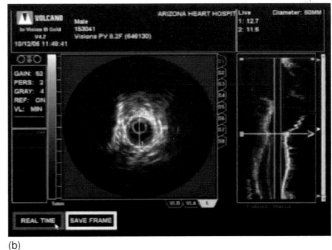

**Figure 3** (a) IVUS demonstrates the area of coarctation with poststenotic dilatation. (b) IVUS poststent deployment demonstrating increased luminal gain.

(a)

(b)

24 mm with a poststenotic dilatation of the distal thoracic aorta measuring 28 mm in diameter. We then exchanged the 9-F sheath to a 65-cm 12-F Keller-Timmermans sheath (Cook Inc., Bloomington, IN). Predilation of the area of coarctation was performed with a 16 mm × 4 cm Maxi LD balloon (Boston Scientific, Natick, MA) (Figure 4a). A post-balloon angioplasty angiogram performed demonstrated an increase in the diameter of the coarctation (Figure 2b). A Palmaz XL 4010 stent was selected and mounted on a 16 mm × 4 cm Maxi LD balloon (Figure 4b). The stent was deployed to the area of coarctation and a repeat angiogram demonstrated an increased luminal gain (Figure 5a). Postdeployment stent balloon angioplasty was performed with

a 25 mm × 4 cm Maxi LD balloon with flaring of the proximal and distal ends of the stent for fixation to the aortic wall. Poststent gradients were less than 10 mm Hg at the completion of the procedure. IVUS performed showed the area of coarctation had doubled to 16 mm (Figure 3b). A completion angiogram showed marked improvement in area of coarctation (Figure 5b). All wires and sheaths were removed; the right common femoral artery was closed in a transverse fashion with restoration of flow. A 6-F angioseal vascular closure device (St. Jude Medical, Inc., St. Paul, MN) was deployed to the left common femoral artery. Patient had bilateral palpable pulses at the end of the procedure and was extubated and transferred to recovery room. Patient was

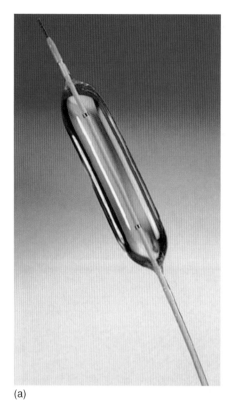

(a)

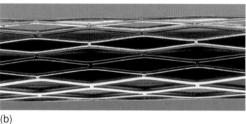

(b)

**Figure 4** (a and b) Maxi LD (Boston Scientific) balloon used to mount a Palmaz XL 4010 stent.

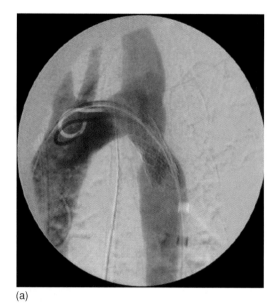

(a)

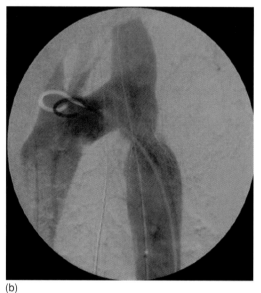

(b)

**Figure 5** (a and b) Pre- and post-Palmaz stent deployment angiograms.

discharged on postoperative day (POD) 2 in satisfactory condition with a CT scan of the chest performed on POD 1 demonstrating satisfactory repair of the primary coarctation with satisfactory stent placement (Figure 6a and 6b).

## Discussion

Adult coarctation is characterized by a shelflike narrowing within the lumen of the aorta with closed ducts forming the ligament arteries. The stated occurrence rate is 0.2–0.6% with a male to female ratio of 2:1 for isolated lesions. Aortic coarctation

results in pre- and poststenotic aortic dilatation. Patients with infantile primary coarctation (preductal coarctation) can be classified into three groups. Group 1 are patients with isolated coarctation of the aorta. Group 2 are patients with an associated ventricular septal defect (VSD) and group 3 patients exhibit complex intracardiac anomalies other than ventral septal defects. Adult group (juxtaductal)

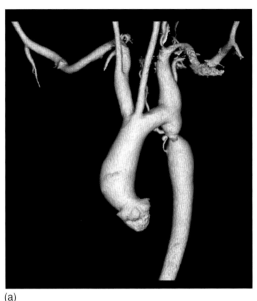

(a)

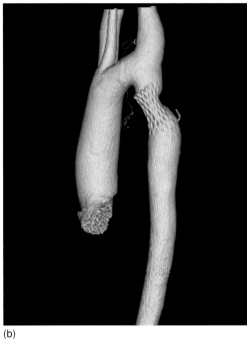

(b)

**Figure 6** (a and b) Pre- and postprocedure 3-D reconstruction models. The presence of a Palmaz stent and a decrease in the severity of the coarctation can be seen in the postimage.

patients may be asymptomatic or they can present with hypertension, chest pain, increased after load on the heart, and or abnormal distal pulses. A residual pressure gradient of 20 mm Hg or lower at rest has been the historical postintervention goal.

Surgical therapy can include resection with an end-to-end anastomosis, prosthetic patch aortoplasty, prosthetic interposition graft, or a subclavian flap aortoplasty. The mortality of such a repair in an adult population is 5%. Potential complications with this type of procedure can include hemorrhage, recurrent laryngeal nerve injury, phrenic nerve injury, Horner's syndrome, chylothorax, hypertension, paraplegia, stroke, aneurysm formation, recoarctation, and left arm ischemia. The data for paraplegia are reported in children so there is the comparison to children. Factors that can increase the rate of paraplegia would be the duration of the cross clamp and the presence of an aberrant right subclavian artery originating from below the area of coarctation [5]. Aneurysmal formation of 13% is reported with the technique of patch aortoplasty in the surgical repair of coarctation [6].

Endovascular management of aortic coarctation involves the deployment of either an uncovered or covered stent at the area of coarctation.

Uncovered stents are usually mounted on a balloon of appropriate size. As the balloon is inflated, the stent will be deployed in unison. The flaring of stent edges may be performed for better apposition to the aortic wall but there is a potential risk for aortic rupture due to sharpness of stent struts or drastic mismatch between compliant aorta and rigid stents may occur. Should the aortic intima become torn, stents have been very effective in stabilizing a focal irregularity. Balloon angioplasty was initially applied to treat recurrent coarctation and native coarctation in critically ill neonates [7, 8]. Aggressive balloon angioplasty can lead to a high prevalence of pseudoaneurysm formation, aortic dissection, and recoarctation/restenosis. Patients with a balloon to coarctation ratio of 3 were found to have the best minimal residual gradient at a 12-month follow-up [9].

Stent implantation has been shown to result in a lower rate of aneurysm and recoarctation than

**Table 1** Summary of our first 6 patients treated with a primary coarctation.

| Age (year) | Indication | History | Treatment | Results (pressure gradient) |
|---|---|---|---|---|
| 52 | Lt UE tingling | CHF, afib | BA/Palmaz 4010/BA | Initial: 60 mm<br>Post: no gradient |
| 29 | No symptoms | Sys and pum HTN, severe AI, ARF, chronic hematuria | BA/Palmaz 4010/BA | Initial: 60 mm<br>Post: 20 mm |
| 48 | Increasing chest pain | MI, NIDDM, HTN, arrhythmia, colitis | BA/Palmaz 4010/BA | Initial: 60 mm<br>Post: no gradient |
| 49 | Exercise intolerance | HTN, DM, obesity, cardiomyopathy, claudication | BA/Palmaz 4010/BA | Initial: 70 mm<br>Post: 5 mm |
| 40 | Increasing dyspnea | HTN | BA/Palmaz 4010/BA | No hemodynamic significance |
| 59 | Chest pain | CAD, PTCA | BA/Palmaz 4010/BA | Post: <10 mm |

Lt, left; UE, upper extremity; CHF, congestive heart failure; afib, atrial fibrillation; sys, systemic; pum, pulmonary; HTN, hypertension; AI, aortic insufficiency; ARF, acute renal failure; MI, myocardial infarction; NIDDM, non-insulin dependent diabetes mellitus; DM, diabetes mellitus; CAD, coronary artery disease; PTCA, percutaneous transluminal coronary angiography; BA, balloon angioplasty.

balloon angioplasty [10, 11]. Aneurysm formation of 6% has been reported with stent implantation after balloon angioplasty [12] and a 1% incidence of aneurysm when stent implantation was performed without preballoon dilatation of the area of coarctation [13]. Neurologic complications of transient ischemic attacks and cerebrovascular accidents have been described with balloon angioplasty and stent implantation [14]. High-pressure angioplasty balloons for stent deployment are associated with a decreased risk of balloon rupture. Stent implantation for primary coarctation may best applied to long diffuse lesions which otherwise require a longer segment of aortic resection or in which balloon angioplasty of such segments would result in aneurysm formation.

Over a 9-year period at our institution, we treated 20 patients (17 males and 3 females) with coarctation, with 9 patients treated for primary coarctation and 11 patients for recurrent coarctation and pseudoaneurysm postsurgical repair of coarctation. A review of the first 6 patients showed that 5 patients were symptomatic from cardiac-related causes and all patients had a cardiac-related history (Table 1). Gradients recorded across the area of coarctation were as high as 70 mm Hg. Technical success was achieved in all patients with a decrease in poststent gradients below 20 mm Hg in all patients with 2 of those patients showing no gradients at all. To date, the first patient in this series is approximately 9 years out from the procedure and has no documented coarctation-related symptoms.

The endovascular management of adult primary aortic coarctation has recently been accepted as a minimally invasive alternative to the open surgical approach. In order to make endovascular management even more attractive, changes need to be made in stent design and sizing to better accommodate to the typical coarctation presentation. Current device designs are often too long in length, have little or no taper between proximal and distal ends, and lack the ability conform to a very tortuous aorta. As with any endovascular treatment, there is little long-term data available and additional studies would be required to determine the ultimate efficacy of endovascular management of primary adult coarctation of the aorta.

# References

1 Craaford C, Nylin G. Congenital coarctation of the aorta and its surgical treatment. *J Thorac Surg* 1945; **14**: 347.
2 Waldhausen JA, Nahrwold DL. Repair of coarctation of the aorta with a subclavian flap. *J Thorac Cardiovasc Surg* 1966; **51**: 532.

3 Zannini L, Lecompte Y, Galli R *et al.* Aortic coarctation with hypoplasia of the arch: description of a new surgical technique. *G Ital Cardiol* 1985; **15**: 1045.

4 Vouhe PR, Trinquet F, Lecompte Y *et al.* Aortic coarctation with hypoplastic arch. Results of extended end-end aortic arch anastomosis. *J Thorac Cardiovasc Surg* 1988; **96**: 557.

5 Lerberg DB, Hardesty RL, Siewers RD *et al.* Coarctation of the aorta in infants and children. 25 years of experience. *Ann Thorac Surg* 1982; **33**: 159–170.

6 Clarkson PM, Brandt PWT, Barrat-Boyes BG *et al.* Prosthetic repair of coarctation of the aorta with particular reference to Dacron onlay patch grafts and late aneurismal formation. *Am J Cardiol* 1985; **56**: 342–346.

7 Lababidi Z. Neonatal transluminal balloon coarctation angioplasty. *Am Heart J* 1983; **106**: 752–753.

8 Fletcher SE, Nihill MR, Grifka RG, O'laughlin MP, Mullins CE. Balloon angioplasty for native coarctation of the aorta: midterm follow-up and prognostic factors. *J Am Coll Cardiol* 1995; **25**: 730–734.

9 Hellenbrand WE, Allen HD, Golinko RJ, Hagler DJ, Lutin W, Kan J. Balloon angioplasty for aortic recoarctation: results of valvuloplasty and angioplasty of congenital Anomalies Registry. *Am J Cardiol* 1990; **65**: 793–797.

10 Rosenthal E, Qureshi SA, Tynan M. Stent implantation for aortic recoarctation. *Am Heart J* 1995; **129**: 1220–1221.

11 Macgee AG, Brzezinska-Rajszys G, Qurshi SA *et al.* Stent implantation for aortic coarctation and recoarctation. *Heart* 1999; **82**: 600–606.

12 Ebeid MR, Preito LR, Latson LA. Use of balloon-expandable stents for coarctation of the aorta: initial results and intermediate term follow up. *Am Coll Cardiol* 1997; **30**: 1847–1852.

13 Thanopoulos BD, Hadjinikolaou L, Konstadopoulou GN, Tsaousis GS, Triposkiadis F, Spirou P. Stent treatment for coarctation of the aorta: intermediate term follow-up and technical considerations. *Heart* 2000; **84**: 65–70.

14 Harrison Da, McLaughlin PR, Lazzam C, Connelly M, Benson LN. Endovascular stents in the management of coarctation of the aorta in the adolescent and adult: one year follow up. *Heart* 2001; **85**: 561–566.

# Endovascular management of the small thoracic aorta with postcoarctation pseudoaneurysm

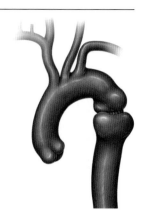

## Introduction

Surgical repair has proven to be an effective treatment for primary aortic coarctation. Traditional surgical approaches include a resection with an end-to-end anastomosis, a subclavian flap aortoplasty, patch aortoplasty, and an interposition graft. Potential complications at long-term follow-up include recurrent coarctation, hypertension, premature coronary artery disease, cerebrovascular disease, and anastomotic pseudoaneurysm [1, 2]. The reported rate of anastomotic pseudoaneurysm has been reported to be between 3 and 38% [3]. Open surgical repair for anastomotic pseudoaneurysm can be associated with high morbidity and mortality. Endovascular management of postcoarctation pseudoaneurysm offers a less invasive treatment approach in high-risk surgical patients.

## Case scenario

A 49-year-old male with a past medical history significant for hypertension had a primary surgical repair for coarctation of the aorta at the age of 20 years. Blood pressure measurements taken in both arms did not identify any significant gradient. An incidental finding of an enlarged thoracic aortic shadow was made on a routine preoperative chest X-ray prior to knee surgery. A contrast-enhanced CT scan of the chest identified a large pseudoaneurysm of the thoracic aorta involving the ostium of the left subclavian artery and extending beyond the site of previous repair (Figure 1a and 1b). Due to the high risk associated with a redo operation, a hybrid repair that consisted of a left carotid artery to left subclavian artery bypass with deployment of a thoracic endoluminal graft was proposed to the patient who agreed to the procedure upon informed consent.

## Technical details (left carotid–subclavian bypass)

A left-sided supraclavicular incision was performed (Figure 2). The platysma was divided and then followed by the clavicular head of the sternocleidomastoid medially to reveal the carotid sheath. The carotid sheath was identified and incised to reveal the common carotid artery and the vagus nerve, which was protected. Next, we divided the omohyoid muscle and identified the scalene fat pad and mobilized it from lateral to medial to reveal the phrenic nerve overlying the scalenus anterior muscle. The phrenic nerve was preserved and the scalenus anterior muscle divided to reveal the aneurysmal ostium of the left subclavian artery. Five thousand units of heparin were administered after which the left subclavian artery was divided between clamps with oversewing of the ostium with a 4-0 Prolene stitch. The distal end of the subclavian artery was sewn in an end-to-end fashion to a 10-mm Gore TAG graft (W.L. Gore & associates, Flagstaff, AZ). The graft was tunneled beneath the internal jugular vein and, after clamping the left common carotid artery proximally and distally, an

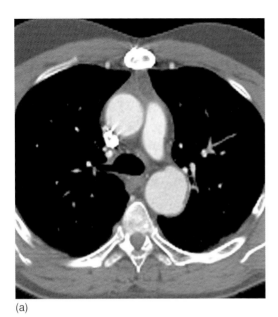

(a)

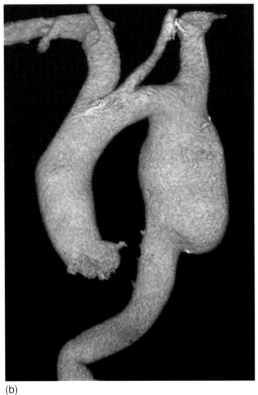

(b)

**Figure 1** (a) An axial CT scan image demonstrating a pseudoaneurysm postcoarctation repair. (b) A 64-slice 3-D reconstruction illustrating the large pseudoaneurysm beginning at the level of the left subclavian artery ostium.

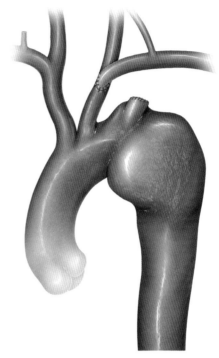

**Figure 2** Left carotid–subclavian transposition.

arteriotomy was made with the graft sewn in an end-to-side fashion with a 5-0 Prolene stitch. De-airing maneuvers were performed prior to unclamping the artery to restore flow. The neck incision was closed and the patient was transferred to the recovery room without any complications.

## Technical details: deployment of a custom assembled endoluminal graft

On the day after the left carotid–subclavian transposition, the patient was returned to the operating room for the deployment of an endoluminal graft to exclude the postcoarctation pseudoaneurysm. Under general anesthesia, open retrograde annulations of the right common femoral artery was performed with an 18-G needle (Cook Inc., Bloomington, IN) and 0.035-in. soft-tip angled glide wire was passed into the aorta and exchanged to a 9-F (French) sheath after 5000 units of heparin were given. Percutaneous access of the left common femoral artery was performed and a 9-F sheath was introduced.

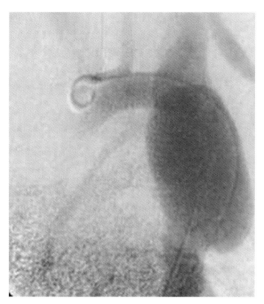

**Figure 3** An angiogram demonstrating a postcoarctation pseudoaneurysm.

A 5-F pigtail angiographic catheter was advanced into the thoracic aorta and an oblique thoracic arch aortogram was performed through the left sheath via a pigtail catheter to delineate the arch and the postcoarctation pseudoaneurysm (Figure 3).

Intravascular ultrasound was performed by introducing an 8.2-F probe (Volcano Therapeutics, Inc., Rancho Cordova, CA) through the right common femoral sheath. The area above the pseudoaneurysm was measured at 20 mm × 21 mm with the area below the pseudoaneurysm slightly larger at 22 mm × 23 mm in diameter. The length of the treatment area to be covered was measured at 14 cm. The smallest thoracic endoprosthesis currently commercially available is 26 mm in diameter and the use of this device would represent a potentially dangerous oversizing of more than 20%, which is currently recommended by the instructions for use for the device. A series of abdominal endoluminal graft components were chosen due to their smaller caliber. A potential stumbling block to the use of these devices was that the delivery catheters would be too short to reach the target area. A Cook (Zenith Graft, Bloomington, IN) iliac limb extensions 22 mm × 55 mm was deployed on the back table and reloaded into a long 20-F Keller-Timmerman introducer sheath (Cook, Inc., Bloomington, IN) and delivered successfully to the target area (Figure 4). This process was repeated a second time with a larger iliac leg extension 24 mm × 55 mm and then finally with a 28 mm × 103 mm bifurcated main body that had been customized

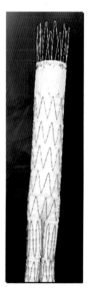

Cook abdominal
bifurcated ELG graft
28 mm × 103 mm

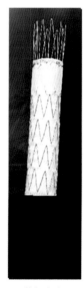

Abdominal
ELG cuff

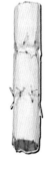

AAA ELG-tapered
iliac limb
22 mm × 24 mm
× 55 mm.

**Figure 4** A Cook Zenith abdominal aortic aneurysm (AAA) endoluminal graft (ELG) main body, cuff, and iliac limb extension components custom assembled for managing a pseudoaneurysm with a small diameter neck.

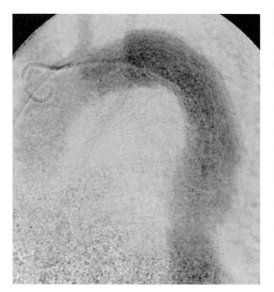

**Figure 5** A completion angiogram demonstrating satisfactory exclusion of pseudoaneurysm.

for this procedure and delivered through a 22-F sheath. Included in this customization was the removal of the suprarenal fixation barbs and the gate area for the limbs. A completion angiogram demonstrated no endoleak with complete exclusion of the

postcoarctation pseudoaneurysm (Figure 5). All wires and sheaths were removed from the right common femoral artery. The artery was closed in a transverse fashion with restoration of flow to the lower extremity. An 8-F angioseal closure device was deployed to the left common femoral artery.

The patient was discharged on the second post operative day (POD 2) in satisfactory condition. A CT scan of the chest performed on POD 1 showed exclusion of the postcoarctation pseudoaneurysm with no endoleak (Figure 6a and 6b). One year has passed since the procedure and he continues to do well with no significant changes in his health or his endoluminal graft.

## Discussion

This case represents a novel approach of customizing off-the-shelf endovascular components for the small thoracic aorta. Until smaller in diameter thoracic endoprostheses are developed, this customized approach is the best solution when an endovascular approach is contemplated. Severe adult type coarctation accounts for 4% of congenital cardiovascular malformations and is usually surgically corrected.

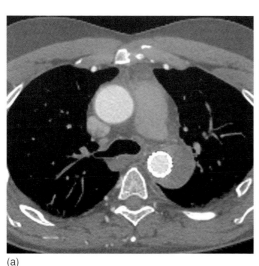

(a)

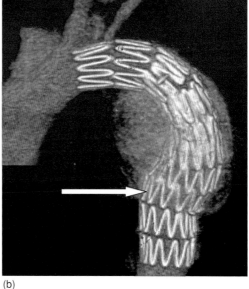

(b)

**Figure 6** (a) An axial CT scan image with endoluminal graft excluding postcoarctation pseudoaneurysm, no endoleak is noted. (b) A 64-slice CT 3-D reconstruction showing the complete exclusion of the aneurysm.

Stent-graft repair of thoracic aneurysm has been shown to be feasible with acceptable mid-term results [4, 5]. Conservative treatment of aneurysms after surgical coarctation repair is associated with a rupture rate of 100% within 15 years in a single center experience [6]. Surgical repair of pseudoaneurysms after coarctation repair is associated with high morbidity and mortality including paralysis of the recurrent laryngeal nerve 13.6–36%, phrenic nerve injury 5–6%, bleeding and paraplegia and death 13.8% [7, 8]. Endovascular management of the small thoracic aorta poses a surgical challenge since the smallest commercially available thoracic endograft is 26 mm in diameter. Customizing off-the-shelf abdominal endoluminal graft components allows for the endovascular repair of the small thoracic aorta. Access can be achieved through the femoral approach or through iliac access via the retroperitoneal approach. The goal of therapy in postcoarctation pseudoaneurysm is to deploy a short stent graft to reduce the potential risk of paraplegia. Should the length of the proximal neck prove to be insufficient, coverage of the left subclavian artery to gain a good proximal landing zone can be performed with minimal associated left upper extremity symptoms [9]. However, a left carotid artery to left subclavian artery bypass should be performed prior to the procedure should imaging indicate the presence of a left internal mammary graft or a dominant left vertebral artery system in the target landing zone. If the left subclavian artery is covered without a vessel bypass, the vessel transposition can be done at any time if there are symptoms of upper extremity ischemia.

In conclusion, off-the-shelf abdominal endoluminal grafts can be customized for use in the small descending thoracic aorta in the absence of commercially available thoracic endoluminal grafts.

## References

1 Webb G. Treatment of coarctation and late complications in the adult. *Semin Thorac Cardiovasc Surg* 2005; **17**: 139–142.

2 Bouchart F, Dubar A, Tabley A *et al.* Coarctation of the aorta in adults: surgical results and long term follow-up. *Ann Thorac Surg* 200; **70**: 1483–1488.

3 von Kodolitsch Y, Aydin MA, Koschyk DH *et al.* Predictors of aneurismal formation after surgical correction of aortic coarctation. *J Am Coll Cardiol* 2002; **39**: 617–624.

4 Wheatley GH, III, Gurbuz AT, Rodriguez-Lopez JA *et al.* Mid-term outcome in 158 consecutive Gore TAG thoracic endoprostheses: single center experience. *Ann Thorac Surg* 2006; **81**(5): 1570–1577; discussion 1577.

5 Cohen M, Fuster V, Steele PM, Driscoll D, McGoon DC. Coarctation of the aorta. Long-term follow-up and prediction of outcome after surgical correction. *Circulation* 1989; **80**: 840–845.

6 Knyshov GV, Sitar LL, Glagola MD, Atamanyuk MY. Aortic aneurysms at the site of the repair of coarctation of the aorta: a review of 48 patients. *Ann Thorac Surg* 1996; **61**: 935–939.

7 Ala-Kulju K, Heikkinen L. Aneurysm after patch graft aortoplasty for coarctation of the aorta: long term results of surgical management. *Ann Thorac Surg* 1989; **47**: 853–856.

8 Greenburg R, Resch T, Nyman U *et al.* Endovascular repair of descending thoracic aneurysms: early experience with immediate term follow-up. *J Vasc Surg* 2000; **31**: 147–156.

9 Hausegger KA, Oberwalder P, Tiesenhausen K *et al.* Intentional left subclavian artery occlusion by thoracic aortic stent grafts without surgical transposition. *J Endovasc Ther* 2001; **8**: 472–476.

# CASE 35

# Recurrent coarctation of the thoracic aorta

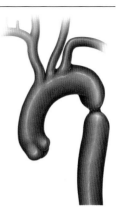

## Introduction

Surgery for recurrent coarctation after a correction of primary coarctation occurs in 16% of survivors [1]. Repeat surgery is much more complicated than the primary repair and only moderately successful [2], prompting the increased use of balloon angioplasty and other adjunctive techniques for the management of recurrent coarctation [3, 4]. The endovascular approach to the treatment of recurrent coarctation results in both intimal and medial tears in the scar tissue of the coarctation, resulting in an increase in the luminal size and a decrease in the systolic pressure. A histological analysis shows that the tears do appear to heal partially or completely. Overaggressive balloon dilatation of the scar tissue may result in transmedial tears, which can increase the risk of pseudoaneurysm formation or aortic dissection [5, 6]. Compared to as little as 10 years ago, the endovascular surgeon has multiple treatment modalities to choose from. The standard repair of balloon angioplasty, uncovered stents, or a combination of both is still present. More cutting-edge techniques include the use of thoracic endoluminal grafts or the off-label use of abdominal graft components (Figure 1a–d). The principal drawback to the newer techniques is the lack of appropriately sized devices and the ability to deliver them in an accurate fashion.

The minimal invasiveness of the endovascular approach is an attractive option for patients who are considered at high risk for a redo operation.

## Casescenario

A 64-year-old male whose primary coarctation repair was conducted 40 years ago presented to his doctor with a tingling sensation that ran down his entire left side. He denied having any chest pain or shortness of breath. On physical examination, he was in sinus rhythm at a rate of 68 beats/min with his blood pressure in the right arm at 148/90 mm Hg and no measurable blood pressure in the left arm. There was no rib notching and the rest of his physical examination was normal. A CT scan of the chest (Figure 2a and 2b) demonstrated a recurrent coarctation with a 70% reduction in the luminal diameter and a poststenotic dilatation of the aorta that diminished the size of the left subclavian and vertebral arteries. A left heart catheterization demonstrated a left ventricular ejection fraction of 55% with normal coronary arteries. The aortogram of the arch showed patent brachiocephalic vessels with a total occlusion of the left subclavian artery with retrograde filling through the left vertebral artery. Due to the increased surgical risk involved with a redo operation and the increased risk of paraplegia, the patient was referred for the endovascular approach which was considered a better, less invasive option.

## Endovascular procedure

Arterial lines were placed in both upper extremities. Under general anesthesia, open retrograde

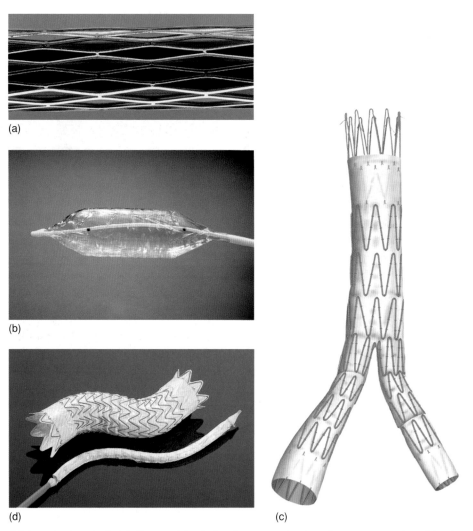

**Figure 1** Palmaz stent, angioplasty balloon, endoluminal graft components adapted to treat coarctation of the thoracic aorta.

cannulation of the right common femoral artery was performed with an 18-G Cook (Cook Inc., Bloomington, IN) needle and 0.035-in. soft-tip angled glide wire was passed in the aorta and exchanged to a 9-F (French) sheath after 5000 units of heparin were given. Percutaneous access of the left common femoral artery was similarly performed and a 5-F sheath was introduced. Oblique thoracic arch aortogram was performed through the left sheath via a 5-F pigtail catheter to delineate the arch and the descending thoracic aorta and identify the area of coarctation (Figure 3). The gradient across the area of coarctation was 65 mm Hg. Intravascular ultrasound (IVUS) was performed using an 8.2-F probe (Volcano Therapeutics, Inc., Rancho Cordova, CA) through the right groin sheath. The diameter of the area at the coarctation was 7 mm in diameter that was 2 cm distal to the left subclavian artery. Measurements of the aorta proximal to the coarctation were 24 mm with a poststenotic dilatation of the distal aorta at 28 mm in diameter. We then exchanged the 9-F sheath to a 65-cm 12-F Cook sheath. Predilation of the coarctation was performed with a 16 mm × 4 cm balloon Maxi LD (Boston Scientific, Natick, MA) (Figure 3). We then selected a Palmaz XL 4010 stent, which

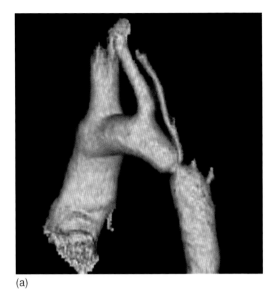

(a)

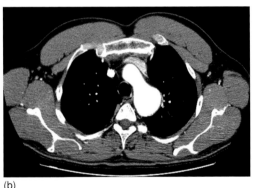

(b)

**Figure 2** (a) A 3-D reconstruction model showing the anatomy. (b) An axial CT scan image of the poststenotic dilation.

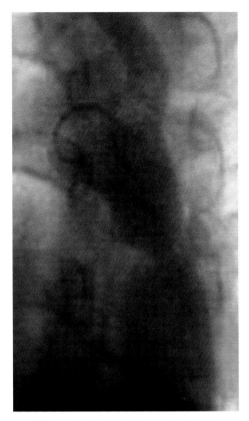

**Figure 3** The pretreatment angiogram showing the recurrent coarctation.

in turn was mounted on a 16 mm × 4 cm balloon Maxi LD. The Palmaz stent was deployed with no incident. Postdeployment balloon angioplasty was performed using a 25 mm × 4 cm Maxi LD balloon. The proximal and distal ends of the stent were flared to allow for greater fixation to the aortic wall. The gradient across the coarctation had been reduced to less than 10 mm Hg. Measurement of the luminal gain by IVUS indicated that the area at the coarctation had increased to 15 mm. A completion angiogram also showed marked improvement in the area of coarctation (Figure 4). The sites of arterial access were closed in the usual fashion. Prior to leaving the operating room, a short neurological and peripheral pulse examination was

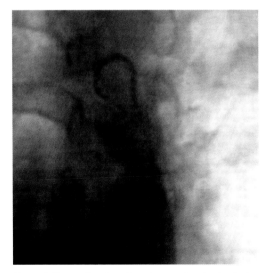

**Figure 4** The posttreatment angiogram showing luminal gain after serial balloon angioplasty accompanied by stent placement.

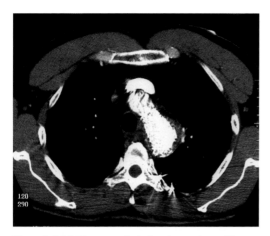

**Figure 5** Axial CT scan conducted postprocedure with improved luminal diameter.

conducted. All examinations were clear with the patient extubated and transferred to the recovery room. Confirming the angiogram, a CT scan conducted prior to discharge showed that luminal gain was achieved with exclusion of the dilation (Figure 5).

## Discussion

Recurrent, or recoarctation, of the aorta is defined as a gradient greater than 20–30 mm Hg across the repaired area. The incidence of recurrent coarctation ranges from 5 to 20% with pseudoaneurysm formation at the previous site of repair estimated to be from 3 to 38% [7–9]. Patients may have primary repair of coarctation at infancy with balloon angioplasty or from a failure of growth at the anastomosis or technical factors such as a short subclavian flap aortoplasty. Other patients may require an operation due to an aneurysmal formation of the patch plasty. Factors associated with recoarctation include an age less than 2–3 months [10] for first repair, weight less than 5 kg at the time of primary repair [11], use of silk suture for primary repair [12], and remaining ductile tissue.

A patient with this condition typically presents with upper body hypertension that can be linked to coronary artery disease, congestive heart failure, and bicuspid aortic stenosis. Preoperative evaluation of this patient includes an echocardiogram to assess left ventricular function and valve function

and a CT scan of the chest with reconstruction or MRA angiography of the arch. IVUS can be a helpful tool inside the operating room. The size of the landing zones can be confirmed and correlated with CT measurements. Most of all, a clear measurement of the coarctation pre- and postintervention can be done immediately to evaluate the procedure's effectiveness. The current gold standard for treatment is an open surgical repair. A surgical repair includes resection of the coarctation with end-to-end anastomosis, subclavian flap aortoplasty, and prosthetic interposition graft. Complications associated with surgical repair include a risk of recurrent laryngeal nerve paralysis (13.1–36%), phrenic nerve injury (5–6%), reexploration for bleeding (3.3%), and death (13.8%) [13, 14].

An endovascular approach to recurrent coarctation is a modality that restores anatomical relief of the obstruction as well as a reduction in an aortic gradient. Both covered and uncovered stents can be used to achieve satisfactory results. Uncovered stents are used mostly for a coarctation with no pseudoaneurym component. Endoluminal grafts are used for pseudoaneuryms at the site of previous surgery. Prior to endoluminal graft deployment, an uncovered stent is deployed to the site for expansion of the stenosis. Generally, uncovered stents have more radial force than endoluminal grafts and are the best choice for opening a vessel. Endoluminal grafts are only meant to exclude pseudoaneurysms. Endoluminal grafts tend to be problematic for this population because the target landing zones can sometimes measure smaller than what the device's instructions for use will allow. Younger patients have not gone through the aging process that will tend to dilate their aorta over time. Customizing abdominal endoluminal grafts, due to their smaller size, is a viable option to overcome this problem. The customized abdominal pieces will need to be reloaded into a longer delivery sheath so that it can reach the target area. In our series, of 11 patients [15] treated for a recoarctation the average size of the aorta was (17–20 mm) (Table 1). The mean age was 47 ± 5 years with a gender distribution of 9 males to 2 females. All patients were able to undergo these procedures in a successful fashion with no perioperative deaths or paraplegia. Two patients with pseudoaneurysm formation at the coarctation site required left carotid–left subclavian bypass

**Table 1** Summary of 11 patients managed by the endovascular approach for recurrent coarctation/pseudoaneurysm.

| Patient | History | Treatment | Complications |
|---|---|---|---|
| 1 | Repair at 7 yr old, HTN, aortic stenosis | BA, Palmaz, BA | None |
| 2 | Repair at 12 yr old, Ross proc, AVR | Palmaz (2) + Cook abdominal (abd) ELG | None |
| 3 | First repair 2004 | Palmaz | Additional Palmaz stent migration of first |
| 4 | Repair at 20 yr old, HTN | Pre S-C bypass, Cook abd. ELG | None |
| 5 | CAD, NIDDM, HTN, Lipids, repaired 28 yr ago | Pre S-C bypass, customized EndoFit, BA Palmaz | Anemia, Gore TAG leak from previous (2 yr post) |
| 6 | 4 surgeries—1 wk, 1 yr, 1993 (BA), 1995 (Palmaz), HTN, CHF | Gore TAG, BA, Palmaz | None |
| 7 | Repair at 36 h, age 16- Palmaz X 2 + BA failed | Palmaz, customized EndoFit | Post S-C bypass (3 wk) |
| 8 | 1° repair at 18 | Gore TAG, coils | Post S-C bypass (1 wk) |
| 9 | Ruptured postcoarctation aneurysm 1998 (open), dissection 6 mo later | Gore TAG | Postimplant syndrome, general weakness |
| 10 | 1° repair at 23 | Gore TAG | None |
| 11 | HTN, lipids, coarctation repair 1957 | Presubclavian carotid bypass, Gore TAG | Left brachial artery occlusion (thrombectomy) |

AVR, aortic valve replacement; CHF, congestive heart failure; ELG, endoluminal graft; HTN, hypertension; NIDDM, non-insulin dependent diabetes mellitus; CAD, coronary artery disease, coronary angiography; BA, balloon angioplasty.

procedures because of left upper extremity ischemia due to coverage of the subclavian artery with an endoluminal graft. The median follow-up was 12.0 ± 4.1 months (range 1–60). There were two reinterventions for endoleak that were successfully managed at 3 and 10 months postprocedure.

In conclusion, recoarctation has been reported to occur up to 16% postprimary repair. Balloon angioplasty, endoluminal graft, and stent implantations are novel techniques for managing recoarctation with minimal morbidity and mortality. The short-term results of this method are encouraging but optimism needs to be tempered. Due to the relatively young age of the patients and the short history of endovascular therapy, it will be the long-term results that will ultimately decide if this type of treatment should be extended to everyone with a recurrent coarctation or only those who meet a high-risk criterion.

# References

1 Toro-Salazar OH, Steinberger J, Thomas WI *et al.* Long-tem follow-up of patients after coarctation of the aorta repair. *Am J Cardiol* 2002; **89**: 541–547.

2 Pollack P, Freed MD, Castaneda AR, Norwood WI. Reoperation for isthmic coarctation of the aorta: follow-up of 26 patients. *Am J Cardiol* 1983; **51**: 1690–1694.

3 Rao PS, Najjar HN, Mardini MK, Solymar L, Thapar MK. Balloon angioplasty for coarctation of the aorta: immediate and long term results. *Am Heart J* 1988; **15**: 657–664.

4 Fawzy ME, Dunn B, Galal O, Wison N, Shaikh A, Sriram R, Duran CM. Balloon coarctation angioplasty in adolescents and adults: early and intermediate results. *Am Heart J* 1992; **24**: 167–171.

5 Erbel R, Bednarczyk I, Pop T *et al.* Detection of dissection of the aortic intima and media after angioplasty of coarctation of the aorta: an angiographic, computer tomographic and echocardiographic comparative study. *Circulation* 1990; **81**: 805–814.

6  Harrison DA, McLaughlin PR, Lazzam C, Connelly M, Benson LN. Endovascular stents in the management of coarctation of the aorta in the adolescent and adult: one year follow-up. *Heart* 2001; **85**: 561–566.

7  Ungerleider RM. Coarctation of the aorta. In: Kaiser LR, Kron IL & Spray TL, eds. *Mastery of Cardiothoracic Surgery.* Lippincott-Raven Publishers, Wickford, RI:, 1998: 704–715.

8  Von Kodolitsch Y, Aydin MA, Koschyk DH *et al.* Predictors of aneurysmal formation after surgical correction of aortic coarctation. *J Am Coll Cardiol* 2002; **39**: 617–624.

9  Knyshov GV, Sitar LL, Glagola MD *et al.* Aortic aneurysms at the site of repair of coarctation of the aorta: a review of 48 patients. *Ann Thorac Surg* 1996; **61**: 935–939.

10 Metzdorff MT, Cobanoglu A, Grunkemeir GL, *et al.* Influence of age at operation on late results with subclavian flap aortoplasty. *J Thorac Cardiovasc Surg* 1985; **89**: 235–241.

11 Sanchez GR, Balsara RK, Dunn JM *et al.* Recurrent obstruction after subclavaian flap repair of coarctation of the aorta in infants. *J Thorac Cardiovasc Surg* 1986; **91**: 738–746.

12 Harlan JL, Doty DB, Brandt B, III, *et al.* Coarctation of the aorta in infants *Thorac Cardiovasc Surg* 1984; **88**: 1012–1019.

13 Cohen M, Fuster V, Steele PM *et al.* Coarctation of the aorta: long-term follow-up and prediction of outcome after surgical correction. *Circulation* 1989; **80**: 840–845.

14 Ala-Kulju K, Heikkinen L. Aneurysm after patch graft aortoplasty for coarctation of the aorta: long term results of surgical management. *Ann Thorac Surg* 1989; **47**: 853–856.

15 Preventza O, Wheatley GH, Williams J *et al.* Endovascular approaches for complex forms of recurrent aortic coarctation. *J Endovasc Ther* 2006; **13**: 400–405.

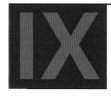

**SECTION IX**

# Thoracic aortobronchial fistula

# CASE 36

# Endovascular management of aortobronchial fistulas

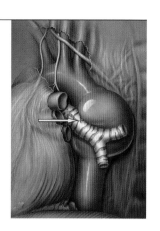

## Introduction

Aortobronchial fistula (ABF) is a rare, life-threatening complication associated with previous thoracic aortic surgery. Patients typically present with hemoptysis and its presence, once confirmed, mandates urgent repair. Progression of atherosclerosis at a previous anastomotic repair results in a weakening of the aortic wall with a resulting break in the aortic wall and subsequent pseudoaneurysm formation. The foreign body reaction to the prosthetic graft and suture, tracheobronchial compression, pulsatile pressure erosion, and localized pulmonary infection are implicated in the pathophysiology of ABF formation. CT scans, aortography, bronchoscopy, and transesophageal echocardiography are the most common modalities used to make the diagnosis. Open surgery of aortobronchial fistulas is associated with respiratory insufficiency, stroke, paralysis, acute renal failure, myocardial infarction, cardiac failure, hemorrhage, secondary graft infection, and a mortality rate ranging from 25 to 41% [1, 2] Endovascular stent grafting provides a less invasive approach to exclude the fistulous tract as well as the pathological aorta with reduced morbidity and mortality [3].

## Case scenario

A 62-year-old female was transferred to our institution with recurrent episodes of hemoptysis. The patient had undergone an open thoracic aortic aneurysm repair with an interposition graft 13 years ago. She had been hospitalized three times in the last 5 months for hemoptysis with no evidence of fistulous tract demonstrated by bronchoscopy. At this presentation, she had massive hemoptysis with pulmonary failure. A chest X-ray (Figure 1) showed a widened mediastinum with a CT scan of the chest (Figure 2a and 2b) demonstrating the pseudoaneurysm of the thoracic aorta with a possible contained rupture. The patient was emergently intubated with a double lumen tube and taken to the operating for immediate intervention.

## Procedure

The procedure was performed under general anesthesia by surgeons in a dedicated endovascular suite with complete fluoroscopic and angiographic capabilities. Intravascular access was obtained through both common femoral arteries as well as the left brachial artery. Preoperative imaging of the access arteries showed that the right common femoral artery was of adequate caliber, with little or no presence of occlusive disease, for advancement of the sheath necessary for device delivery. The patient was given 5000 units of intravenous heparin for anticoagulation. An arteriographic 5-F (French) pigtail catheter was advanced through the right common femoral artery 9-F groin sheath. Aortography and intravascular ultrasonography were performed to measure the dimensions of the thoracic aorta and distances from the brachiocephalic and visceral vessels as well as to demonstrate the fistulous tract. Transesophageal echocardiography (Figure 3) was used to delineate the exact position of the fistula (Figure 4a and 4b). A 24-F Keller-Timerman sheath (Cook Inc., Bloomington, IN) was inserted through the right common femoral artery over a stiff

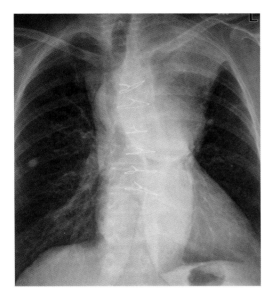

**Figure 1** Chest X-ray demonstrating a widened mediastinum.

0.035-in. Amplatz guide wire (Boston Scientific-Meditech, Watertown, MI) to the level of the thoracic aorta. A 37 mm × 20 cm Gore TAG device (W.L. Gore & Associates, Flagstaff, AZ) was inserted into the sheath. The device was advanced under fluoroscopic and TEE guidance to the designated proximal landing zone. The endoluminal graft was deployed in the distal arch of the aorta with coverage of the left subclavian artery to achieve a good proximal landing zone. Postdeployment balloon angioplasty was performed at both the proximal and distal landing zones to secure fixation of the graft. Completion arteriography and TEE were performed to assess accurate placement with no endoleak detected. The patient was kept in the intensive care unit overnight. Postoperative CT scanning of the chest (Figure 5) was performed the next day with the graft in good position and no evidence of an endoleak. At 24-month postprocedure, the patient continues to do well with serial imaging showing regression of the pseudoaneurysm sac, resolution of hemoptysis, and no change in device integrity or position (Figure 6a–6c).

## Discussion

Thoracic endografting has recently been approved for the management of descending thoracic

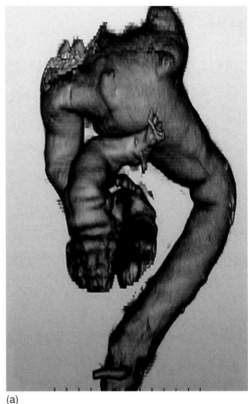

(a)

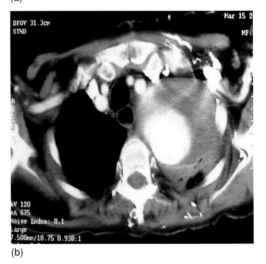

(b)

**Figure 2** (a) A 3-D reconstruction of the chest demonstrating a large pseudoaneurysm. (b) An axial CT image demonstrating a large pseudoaneurysm with mural thrombus.

aneurysms with encouraging mid-term results [4, 5]. Endovascular techniques offer an alternative

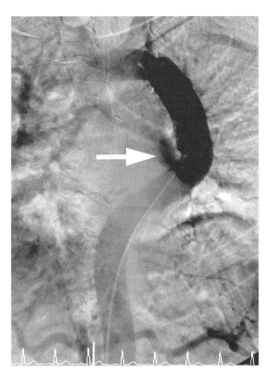

**Figure 3** An angiogram showing an aortobronchial fistula. The arrow shows the fistulous tract.

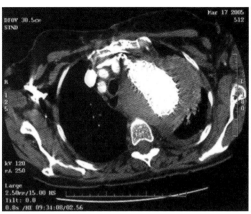

**Figure 5** An axial CT image demonstrating exclusion of ABF by thoracic endoluminal stent graft.

and less invasive repair of ABF particularly in patients with prohibitive surgical risks [6–8]. A differential diagnosis of an aortobronchial fistula should be given serious consideration if a patient presents with hemoptysis and a history of thoracic aortic surgery. Chest radiography, CT scan of chest, aortography, bronchoscopy, chest magnetic imaging, transesophageal echocardiogram, and intravascular ultrasound are all imaging modalities that

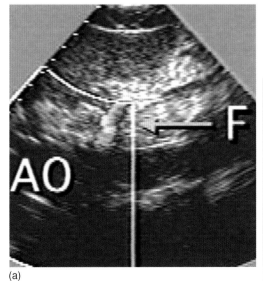

(a)

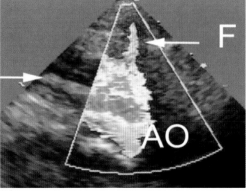

(b)

**Figure 4** (a) Intraoperative transesophageal echocardiogram (TEE) in longitudinal view demonstrating extraluminal flow from the aortic lumen (AO) through the fistulous tract (F) (yellow arrow). (b) Intraoperative TEE in longitudinal view demonstrating extraluminal flow from the aortic lumen (AO) through the fistulous tract (F) prior to endoluminal graft deployment.

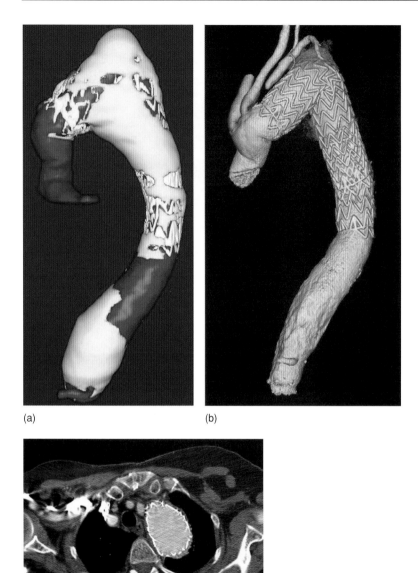

(a)                                        (b)

(c)

**Figure 6** (a–c) Axial and reformatted CT scan of the chest showing the thoracic arch with the start of the defect highlighted along with the accompanying 3-D reconstruction at the 18-month follow-up visit.

have been used to detect a fistulous tract. All the imaging modalities have their limitations. The risk of open operation for ABF is high due to emergency conditions, difficult redo operations, and the possibility of infectious complications. In ABF, there is usually a communication between the previous aortic graft and the tracheobronchial tree. Conventionally, open surgical correction involves a thoracotomy and carries a fairly high morbidity and mortality due to the difficulty of operative dissection. Physiologic stresses of an open repair can be complicated by active hemorrhage and pulmonary compromise, paralysis, renal failure, and cardiac events. In a 2002 literature review, Piciche *et al.* [9] found 76 cases of ABF; 52 were treated with conventional open graft repair (15.3% mortality) and 15 were treated with a stent graft (6.6% mortality). The specter of reoperation when added to the extensive list of patient comorbidities and potential complications of the open procedure makes an endovascular route look more attractive. In our experience, we have treated 7 patients with ABF with no perioperative mortality. Intraoperative TEE proved to be an invaluable tool due to its ability to demonstrate a breach of blood flow from the aortic graft into the pseudoaneurysm as well as the fistulous tract in all our patients. TEE was our most reliable imaging test for our patients and also permitted us to guide the device into accurate placement [10]. Cultures in all our patients have been negative. The role of long-term antibiotics for postprocedure endoluminal graft patients is a topic of hot debate due to the possibility of graft infection. Our current philosophy is an extended course of antibiotics for 6 weeks postprocedure.

Although long-term results of endovascular repair are lacking, stent-graft repair of ABF is our preferred treatment due to the avoidance of aortic cross clamping, thoracotomy, extracorporeal circulation as well as the potential hemodynamic instability that is inherent with an open repair.

## References

1 Leobon B, Roux D, Mugniot A *et al.* Endovascular treatment of thoracic aortic fistulas. *Ann Thorac Surg* 2002; **74**: 247–249.

2 Macintosh EL, Parrott JC, Unruh HW. Fistulas between the aorta and tracheobronchial tree. *Ann Thorac Surg* 1991; **51**: 515–519.

3 Svenson LG, Patel V, Robinson MF. Variables predictive of outcome in 832 patients undergoing repairs of the descending thoracic aorta. *Chest* 1993; **104**: 1248–1253.

4 Makaroun MS, Dillavou ED, Kes ST *et al.* Endovascular treatment of thoracic aortic aneurysms: results of the phase II multicenter trial of the Gore TAG thoracic endoprosthesis. *J Vasc Surg* 2005; **41**: 1–9.

5 Greenberg R, Resch T, Nyman U *et al.* Endovascular repair of descending thoracic aortic aneurysm: an early experience with intermediate-term follow-up. *J Vasc Surg* 2000; **31**: 147–156.

6 Karmy-Jones R, Lee CA, Nicholls SC, Hoffer E. Management of aortobronchial fistula with an aortic stent-graft. *Chest* 1999; **116**: 255–257.

7 Chuter TA, Ivancev K, Lindblad B, Brunkwall J, Aren C, Risberg B. Endovascular stent-graft exclusion of an aortobronchial fistula. *J Vasc Interv Radiol* 1996; **7**: 357–359.

8 Von Segesser LK, Tkebuchava T, Niederhauser U *et al.* Aortobronchial and aortoesophageal fistulae as risk factors in surgery of descending thoracic aortic aneurysms. *Eur J Cardiothorac Surg* 1997; **12**: 195–201.

9 Piciche M, DePaulis R, Fabbri A *et al.* Postoperative aortic fistulas into the airways: etiology, pathogenesis, presentation, diagnosis and management. *Ann Thorac* 2003; **75**: 1998–2006.

10 Thomson CS, Ramaiah VG, Rodriguez-Lopez JA *et al.* Endovascular stent graft repair of aortobrochial fistula. *J Vasc Surg* 2002; **35**: 387–391.

## SECTION X

# Complications of thoracic aortic endografting

# Endovascular management of a type I endoleak

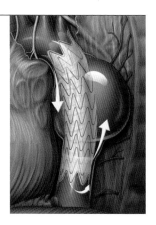

## Introduction

Endoleaks are defined as blood flow outside the lumen of the stent graft but within the aneurysm sac. Risk factors for developing endoleaks include an aortic implantation zone of less than 2 cm from the left subclavian artery and existence of an entry tear at the lesser curvature of the arch aorta [1]. Development of a type I endoleaks after thoracic aortic aneurysm (TAA) repair is associated with aneurysmal sac expansion and a potential rupture of the sac.

## Case scenario

A 76-year-old asymptomatic man had an endoluminal graft placed for a TAA measuring 6.0 cm approximately 2 years ago. Following a set follow-up schedule, the patient underwent periodic CT scans of the chest with and without contrast dye. At his last visit CT scan, flow was identified within the aneurysm sac and the maximum diameter had increased to 6.4 cm. With the combination of these two high-risk factors, he was scheduled for an elective repair of the distal type I endoleak (Figure 1a and 1b) as demonstrated on 64-slice CT images.

## Procedure

Under general anesthesia, open retrograde cannulation of the right common femoral artery was performed with an 18-G (Cook Inc., Bloomington, IN) needle and 0.035-in. soft-tip angled glide wire (Medi-tech/Boston Scientific, Natick, MA) was

passed into the aorta and exchanged to a 9-F (French) sheath after 5000 units of heparin were given.

Percutaneous access of the left common femoral artery was similarly performed and a 9-F sheath was introduced. A 5-F pigtail angiographic catheter was advanced through the left groin sheath into the thoracic aorta. The fluoroscopic C-arm was positioned in a left anterior oblique angle and an oblique thoracic arch aortogram was performed to visualize the orifices of the arch vessels and the descending TAA. An oblique thoracic arch aortogram performed demonstrated the type I distal endoleak (Figure 2). An adequate landing zone was identified distal to the endograft for possible deployment of a short endograft up to the level of the celiac trunk. Intravascular ultrasound (IVUS) was performed using an 8.2-F probe (Volcano Therapeutics, Inc., Rancho Cordova, CA) through the right groin sheath to determine the distal landing zone diameter. A distal neck of 37 mm was measured. The IVUS probe was exchanged for an extra-stiff Lunderquist wire (Cook Inc., Bloomington, IN). Based on the IVUS measurements, a 40 mm × 10 cm Gore TAG graft (W.L. Gore & Associates, Flagstaff, AZ) was chosen to be deployed distal to the previously placed endoluminal graft.

The right 9-F sheath was exchanged for a 24-F sheath and a 40 mm × 10 cm Gore TAG stent-graft device was advanced through the Gore sheath. An anterior–posterior thoracic aortogram was performed and a road map obtained with a guiding needle placed at the level of the celiac trunk. A 40 mm × 10 cm Gore TAG graft was deployed distally

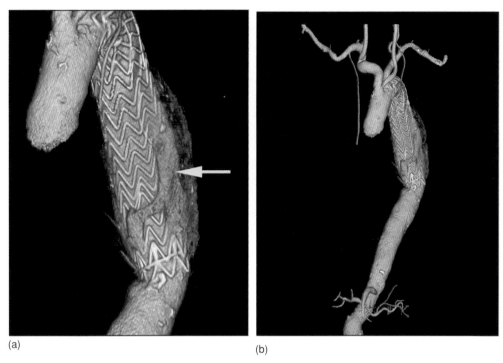

(a)

(b)

**Figure 1** (a and b) Reconstruction of a 64-slice CT scan of the chest shows the placement of the endoluminal graft with a type I distal endoleak (arrow).

making sure we had about 5 cm of overlap between grafts and also making sure the celiac trunk was not covered. A Gore trilobe balloon was exchanged for the device's delivery catheter through the right groin

sheath and a postdeployment balloon angioplasty was conducted. A completion angiogram showed complete exclusion of the aneurysm (Figure 3). All wires and sheaths were removed from the right

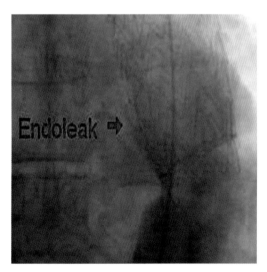

**Figure 2** An angiogram demonstrates a type I distal endoleak.

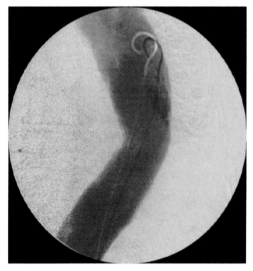

**Figure 3** A completion angiogram demonstrates resolution of distal endoleak.

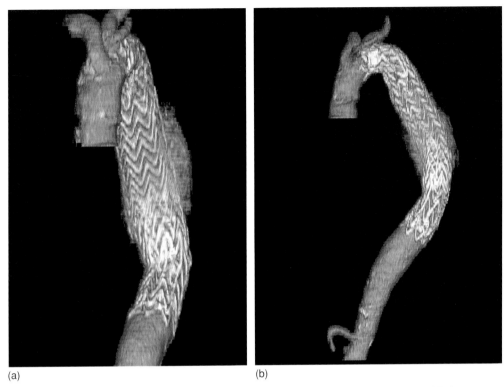

(a)                                                    (b)

**Figure 4** (a and b) 3-D reconstruction images demonstrate satisfactory exclusion of the type I distal endoleak.

common femoral artery, with the artery closed in a transverse fashion with restoration of flow. A 6-F angioseal vascular closure device (St. Jude Medical, Inc., St. Paul, MN) was deployed to the left common femoral artery. Patient who had bilateral palpable pulses at the end of the procedure was extubated and transferred to recovery room. A CT scan conducted prior to discharge showed resolution of the type I endoleak with satisfactory exclusion of TAA (Figure 4a and 4b).

## Discussion

Open surgical repair of thoracic aortic pathologies requires aortic cross clamping, use of extracorporeal circulation, hypothermia, and sometimes circulatory arrest. The morbidity and mortality associated with open surgical repair may be higher in high-risk patients and the elderly requiring alternative less invasive approach. The use of an endoluminal graft for the treatment of thoracic aortic pathologies is associated with a decrease in morbidity, mortality, and

paraplegia when compared to open surgical repair [2–6]. In March 2005, the Federal Drug Administration approved the use of endoluminal grafts for the treatment of TAAs. Although minimal imaging is required after open surgical repair, patients undergoing endovascular TAA repair require lifelong postoperative surveillance imaging with CT scans [2–7] to evaluate for the diameter of the aneurysm, the detection of stent-graft migration or fracture, and the presence of endoleaks [8, 9].

Type I endoleaks represent the most common type of endoleak seen after endovascular TAA repair and its reported incidence varies from 0 to 44% [10–12]. This type of endoleak represents a failure for the endoluminal graft to be fully apposed to the arterial wall. When this happens, active arterial flow is able to seep into the aneurysm sac and keep it somewhat pressurized. Computed tomography angiography (CTA) has been the primary imaging modality for postoperative surveillance of endoleaks. At our institution, CTA is performed at 30 days, 6 months, and then annually for the life of the patient. Magnetic resonance angiography may also be used for postprocedure surveillance when magnetic resonance compatible stent grafts are used for the TAA repair.

Type I endoleaks are classified on CTA according to the location of the endoleak in contiguity with the proximal or distal attachment site, as well as their ability to fill the aneurysm sac. Catheter angiography can be performed to confirm the diagnosis. Type I endoleaks are more prevalent in the thoracic aorta than in the abdominal aorta due to the angled nature of the proximal attachment in the aortic arch and the frequently short attachment zones, which present a sealing challenge. Type I leaks are often seen during completion angiography or on the initial CT scan after operative repair. They can appear later as a result of migration or failure of the metallic elements within the attachment.

The importance of type I endoleaks are still debatable, as some authors believe there is spontaneous healing of type I endoleaks. Lepore *et al.* [12] reported 7 patients (16%) with a type I endoleak among 43 thoracic aortic stent grafts. Three patients were treated with additional stent grafts and the rest resolved spontaneously at the 1-month follow-up. Shimono *et al.* also reported an 80% spontaneous resolution of type I endoleaks in 37 stent grafts for aortic dissections [13]. The current consensus of authors [14–16] believe that failure of proximal or distal sealing can be expected to result in the persistence of systemic pressure to the aneurysm sac, with less sac regression thus leaving the patient unprotected from the possibility of fatal rupture of the aneurysm. Type I endoleaks can be corrected by securing the attachment sites. Initial attempts at type I endoleak repairs are initially made with angioplasty balloons. These large-diameter balloons are used to ensure that the stents are fully expanded at both their proximal and distal fixation points, thus encouraging them to conform to the vessel wall. Balloon inflation within the thoracic aorta produces significant hemodynamic shifts and requires careful monitoring and regulation of the blood pressure during the inflation interval. The use of a balloon that does not tamponade flow through the aorta by the means of its trilobe design is the Gore trilobe balloon (W.L. Gore & Associates, Flagstaff, AZ). It can decrease this hemodynamic effect but it does not totally eliminate it. We also use the Cook Coda balloon in our

operating rooms due its ability to be quickly inflated and deflated minimizing the effect of circulatory occlusion. Balloon-mounted bare metal stents or stent-graft extensions can be used to secure the proximal or distal attachment sites (Figure 1). If there is persistence of a type I endoleak despite balloon angioplasty of the fixation points of the endoluminal grafts, then the use of bare stents can be a useful option when the device position is acceptable in the sealing zone, but the vessel wall contact is insufficient. Bare stents are useful when the device position is acceptable in the sealing zone, but the vessel wall contact is insufficient. Balloon expandable stents provide greater radial force than do self-expanding stents, which are contained in the stent graft itself. If, conversely, the device does not fully cover the allotted seal zone, the use of a supplemental extension stent graft is preferred to take full advantage of the entire available aorta in which a seal may be accomplished. Because of the lack of available large-diameter balloon-expandable bare stents, the placement of stent grafts of large diameter within each other can also be performed to increase the sealing force of a failed attachment zone. If the type I endoleak cannot be resolved by endovascular means, open conversion should be considered, because this leak is considered virulent and the patient would not be expected to be protected against aneurysm rupture.

## References

1 Palmer RS, Kotsis T, Gorich J, Kapfer X, Orend KH, Plassman LS. Complications after endovascular repair of type B aortic dissection. *J Endovasc Ther* 2002; **9**: 822–828.

2 Morishita K, Kurimoto Y, Kawaharada N et al. Descending thoracic aortic rupture (role of endovascular stent-grafting). *Ann Thorac Surg* 2004; **78**: 1630–1634.

3 Makaroun M, Dillavou E, Kee S et al. Endovascular treatment of thoracic aortic aneurysms (results of the phase II multicenter trial of the GORE TAG thoracic endoprosthesis). *J Vasc Surg* 2005; **41**: 1–9.

4 Leurs L, Bell R, Degrieck Y, Thomas S, Hobo R, Lundbom J. Endovascular treatment of thoracic aortic diseases (combined experience from the EUROSTAR and United Kingdom Thoracic Endograft registries). *J Vasc Surg* 2004; **40**: 670–680.

5 Bortone A, DeCillis E, D'Agostino D, de Luca TSL. Endovascular treatment of thoracic aortic disease, four years

of experience. *Circulation* 2004; **110**(Suppl 2): II262–II267.

6 Brandt M, Hussel K, Walluscheck K *et al.* Stent-graft repair versus open surgery for the descending aorta (a case-control study). *J Endovasc Ther* 2004; **11**: 535–538.

7 Hansen C, Bui H, Donayre C *et al.* Complications of endovascular repair of high-risk and emergent descending thoracic aortic aneurysms and dissections. *J Vasc Surg* 2004; **40**: 228–234.

8 Grabenwoger M, Fleck T, Ehrlich M *et al.* Secondary surgical interventions after endovascular stent-grafting of the thoracic aorta. *Eur J Cardiothorac Surg* 2004; **26**: 608–613.

9 Barkhordarian R, Kyriakides C, Mayet J, Clark M, Cheshire N. Transoesophageal echocardiogram identifying the source of endoleak after combined open/endovascular repair of a type III thoracoabdominal aortic aneurysm. *Ann Vasc Surg* 2004; **18**: 264–269.

10 Czemark V, Waldenerger P, Perkmann R *et al.* Placement of endovascular stent grafts for emergency treatment of acute diseases of the descending thoracic aorta. *Am J Roentgenol* **179**: 337–345.

11 Gorich J, Asquan Y, Seifarth H. Initial experience with intentional stent graft coverage of the subclavian artery during endovascular thoracic aortic repairs. *Endovasc Ther* 2002; **9**(Suppl): 1139–1143.

12 Lepore V, Loonn L, Delle M *et al.* Endograft therapy for diseases of the descending thoracic aorta: results in 43 high risk patients. *Endovasc Ther* 2002; **9**: 829–837.

13 Shimono T, Kato N, Yasuda F *et al.* Transluminal stent graft placement for the treatment of acute onset and chronic aortic dissections. *Circulation* 2002; **106**(Suppl): 1241–1247.

14 Parmer SS, Carpenter JP, Stavropoulos W *et al.* Endoleaks after endovascular repair of thoracic aortic aneurysms. *J Vasc Surg* 2006; **44**: 447–452.

15 Veith FJ, Baum RA, Ohki T *et al.* Nature and significance of endoleaks and endotension (summary of opinions expressed at an international conference). *J Vasc Surg* 2002; **35**: 1029–1035.

16 Mennander A, Pimenoff G, Heikkinen M, Partio T, Zeitlin R, Salenius JP. Nonoperative approach to endotension. *J Vasc Surg* 2005; **42**: 194–198.

# Endovascular management of a type II endoleak

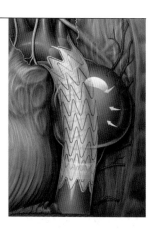

## Introduction

Endoleaks are defined as blood flow outside the lumen of a stent graft but within the aneurysm sac. Type II endoleaks can result from retrograde flow from a covered artery (i.e., left subclavian artery) into the aneurysm sac or when blood travels through branches from the nonstented portion of the aorta through anastomotic connections into vessels with a direct communication with the aneurysm sac. When compared to the endoleak percentages of abdominal endoluminal grafts, the type II endoleak of the thoracic grafts is less common. Type II endoleaks can be classified with computed tomography angiography if the endoleak sac cannot be seen communicating with the distal or the proximal attachment site or if there was delayed enhancement of the aneurysm sac.

## Case scenario

This is a 68-year-old woman who recently underwent a hybrid debranching of the left common carotid and innominate artery followed by deployment of an endoluminal graft to exclude an arch pseudoaneurysm. A CT scan conducted approximately 1 month after the procedure indicated the possibility of a type II endoleak. Images from the CT scan were put through an imaging software program that allowed a 3-D model to be built. Upon studying the model, it was definitive that the leak was coming from the covered left subclavian artery (Figure 1a and 1b). Doctors were hopeful for a spontaneous resolution of the endoleak. A repeat CT scan done 2 months later showed that the leak was still present and that no regression of the aneurysm sac size had taken place. She was referred to surgery to fully exclude the aneurysm from pressurized arterial blood flow.

## Procedural details

Bilateral radial arterial lines were placed with both arterial lines demonstrating no gradient. The patient was subsequently placed under general anesthesia.

A left open retrograde approach was used to cannulate the left brachial artery with a 35-cm 6-F (French) sheath. Heparin was given to achieve an activated time greater than 200 seconds. A 5-F pigtail catheter was advanced over a 180-cm soft-tip angled glide wire trough the left brachial sheath and a selective left subclavian artery arch angiogram demonstrated the type II endoleak (Figure 2). A Bereinstein catheter was exchanged for the 5-F angiographic pigtail catheter and a couple of 15 mm × 15 cm Cook coils (Cook Inc., Bloomington, IN) were deployed in the ostium of the left subclavian artery with care not to coil embolize the left vertebral artery in the process. Upon embolization, there was a noticeable drop in the left radial arterial line pressure with flattening of the pressure wave form. A completion angiogram demonstrated satisfactory repair of the type II endoleak from the left subclavian artery origin (Figure 3). A postoperative CT scan confirmed these results (Figure 4a and 4b).

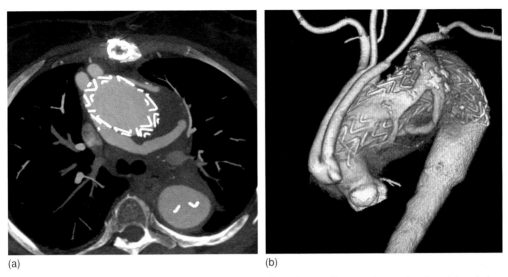

(a)                              (b)

**Figure 1** (a and b) An axial and 3-D reconstruction image taken from the scan illustrates how a virtual model can help evaluate the etiology of endoleaks.

## Discussion

The occurrence of endoleaks after endovascular repair of thoracic aortic aneurysms remains one of the principal concerns of thoracic endografting. Endoleak detection requires rigorous follow-up with high-quality imaging. A CT scan is currently the most widely used imaging modality for endoleak detection, although magnetic resonance angiography and transesophageal echocardiogram also play a significant role in device surveillance.

Most type II endoleaks are recognized early on the initial postintervention CT scan with late

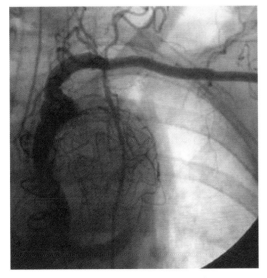

**Figure 2** A selective left subclavian artery angiogram demonstrating retrograde filling of the aneurysm sac compatible with the definition of a type II endoleak.

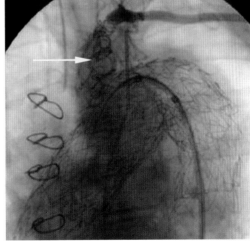

**Figure 3** An angiogram showing a series of embolization coils that were deployed to treat the type II endoleak.

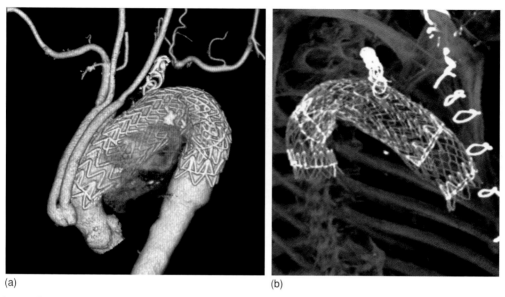

(a)                                                                                           (b)

**Figure 4** (a and b) A 3-D model created after the endoleak repair shows a significant improvement in the exclusion of the aneurysm sac.

appearance of type II endoleaks a rarity. Most type II endoleaks will spontaneously thrombose resulting in increased stability or regression of the aneurysmal sac [1–9]. Common criteria for determining if action is warranted for an endoleak would be signs of aneurysm expansion or increased endotension. Fortunately, the majority of endoleaks can be fixed through an endovascular means and rarely require an open conversion. The preferred method for the treatment of a confirmed type II endoleak is a coil embolization of the offending artery. Coil embolization using coils and *n*-butyl cyanoacrylate (Trufill, Cordis, Miami, FL) can be performed percutaneously through a transthoracic approach if a safe window into the aneurysm can be identified.

Transarterial and transthoracic embolization are additional techniques that can be used to treat type II endoleaks. Conducting a direct transthoracic puncture is a procedure that comes with risks that are not limited to a pneumothorax or some other lung injury that makes this method riskier when compared to a translumbar puncture and embolization. This finding was documented in the abdominal endoluminal graft population [9, 10].

For specific type II endoleaks involving the left subclavian artery, a new series of products are becoming available to use. Embolization coils rely on decreasing the circulation of the blood to the point where the blood will begin to clot. The use of coils usually takes multiple administrations. The danger with coil embolization is that a stray coil may migrate and cause problems downstream from the intended target site. Larger-diameter vessels now can be treated with a class of products called vascular plugs. Originally used to occlude iliac arteries when used in combination with aortomonoiliac endoluminal grafts, these products essentially dam the blood from getting past them. Current vascular plugs available on the commercial market come from AGA Medical (Amplatzer) or from Cook Medical in their Zenith accessory kit.

Complications from thoracic endoluminal grafts that involve the continued pressurization of an aneurysm are a topic for great concern. The diagnosis of one type of endoleak, the type II accessory vessel leak, requires high-quality imaging and a thorough understanding of the anatomy. The presence of the leak is not one of great concern but of careful surveillance. Should clinical measurements or a patient request mandate treatment, the treatment of such an endoleak can be done through the preferred endovascular method.

# References

1  Makaroun M, Dillavou E, Kee S *et al.* Endovascular treatment of thoracic aortic aneurysms (results of the phase II multicenter trial of the GORE TAG thoracic endoprosthesis). *J Vasc Surg* 2005; **41**: 1–9.

2  Leurs L, Bell R, Degrieck Y, Thomas S, Hobo R, Lundbom J. Endovascular treatment of thoracic aortic diseases (combined experience from the EUROSTAR and United Kingdom Thoracic Endograft registries). *J Vasc Surg* 2004; **40**: 670–680.

3  Farber M, Criado F, Hill C. Endovascular repair of nontraumatic ruptured thoracic aortic pathologies. *Ann Vasc Surg* 2005; **19**: 167–171.

4  Bortone A, DeCillis E, D'Agostino D, de Luca TSL. Endovascular treatment of thoracic aortic disease, four years of experience. *Circulation* 2004; **110**(Suppl 2): II262–II267.

5  Brandt M, Hussel K, Walluscheck K *et al.* Stent-graft repair versus open surgery for the descending aorta (a case-control study). *J Endovasc Ther* 2004; **11**: 535–538.

6  Hansen C, Bui H, Donayre C *et al.* Complications of endovascular repair of high-risk and emergent descending thoracic aortic aneurysms and dissections. *J Vasc Surg* 2004; **40**: 228–234.

7  Grabenwoger M, Fleck T, Ehrlich M *et al.* Secondary surgical interventions after endovascular stent-grafting of the thoracic aorta. *Eur J Cardiothorac Surg* 2004; **26**: 608–613.

8  Barkhordarian R, Kyriakides C, Mayet J, Clark M, Cheshire N. Transoesophageal echocardiogram identifying the source of endoleak after combined open/endovascular repair of a type 3 thoracoabdominal aortic aneurysm. *Ann Vasc Surg* 2004; **18**: 264–269.

9  Baum R, Stavropoulos S, Fairman R, Carpenter J. Endoleaks after endovascular repair of abdominal aortic aneurysms. *J Vasc Interv Radiol* 2003; **14**: 1111–1117.

10  Veith FJ, Baum RA, Ohki T *et al.* Nature and significance of endoleaks and endotension (summary of opinions expressed at an international conference). *J Vasc Surg* 2002; **35**: 1029–1035.

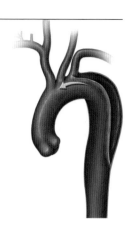

# Retrograde dissection following endovascular management of thoracic aortic aneurysm

## Introduction

Thoracic endografting has recently been approved by the Food and Drug Administration in the United States for the treatment of thoracic aortic aneurysms (TAAs) (1). The first thoracic stent graft for the treatment of TAA was reported by Dake *et al.* (2). A 30-day analysis on the use of endoluminal grafts revealed a statistically significant lower incidence of the following complications in the endovascular cohort versus the surgical cohort: spinal cord ischemia respiratory failure, renal insufficiency, and peripheral vascular complications (3). Retrograde dissection is a rare but fatal complication from stent grafting. Possible etiologies may include balloon dilation, stent oversizing, and the use of bare spring semirigid stents. We describe a case of retrograde dissection following stent-graft therapy for a thoracic aneurysm.

## Case scenario

A 73-year-old female with a past medical history significant for hypertension and coronary artery disease presented with a 5.8-cm TAA. Due to multiple surgical comorbidities, she was felt to be at an increased risk for open surgical repair. She was therefore felt to be a good candidate for a thoracic endoluminal graft. A CT scan of the chest was conducted to evaluate her candidacy for the procedure and take measurements for the sizing of then endoluminal graft (Figure 1a–1c). The area above the

aneurysm was measured in an oblique, cross section view using a 3-D reconstruction program to negate the effect of angulation. Measurements from this modality showed that the aorta was approximately 29 mm in diameter. Intravascular ultrasound conducted in the operating room measured the same area to be 34 mm in width. With conflicting measurements, the larger measurement was used and a 37 mm × 20 cm endoluminal graft was deployed.

## Technical details of endoluminal graft deployment

Open retrograde cannulation of the right common femoral artery using an 18-G needle was performed; a 9-F (French) sheath was introduced over a 0.035-in. soft-tip angled glide wire. Percutaneous retrograde access of the left common femoral artery was similarly performed and a 5-F sheath was introduced. An oblique thoracic aortogram was performed using a pigtail from the 5-F sheath which demonstrated the TAA (Figure 2). Intravascular ultrasound performed through the 9-F sheath was used to determine the proximal neck diameter which we measured 34 mm. This was in contrast to the 29-mm measured on axial CT scan (Figure 1a). All device manufacturers require that measurements for their devices be done off CT scans. Intravascular ultrasound is a relatively new modality that can be subjective and needs further validation before it becomes as widely accepted as CT

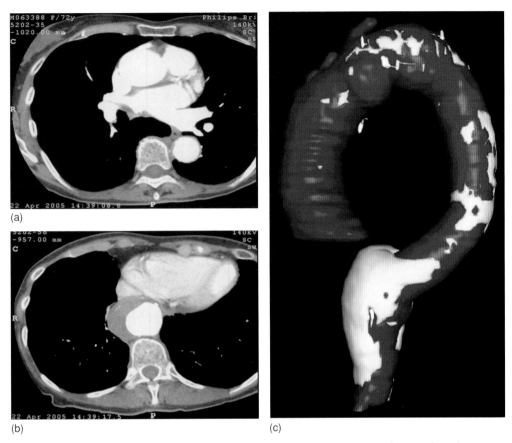

**Figure 1** (a) A preoperative CT scan chest demonstrating an aortic diameter of about 29-mm diameter above the aneurysm. (b) Axial CT images demonstrating an aneurysm measuring 5.8 cm. (c) A 3-D reconstruction of the thoracic aorta.

scans for measurements. Based on our site's familiarity with this technology, the device was sized off the ultrasound's measurements. A 9-F sheath in the right common femoral artery was exchanged to a 24-F Gore sheath. A 37 mm × 15 cm Gore TAG device (W.L. Gore & Associates, Flagstaff, AZ) was deployed to exclude the aneurysm. A completion aortogram demonstrated no endoleak. Wires and sheaths were removed and the right common femoral artery was repaired with a closure device deployed to the left common femoral artery.

On the first postoperative day, the patient started to complain of severe chest pain with her blood pressure continuing to be hypotensive in nature. A CT scan of the chest was immediately performed showing the retrograde dissection into the arch and ascending aorta (Figure 3a–3c). The patient went into cardiac arrest on her way to surgery and could not be successfully revived.

## Discussion

Retrograde dissection following stent grafting for repair of TAA is a rare complication. Most reported cases to date show a strong association with stent-graft treatment of type B dissection (4–10). Possible etiologic factors in the treatment of TAA may include stent oversizing greater than 10% of indication for use. Oversizing of stent grafts is necessary to produce enough radial force for stent-graft apposition to the aortic wall. If the measurements from the CT scan in this particular case were indeed accurate, then the endoluminal graft would have been oversized by 27.4% for the area above the aneurysm. The amount of the oversizing would have well

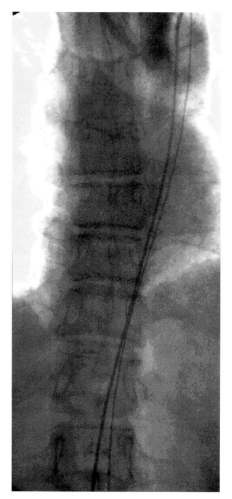

**Figure 2** An angiogram demonstrates a TAA.

exceeded the device manufacturer's guidelines. Events like this one may cause intimal tears in patients with fragile aortic walls or may promote the collapse of the graft (Figure 4).

Procedure-related complications from wires and sheath manipulation in the aortic arch during the endovascular procedure may cause localized intimal tears which could propagate to frank dissection. Device-related complications may arise from the use of semirigid designed grafts not able to adapt perfectly to the aortic curve in an angulated aortic arch. Stent grafts with bare springs used for anchoring at their proximal ends can create new intimal tears (11). Aggressive balloon dilatation of the aorta may cause intimal injuries which again can be a precursor for frank dissection.

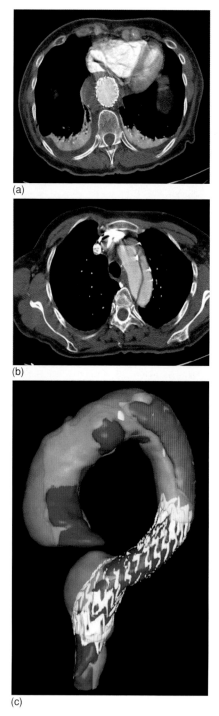

**Figure 3** (a and b) A CT scan taken on the first postoperative day showing endoluminal exclusion of the aneurysm with a retrograde dissection involving the arch. (c) Reconstructed image demonstrates retrograde type B dissection from an exclusion of a TAA with an endoluminal graft.

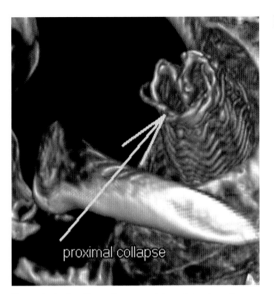

**Figure 4** Graft collapse from oversizing of stent graft.

Mortality as a result of retrograde dissection is high. Between 1998 and 2007, we treated 512 patients with thoracic stent grafts, 8 patients developed a retrograde dissection with 6 patients treated for a type dissection and only 1 patient treated for a TAA. The mortality was 62.5% ($n = 5$), with 3 patients dying perioperatively. The 3 survivors required replacement of the ascending aorta.

Better patient selection, precise stent-graft deployment, avoidance of oversizing, and less aggressive balloon dilation whenever possible may help to prevent these complications. This study also highlights the importance of serial surveillance following endoluminal graft repair of the descending thoracic aorta.

## References

1 Makaroun MS, Dillavou ED, Kes ST *et al.* Endovascular treatment of thoracic aortic aneurysms: results of the phase II multicenter trial of the Gore TAG thoracic endoprosthesis. *J Vasc Surg* 2005; **41**: 1–9.

2 Dake MD, Miller DC, Semba CP *et al.* Transluminal placement of endovascular stent-grafts for the treatment of descending thoracic aortic aneurysms. *N Engl J Med* 1994; **331**: 1729–1734.

3 Kasirajan K, Milner R, Chaikof E. Late complications of thoracic endografts. *J Vasc Surg* 2006; **43**: 94A–99A.

4 Totaro M, Miraldi F, Fanelli F *et al.* Emergency surgery for retrograde extension of type B dissection after endovascular stent graft repair. *Eur J Cardiothorac Surg* 2001; **20**: 1057–1058.

5 Fanelli F, Salvatori FM, Marcelli G *et al.* Type A aortic dissection developing during endovascular repair of an acute type B dissection. *J Endovasc Ther* 2003; **10**: 254–259.

6 Nienaber CA, Eagle KA. Aortic dissection: new frontiers in diagnosis and management. Part II: Therapeutic management and follow-up. *Circulation* 2003; **108**: 772–778.

7 Pasic M, Bergs P, Knollmann F *et al.* Delayed retrograde aortic dissection after endovascular stenting of the descending thoracic aorta. *J Vasc Surg* 2002; **36**: 184–186.

8 Grabenwoger M, Fleck T, Ehrlich M *et al.* Secondary surgical interventions after endovascular stent-grafting of the thoracic aorta. *Eur J Cardiothorac Surg* 2004; **26**: 608–613.

9 Bethuyne N, Bove T, Van den Brande P *et al.* Acute retrograde aortic dissection during endovascular repair of a thoracic aortic aneurysm. *Ann Thorac Surg* 2003; **75**: 1967–1969.

10 Misfeld M, Notzold A, Geist V *et al.* Retrograde type A dissection after endovascular stent grafting of type B dissection [in German]. *Z Kardiol* 2002; **91**: 274–277.

11 Criado FJ. Bare springs thoracic endograft: the balloon stops here. *J Endovasc Ther* 2003; **10**: 932.

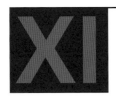

## SECTION XI

# Ascending aortic pathologies

# Endovascular management of an ascending aortic pseudoaneurysm

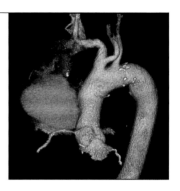

## Introduction

Ascending aorta pseudoaneurysms are rare and occur infrequently from traumatic causes, infectious causes, anastomotic dehiscence of suture lines, and cannulation sites from previous aortic surgery [1]. Pseudoaneurysms of the ascending aorta are occasionally picked up on routine imaging for other causes. Computed tomography and angiography are the most common forms of diagnosis. A recent magnetic resonance imaging study found a pseudoaneurysm incidence of 13% associated with ascending aortic replacement [2]. Pseudoaneurysms of the ascending aorta are prone to rupture with fatal complications including death from pericardial tamponade, free rupture into the mediastinum, compressive symptoms of dyspnea, vocal cord paresis or paralysis, and pain. Indications for repair include compressive symptoms relating to the size of aneurysm and a maximum diameter of greater than 5.0 cm. The standard treatment involves replacing the diseased portion of the aorta with a Dacron patch that can sometimes require cardiopulmonary bypass. A redo median sternotomy offers a higher surgical risk to the patient and may be associated with a higher morbidity and mortality. Hybrid interventions involving both open surgical and endovascular techniques have been reported [3–10] to treat high-risk surgical patients with success. A complete endovascular repair of ascending aortic pseudoaneurysms is an attractive option that can be offered in high-surgical-risk patients with suitable indications and amenable anatomy.

## Case scenario

A 74-year-old male with a past medical history significant for atrial fibrillation and pacemaker insertion was referred to our clinic to explore his options of an endovascular repair of his condition. After the pacemaker implant, he developed an infective endocarditis of his mitral valve apparatus requiring replacement with mechanical valve prosthesis. His postoperative course was complicated by sternal wound dehiscence requiring extensive debridement of the sternum with a pectoral muscle flap reconstruction. Approximately 2 months after his mitral valve replacement, he developed fever and chills with blood cultures coming back positive. He was again diagnosed with a prosthetic valve infective endocarditis. A second mitral valve replacement was conducted using a porcine valve through a right thoracotomy with his postoperative course uneventful until 5 months after this most recent procedure. The patient was starting to complain of periodic episodes of chest discomfort. A chest X-ray revealed a mass on the ascending aorta suspicious for a pseudoaneurysm. A CT scan of the chest was performed which demonstrated a large pseudoaneurysm arising from the anterior aspect of the ascending aorta (Figure 1). The pseudoaneurysm measured 7.6 cm × 8.0 cm and was thought to have originated from the cardioplegia site. Using reconstruction software, the specific defect was identified with its width measuring 8 mm. He was felt to be at an extreme risk for an open surgical repair and was consented for the use of an endovascular device in an off-label fashion.

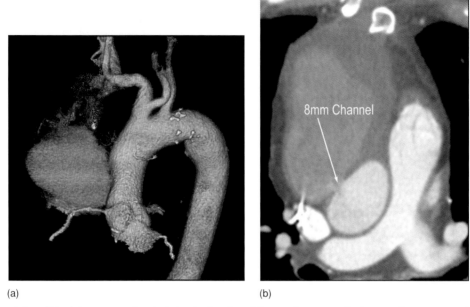

(a)                                          (b)

**Figure 1** (a and b) A 3-D reconstruction depicting the location of the pseudoaneurysm in the ascending aorta. An oblique view of the same region shows the measurement of the defect.

## Endovascular approach

The left common femoral artery was exposed and open retrograde cannulation using an 18-G needle was done. The patient was heparinized and a sheath inserted to maintain wire access. Percutaneous retrograde cannulation of the right common femoral artery was performed with an 18-G needle and similarly a 0.035-in. soft-tip angled glide wire was advanced into the thoracic aorta and a 5-F sheath exchanged. A 5-F pigtail angiographic catheter was advanced to the ascending aorta where the anatomy was documented with an aortogram (Figure 2a). The glide wire was maneuvered so that

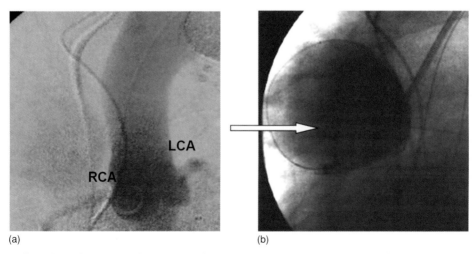

(a)                                          (b)

**Figure 2** (a and b) Dual angiograms demonstrating the ascending aorta pseudoaneurysm (arrow) as well as the right (RCA) and left coronary (LCA) arteries.

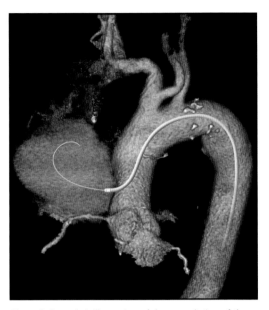

**Figure 3** An artist's illustration of the cannulation of the pseudoaneurysm.

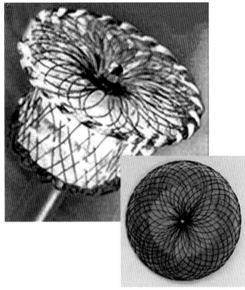

**Figure 4** An Amplatzer septal occluder used to close the neck of the pseudoaneurysm.

it transversed the defect and was now in the pseudoaneurysm sac. An aortogram of the sac was conducted to document all potential entry and exit points (Figure 2b). An intravascular ultrasound (IVUS) probe was loaded on the wire and the probe advanced to the area of the defect. The width of the defect as measured by IVUS was in agreement with measurements from the CT scan (Figure 3). The defect was 2-cm away from the right coronary artery, and with the confirmed neck diameter of 8 mm the patient was evaluated to be eligible to receive a septal occluder to exclude the pseudoaneurysm sac. From the left groin, an Amplatzer septal occluder (AGA Medical Corporation, Golden Valley, MN) was advanced and deployed across the aortic pseudoaneurysm under fluoroscopic control (Figure 4). The completion aortogram showed good position of the occluder device and minimal leak through the device (Figure 5). The bilateral groins were closed in the usual fashion and the patient was transferred to the recovery room. His postoperative CT scans revealed complete occlusion of the neck of the pseudoaneurysm (Figure 6a, 6b, and 6c). He was discharged home in stable condition. Since the surgery, he has not had any complications or significant medical events. Surveillance imaging

indicates that the pseudoaneurysm is starting to regress in size with no evidence of arterial filling (Figure 7).

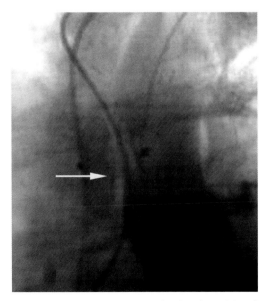

**Figure 5** A completion angiogram showing the position of the Amplatzer with a slight blush of contrast in the pseudoaneurysm sac.

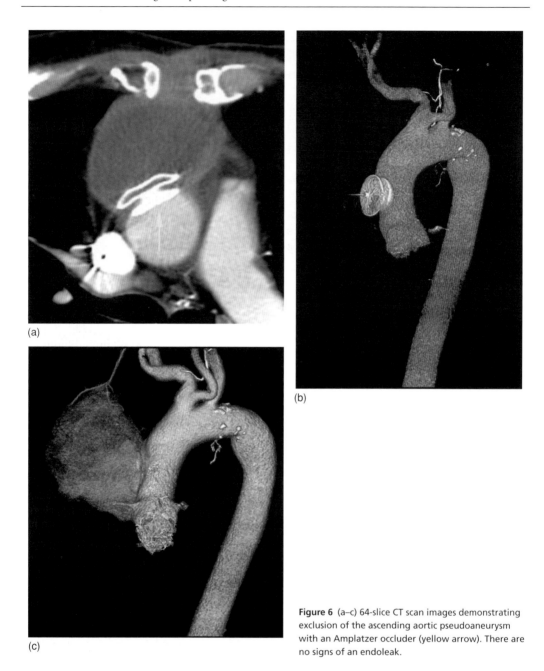

(a)

(b)

(c)

**Figure 6** (a–c) 64-slice CT scan images demonstrating exclusion of the ascending aortic pseudoaneurysm with an Amplatzer occluder (yellow arrow). There are no signs of an endoleak.

## Discussion

Pseudoaneurysms of the ascending aorta can arise from cannulation sites from aortic perfusion catheters, cardioplegia cannulation sites, origin of saphenous vein grafts conduits, and aortotomy sites from aortic valve replacement during cardiopulmonary bypass. Pseudoaneurysms of the ascending aorta and aortic arch are difficult to treat with open surgical techniques associated with considerable morbidity and mortality due to the redo median sternotomy. The application of thoracic aortic endografting to treat thoracic aortic disease has been associated with decreases in morbidity and

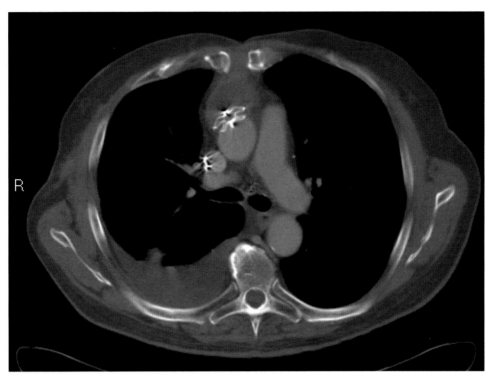

**Figure 7** Axial CT scan image 9-month postprocedure demonstrates marked regression of the pseudoaneurysm.

mortality, paraplegia, hospital and ICU stay, blood transfusions, and a more rapid recovery compared to that of open surgical techniques [11–13].

Total endovascular management of the ascending aorta while an attractive option is still in its infancy [14] and requires an in-depth knowledge of the surgical anatomy. The complex anatomy of the sinotubular junction, the variations in the aortic pathology, and the presentation of disease require a unique approach to each patient. The majority of ascending aortic aneurysms are atherosclerotic that will eventually require an elective replacement when the diameter is 6.0 cm or greater. There is no commercially available endoluminal graft for the management of ascending aortic pathology. Application of endoluminal graft technology to the ascending aorta has to take into account the short landing zones and the possibility of flow obstruction to both coronary artery circulation and the brachiocephalic vessels. In the past, customized grafts incorporating Gianturco Z stents and poly(tetrafluoroethylene) have been constructed to create grafts of varying diameters and lengths suitable for use in the ascending aorta.

Hybrid interventions of the ascending aorta [3–10] that comprise both the open surgical and the endovascular techniques have been applied to solve the anatomic pitfalls of endovascular stent grafting of the ascending aorta. The use of these techniques has lessened the morbidity and mortality of the procedure, but they have not equaled the rates of a total endovascular repair. Combination of endovascular techniques using coil embolization [15], endoluminal grafts, and septal occluders [16] can be used to treat pseudoaneurysms of the ascending aorta. The application of the Amplatzer atrial septal occluder device to exclude a pseudoaneurysm of the ascending aorta is a novel technique which requires a discrete neck for deployment. IVUS approved to be a useful tool in determining or confirming the exact diameter of the neck for careful selection of the appropriately sized device.

In conclusion, the continued evolution of medical imaging and with improvements in device technology may make the ascending aorta more amenable to a total endovascular repair. Endograft design would need to address the challenges presented by the origin of the coronary arteries, the innominate artery, and the aortic valve. A concept device for the future would have components that would allow side branches for coronary artery perfusions and a method to affix the graft to the aortic wall, perhaps with the use of endostaples. For now, simple endovascular repair of the ascending aorta will remain a rare occurrence until the technological hurdles are beaten.

# References

1 Sullivan KL, Steiner RM, Smullens SN, Griska L, Meister SG. Pesudoaneurysm of the ascending aorta following cardiac surgery. *Chest* 1988; **93**: 138–143.

2 Hatfield DR, Fried AM, Ellis GT, Mattingly WT, Jr, Todd EP. Intraoperative control of an ascending aortic pseudo aneurysm by Fogarty balloon catheter: a combined radiologic and surgical approach. *Radiology* 1980; **135**: 515–517.

3 Kato M, Kuratani T, Kaneko M *et al*. The results of total arch graft implantation with open stent-graft placement for type A aortic dissection. *J Thorac Cardiovasc Surg* 2002; **124**: 531–540.

4 Naganuma J, Ninomiya M, Miyairi T *et al*. Total aortic arch aneurysm repair using a stent graft without cardiac or cerebral ischemia. *Jpn J Thorac Cardiovasc Surg* 2002; **50**: 298–301.

5 Schumacher H, Bockler D, Bardenheuer H *et al*. Endovascular aortic arch reconstruction with supra aortic transposition for symptomatic contained rupture and dissection: early experience in 8 high risk patients. *J Endovasc Ther* 2003; **10**: 1066–1074.

6 Melissano G, Civilini E, Maisano F *et al*. Off-pump endovascular treatment of aortic arch aneurysms [in Italian]. *Ital Heart J Suppl* 2004; **5**: 727–734.

7 Diethrich EB, Ghazoul M, Wheatley GH *et al*. Surgical correction of an ascending type A dissection: simultane-

ous endoluminal exclusion of the arch and distal aorta. *J Endovasc Ther* 2005; **12**: 660–666.

8 Diethrich EB, Ghazoul M, Wheatley GH *et al*. Great vessel transposition for antegrade delivery of the TAG endoprosthesis in the proximal aortic arch. *J Endovasc Ther* 2005; **12**: 583–587.

9 Shah A, Coulon P, de Chaumaray T *et al*. Novel technique: staged hybrid surgical and endovascular treatment of acute type A aortic dissections with aortic arch involvement. *J Cardiovasc Surg (Torino)* 2006; **47**(5): 497–502.

10 Zhou W, Reardon M, Peden EK, Lin PH, Lumsden AB. Hybrid approach to complex thoracic aortic aneurysms in high risk patients: surgical challenges and clinical outcomes. *J Vasc Surg* 2006; **44**(4): 688—693.

11 Makaroun MS, Dillavou ED, Kes ST *et al*. Endovascular treatment of thoracic aortic aneurysms: results of the phase II multicenter trial of the Gore TAG thoracic endoprosthesis. *J Vasc Surg* 2005; **41**: 1–9.

12 Bavaria JE, Appoo JJ, Makaroun MS, Verter J, Zi-Fan Yu, Scott Mitchell RS. Endovascular stent grafting versus open surgical repair of descending thoracic aortic aneurysms in low-risk patients: a multicenter comparative trial. *J Thorac Cardiovasc Surg* 2007; **133**: 369–377.

13 Wheatley GH, III, Gurbuz AT, Rodriguez-Lopez JA *et al*. Midterm outcome in 158 consecutive Gore TAG thoracic endoprostheses: single center experience. *Ann Thorac Surg* 2006; **81**(5): 1570–1577; discussion 1577.

14 Mussa FF, Le Maire SA, Bozinovski J, Coselli JS. An entirely endovascular approach to the repair of an ascending aortic pseudo aneurysm. *J Thorac Cardiovasc Surg* 2007; **133**: 562–563.

15 Lin PH, Busch RL, Tong FC, Chaikof E, Martin LG, Lumsden AB. Intra-arterial thrombin injection of an ascending aortic pseudo aneurysm complicated by transient ischemic attack and rescued with systemic abciximab. *J Vasc Surg* 2001; **34**: 939–942.

16 Komanapalli CB, Burch G, Tripathy U, Slater MS, Song HK. Percutaneous repair of an ascending aortic pseudoaneurysm with a septal occluder device. *J Thorac Cardiovasc Surg* 2005; **130**: 603–604.

# Endovascular management of aneurysm of a right coronary vein graft using an ascending aorta endoluminal graft

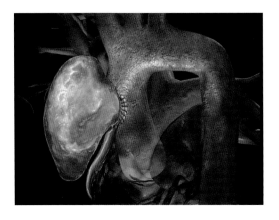

## Introduction

Aneurysms and dissections are the most common diseases which affect the ascending aorta. When aneurysms or dissections involve the ascending aorta, there is a loss of aortic wall integrity with potential lethal complications of severe hemorrhaging and cardiac tamponade. A compromise of the coronary circulation may result in an acute myocardial infarction with possible cardiogenic shock. Should the aortic valve be compromised, there is a risk of severe aortic insufficiency. The ascending aorta is a target for many types of procedures including vein bypass grafts, perfusion catheters, cardioplegic catheters, and as an entry to access the aortic valve during cardiopulmonary bypass. The trauma done to the artery during these procedures makes it a risk for pseudoaneurysm formation that can present immediately after a procedure or take a couple of years to form. The standard operative approach to the ascending aorta involves, in most instances, a median sternotomy, a partial upper median sternotomy, and a right second intercostals space approach. Endovascular repair of thoracic aortic aneurysms has been associated with a lower morbidity and mortality than open surgical repair [1–3]. The application of this technology to the ascending aorta has been limited to few case reports. Pseudoaneurysms of the ascending aorta and saphenous vein grafts may be amenable to endovascular therapy in carefully selected patients. A detailed review of the anatomy must be done to identify the sinotubular junction, the origins of the coronary arteries, and the ostium of the brachiocephalic trunk.

## Case scenario

A 48-year-old male with a previous history of coronary artery disease underwent five-vessel coronary bypass graft surgery, including an internal mammary artery to left anterior descending artery bypass graft for the management of his coronary artery disease in 1987. In 1997, he developed recurrent chest pain and was found to have an occlusion of the right saphenous vein graft from the ascending aorta to the distal right coronary artery requiring a redo one-vessel coronary artery bypass operation with grafting of the distal right coronary artery with a gastroepiploic artery graft. He again became symptomatic 5 years after his last intervention. Conducted imagery showed an occlusion of all the vein grafts including a pseudoaneurysm of the right saphenous vein bypass. The maximum diameter was measured to be 9 cm. Percutaneous coronary angioplasty and stent deployment was performed on the circumflex branch of his coronary artery for a 90% stenosis with successful results. Attempts at coiling the pseudoaneurysm was also performed with only one coil successfully deployed. The follow-up CT scan examination performed at 4 months for chest discomfort demonstrated enlargement of the pseudoaneurysm to 11 cm in diameter (Figure 1). The patient, however, remained asymptomatic from coronary artery disease. An endovascular approach was recommended to the patient so that an open procedure could be avoided.

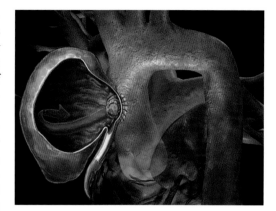

**Figure 2** An Illustrative diagram demonstrating the pseudoaneurysm of the right vein bypass graft. Flow is still present even with the presence of embolization coils.

## Technical details

Under general anesthesia, open retrograde cannulation of the left common femoral artery was performed with an 18-G Cook needle (Cook Inc., Bloomington, IN) and 0.035-in. soft-tip angled glide wire was passed in the aorta and exchanged to a 9-F (French) sheath after 5000 units of heparin were given.

Percutaneous access of the right common femoral artery was similarly performed and a 9-F sheath was introduced over a 0.035-in. soft-tip angled glide wire. A 5-F pigtail angiographic catheter was advanced through the right groin sheath up to the ascending aorta. The fluoroscopic C-arm was positioned in a left anterior oblique angle and an oblique thoracic arch aortogram was performed demonstrating the large pseudoaneurysm of the right saphenous vein graft bypass to the distal right coronary artery (Figure 2). Intravascular ultrasound (IVUS) was performed using an 8.2-F probe (Volcano Therapeutics, Inc., Rancho Cordova, CA) through the left groin sheath to determine the diameter of the proximal and distal landing zone in the ascending aorta where we planned deploying an endograft to exclude flow to the right sapheonous vein graft. The diameter of the landing zone was 28 mm and the length of aorta to be covered without obstructing flow to the coronary arteries and the innominate artery was measured to be 5 cm. An End-oFit customized endoluminal graft (LeMaitre Vascular, Inc., Burlington, MA) measuring 32 mm ×

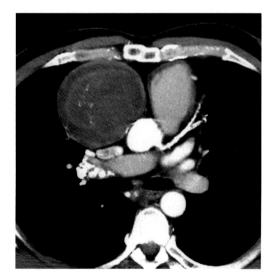

**Figure 1** A CT scan demonstrating an 11-cm pseudoaneurysm of the right saphenous vein bypass graft to the right distal coronary artery.

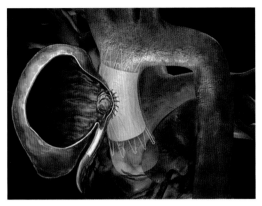

**Figure 3** An Illustrative diagram demonstrating exclusion of pseudoaneurysm with a customized ascending aortic endoluminal graft.

5 cm was felt to be an appropriate device to achieve exclusion of the right saphenous vein bypass graft. The IVUS probe was subsequently exchanged for a 260-cm Lunderquist wire through the left groin sheath. The left 9-F sheath was exchanged for a long 20-F Keller-Timmermans introducer sheath (Cook Inc., Bloomington, IN) and the EndoFit device was advanced through the 20-F sheath (Figure 3) and subsequently deployed in the ascending aorta. Care was taken not to obstruct the coronary arteries and to compromise the origin of the innominate. Completion angiogram demonstrated exclusion of the pseudoaneurysm with no endoleak (Figure 4). A transesophageal echocardiogram was performed which confirmed absence of flow in the pseudoaneurysm with an acute shrinkage in the aneurysm sac. All wires and sheaths were removed; the left common femoral artery was closed in a transverse fashion with restoration of flow. A 6-F angioseal vascular closure device (St. Jude Medical, Inc., St. Paul, MN) was deployed to the left common femoral artery. Patient had bilateral palpable pulses at the end of the procedure was extubated and transferred to recovery room. A postoperative axial CT scan of the chest (Figure 5) demonstrated complete exclusion of pseudoaneurysm with no identifiable endoleak.

## Discussion

Ascending aortic aneurysms and type A dissections are the most common aortic pathologies encoun-

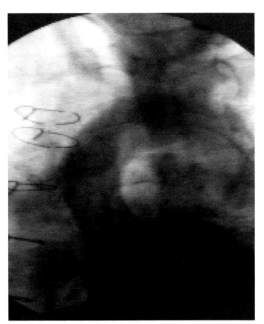

**Figure 4** A completion angiogram demonstrating exclusion of the pseudoaneurysm with a customized endoluminal graft.

tered. Open surgical management of ascending aortic pathologies requires a median sternotomy, partial upper median sternotomy or second right intercostals space thoracotomy incision associated with cardiopulmonary bypass, and sometimes hypothermic circulatory arrest if the arch requires replacement. Medical management of type A dissection is rarely indicated and is often associated with close to

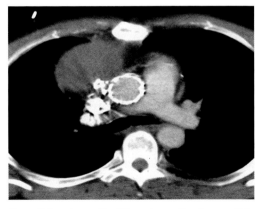

**Figure 5** A postoperative CT scan image showing complete exclusion of the pseudoaneurysm.

100% mortality at 3 months postdiagnosis. Deaths resulting from acute rupture with bleeding, cardiac tamponade, myocardial infarction from dissection involving coronary arteries, and acute aortic insufficiency have been reported for these dissections. Results with endovascular management of the descending thoracic aorta have been encouraging with shorter operating time, reduced blood loss, and more rapid recovery when compared to open surgical techniques. Hybrid techniques that combine open and endovascular procedures have been described and provide a less invasive approach to management of complicated ascending aortic and arch pathologies [4–11].

Total endovascular approaches to the management of the ascending aorta are limited [12–14] and have to be individualized due to the complex anatomy of the sinotubular junction and the variation in the pathological presentation of aortic disease and the lack of any commercially available product. Pathologies of the ascending aorta that could be amenable to endovascular therapy include pseudoaneurysms, vein bypass graft aneurysms, aortic perfusion catheters cannulation sites for cardiopulmonary bypass, cardioplegic cannulation sites, and access avenues for the aortic valve. Type A dissections involving the ascending aorta could potentially be amenable to customized endoluminal grafts provided that the entry point is excluded and there is no extension of the dissection flap into the sinotubular junction. There are no endoluminal grafts approved for the ascending aorta and current commercially available endografts have a large diameter delivery system. A weakness in these current delivery sytems is that the large bore sheaths are not flexible enough to tract around the aortic arch. If the devices cannot maneuver to the target area or the sheaths tear the aorta in the process of advancing, the patient would need an open surgical repair. Some of the current endoluminal grafts are very stiff by nature and cannot fully conform to a tortuous aorta. Endoluminal grafts for the management of the ascending aorta would require grafts to be shorter in lengths with the possibility of an uncovered proximal and distal portion to prevent covering the ostium of the coronary and innominate arteries. Special care must be taken to prevent migration proximally that may interfere with the left ventricular outflow tract resulting in aortic insufficiency

from a prolapse of the aortic valve leaflets. Distal migration of the device could impinge or entirely cover the innominate artery cutting off circulation to the head.

We have used customized grafts incorporating Gianturco stents and PTFE to construct devices of varying diameters and lengths for use in the ascending aorta. Using available commercial components as a foundation, physicians have the ability to customize these devices in order to treat their patients. Modifications such as barb removals or trimming the devices to fit a particular length would fall under this medical provision. These customizations allow patients to be treated earlier without having to wait for the technology or device manufacturers to fulfill a medical need. It is important to remember that the implanting surgeon bears the full responsibility of the customized device and will ultimately answer for it should something go wrong.

In conclusion, hybrid interventions combining endovascular and open techniques currently provide a less invasive approach to the management of ascending aortic and arch pathologies. As technology advances, endoluminal grafts dedicated to the treatment of the ascending aorta will become possible with the work that is being done today by innovative surgeons and engineers. Current innovation in the use of side branches to maintain vascularization of covered vessels or the use of endostaples as a fixation adjunct could help make the next generation of thoracic endoluminal grafts a reality.

## References

1 Makaroun MS, Dillavou ED, Kes ST *et al*. Endovascular treatment of thoracic aortic aneurysms: results of the phase II multicenter trial of the Gore TAG thoracic endoprosthesis. *J Vasc Surg* 2005; **41**: 1–9.

2 Bavaria JE, Appoo JJ, Makaroun MS, Verter J, Zi-Fan Yu, Scott Mitchell RS. Endovascular stent grafting versus open surgical repair of descending thoracic aortic aneurysms in low-risk patients: a multicenter comparative trial. *J Thorac Cardiovasc Surg* 2007; **133**: 369–377.

3 Wheatley GH, III, Gurbuz AT, Rodriguez-Lopez JA *et al*. Midterm outcome in 158 consecutive Gore TAG thoracic endoprostheses: single center experience. *Ann Thorac Surg* 2006; **81**(5): 1570–1577; discussion 1577.

4 Kato M, Kuratani T, Kaneko M *et al*. The results of total arch graft implantation with open stent-graft placement

for type A aortic dissection. *J Thorac Cardiovasc Surg* 2002; **124**: 531–540.

5 Naganuma J, Ninomiya M, Miyairi T *et al*. Total aortic arch aneurysm repair using a stent graft without cardiac or cerebral ischemia. *Jpn J Thorac Cardiovasc Surg* 2002; **50**: 298–301.

6 Schumacher H, Bockler D, Bardenheuer H *et al*. Endovascular aortic arch reconstruction with supra aortic transposition for symptomatic contained rupture and dissection: early experience in 8 high risk patients. *J Endovasc Ther* 2003; **10**: 1066–1074.

7 Melissano G, Civilini E, Maisano F *et al*. Off-pump endovascular treatment of aortic arch aneurysms [in Italian]. *Ital Heart J Suppl* 2004; **5**:727–734.

8 Diethrich EB, Ghazoul M, Wheatley GH *et al*. Surgical correction of an ascending type A dissection: simultaneous endoluminal exclusion of the arch and distal aorta. *J Endovasc Ther* 2005; **12**: 660–666.

9 Diethrich EB, Ghazoul M, Wheatley GH *et al*. Great vessel transposition for antegrade delivery of the TAG endoprosthesis in the proximal aortic arch. *J Endovasc Ther* 2005; **12**: 583–587.

10 Shah A, Coulon P, de Chaumaray T *et al*. Novel technique: staged hybrid surgical and endovascular treatment of acute type A aortic dissections with aortic arch involvement. *J Cardiovasc Surg (Torino)* 2006; **47**(5): 497–502.

11 Zhou W, Reardon M, Peden EK, Lin PH, Lumsden AB. Hybrid approach to complex thoracic aortic aneurysms in high risk patients: surgical challenges and clinical outcomes. *J Vasc Surg* 2006; **44**(4): 688–693.

12 Mussa FF, Le Maire SA, Bozinovski J, Coselli JS. An entirely endovascular approach to the repair of an ascending aortic pseudo aneurysm. *J Thorac Cardiovasc Surg* 2007; **133**: 562–563.

13 Lin PH, Busch RL, Tong FC, Chaikof E, Martin LG, Lumsden AB. Intra-arterial thrombin injection of an ascending aortic pseudo aneurysm complicated by transient ischemic attack and rescued with systemic abciximab. *J Vasc Surg* 2001; **34**: 939–942.

14 Komanapalli CB, Burch G, Tripathy U, Slater MS, Song HK. Percutaneous repair of an ascending aortic pseudo aneurysm with a septal occluder device. *J Thorac Cardiovasc Surg* 2005; **130**: 603–604.

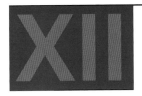

# SECTION XII

# Supra-aortic thoracic aortic aneurysms

# CASE 42

# Hybrid approach to the management of a type C innominate artery aneurysm

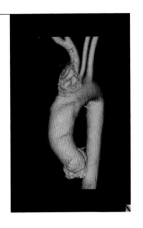

## Introduction

Innominate artery aneurysms are uncommon and account for 1% of peripheral artery aneurysms. Atherosclerosis comprises 50% of the etiologies for this condition with trauma, infection, arteritis, and aberrant anatomy accounting for the remainder of the cases. Treatment of these aneurysms is deemed necessary due to the risk of aneurysm rupture, ischemia from thrombembolism, transient ischemic attacks, and compression of surrounding structures. The majority of patients are asymptomatic in nature with aneurysm detection as an incidental finding on routine imaging. Compressive symptoms from an enlarging innominate artery aneurysm may result in hoarseness from recurrent laryngeal nerve compression, dyspnea from tracheal compression, and dysphagia. An open surgical approach for a type C innominate artery aneurysm requires a median sternotomy, extracorporeal circulation with hypothermic circulatory arrest, and prosthetic arch or innominate artery graft replacement. Mortality rates of up to 11% are reported for this procedure [1]. A hybrid approach, which consists of a debranching of the innominate artery and left carotid artery with deployment of an endoluminal graft, is a less invasive procedure that can be performed without extracorporeal circulation with decreased morbidity and mortality.

We present a hybrid approach to the management of a type C innominate artery aneurysm.

## Case scenario

A 41-year-old male developed a productive cough with no fevers and was subsequently treated with a week's course of antibiotics. A review of the patient's medical history and physical examination did not produce any significant findings. Despite completing full course of antibiotics, he continued to have a productive cough. A chest X-ray was obtained that was suspicious for a hilar mass. A 64-slice CT scan of the chest (Figure 1a and 1b and Figure 2) with virtual angioscopy (Figure 3) was performed demonstrating the presence of a large innominate artery aneurysm with a diameter 4.5 cm at the ostium of the vessel. To exclude this aneurysm with an endoluminal graft, a debranching procedure would be required to circumvent arterial circulation to both the innominate and left carotid arteries.

## Technical details

A median sternotomy incision approximately 8 cm long was made for exposure of the ascending aorta and arch vessels (Figure 4a). The ascending aorta and the origins of the innominate and left common carotid arteries were mobilized. A woven Dacron graft was selected based upon the diameter of the ascending aorta and the branch arteries to be bypassed. For this specific care, an 18 mm × 9 mm Hemashield Dacron bifurcated graft (Boston Scientific, Natick, MA) was used. A 10-mm straight

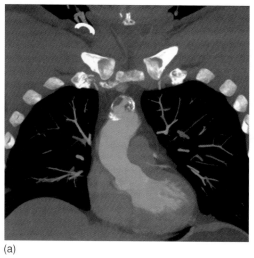 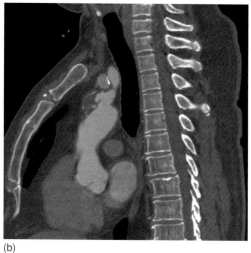

(a)                                                    (b)

**Figure 1** (a and b) Reformatted CT scan images demonstrating the aneurysm at the base of the innominate artery.

graft was cut obliquely (60°) and anastomosed to the heel of the bifurcated graft using 5-0 Prolene suture (Figure 4b). This can be used as a delivery conduit for antegrade deployment of the endoluminal graft across the aortic arch. A partially occluding clamp was applied to the lateral curve of the ascending aorta and the bifurcated conduit graft was anastomosed with 4-0 Prolene suture. After 2000 to 3000 units of heparin had been administered, the left common carotid artery was clamped, transected at the arch, and sutured proximally. The lateral limb of the graft was anastomosed in an end-to-end configuration (Figure 4c). The innominate artery was similarly addressed (Figure 4c). After each anastomosis, the graft was flushed to eliminate any thrombus or air. All clamps were removed and the integrity of the suture line confirmed.

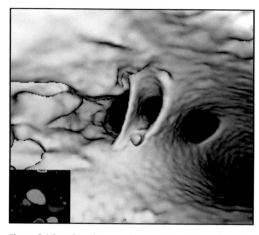

**Figure 2** A 3-D reconstruction demonstrating a type C innominate artery.

**Figure 3** Virtual angioscopy demonstrating the ostium of the innominate artery with plaque calcification. The ostia of the two other arch vessels can also be visualized.

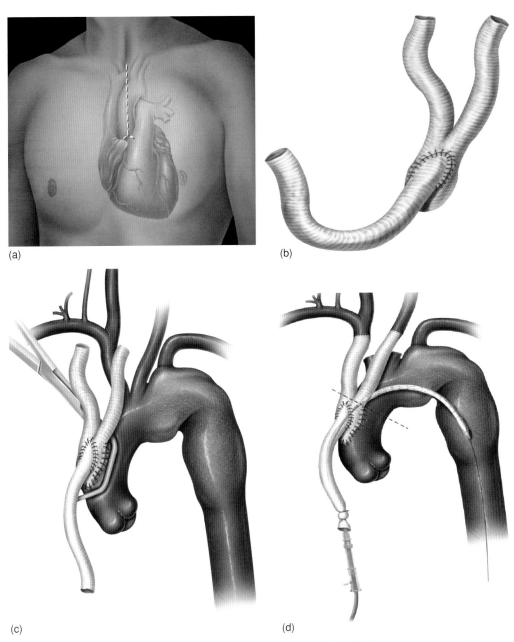

(a)

(b)

(c)

(d)

**Figure 4** (a) The ascending aorta is exposed through a short upper median sternotomy. (b) A 10-mm graft is anastomosed obliquely to a 18 mm × 9 mm bifurcated prosthesis. (c) The bifurcated conduit graft is anastomosed to the ascending aorta, and the common carotid and innominate arteries are transected and anastomosed end-to-end to the limbs of the bifurcated graft. (d) The delivery sheath is inserted through the conduit and passed across the aortic arch. (e) The endoluminal graft is positioned and deployed. (f) A completion angiogram demonstrating the successful deployment of an endoluminal graft. Flow to the supra-aortic vessels is supplied by a 18 mm × 9 mm bifurcated graft off the ascending aorta (arrow). (g) The attachment site of the bypass graft.

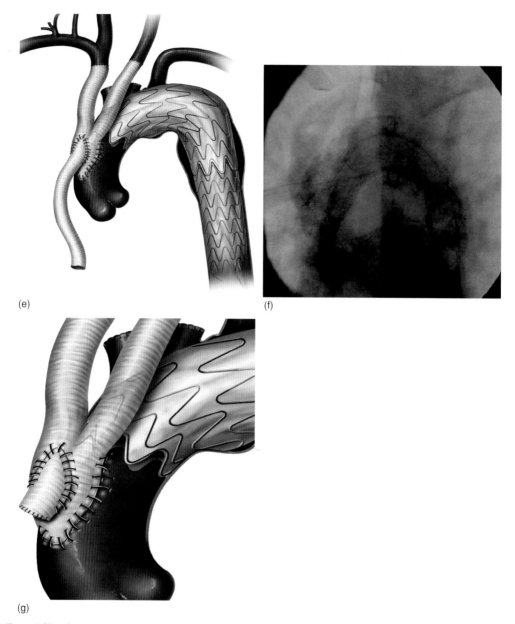

(e)

(f)

(g)

**Figure 4** (*Cont.*)

Percutaneous access of the right common femoral artery was performed with a 9-F (French) sheath. Similarly, the left common femoral artery was percutaneously accessed with an 18-G needle and a 5-F sheath introduced. A 9-F sheath was secured in the conduit and a 260-cm angled hydrophilic guide wire was passed to the right iliac artery. The wire was captured with a snare and exteriorized through the right femoral sheath. The conduit was clamped, and the stent-graft delivery sheath substituted for the 24-F sheath. An opaque marker string, clips, or a sternal wire can be placed at the proximal portion of the conduit to assure that the stent-graft's deployment is just beyond the limb origins of the bifurcated graft. The endoluminal graft was introduced through the 24-F sheath attached to the

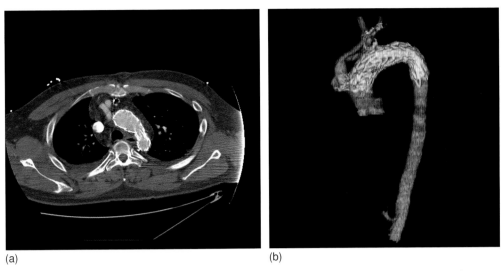

(a)                                                    (b)

**Figure 5** (a) An axial CT scan image depicting the full exclusion of the innominate artery. (b) A 3-D reconstruction showing the bifurcated graft coming off the ascending aorta supplying both the innominate and left carotid artery.

10-mm conduit across the aortic arch with constant tension placed on the conduit–femoral artery wire (Figure 4d). Once in the desired position, the 40 mm × 20 cm Gore TAG endoprosthesis (W.L. Gore & Associates, Flagstaff, AZ) was introduced and positioned at the marker. The sheath was withdrawn into the conduit upon deployment of the endoluminal graft (Figure 4e). A final completion angiogram of the aortic arch was performed through a 5-F pigtail angiographic catheter that had been introduced through the contralateral left femoral artery sheath (Figure 4f). The delivery sheath was removed with the conduit transected and oversewn (Figure 4g). Heparinization was reversed and the sternotomy incision closed with one mediastinal tube placed for drainage. A postoperative CT scan of the chest was performed which demonstrated complete exclusion of the innominate aneurysm with no identifiable endoleak and patent flow to the debranched innominate artery and the left common carotid artery (Figure 5a and 5b).

## Discussion

Innominate artery aneurysms, unlike atherosclerotic aortic aneurysms, are more likely to present with cerebral emboli. Kieffer *et al.* reported that approximately 25.9% of their patients who present with this type of aneurysm have cerebral emboli.

Management of innominate artery aneurysms depends on the origin of the aneurysm. A classification of innominate aneurysms described by Kieffer is based on the extent of aneurysmal disease. Type A involves the innominate artery only beginning distal to the origin. Type B, which is the most common, involves the innominate artery and its origin, while type C involves both the innominate artery and the ascending aorta. Treatment of type A and B innominate artery aneurysms require a median sternotomy with the proximal graft originating from the native ascending aorta proximal to the innominate origin. The graft extends to the normal distal innominate artery. The origin of the innominate is closed by a running suture or patch angioplasty of the aorta. Treatment of type C innominate artery aneurysms, which may require cardiopulmonary bypass and hypothermic circulatory arrest, includes aortic arch and innominate artery prosthetic graft replacement. Patients with true aneurysms are often elderly, have multiple comorbidities, and may present emergently with rupture or dissection. Additional relative contraindications to open repair include patients with severely compromised pulmonary function, prior sternotomy or left thoracotomy, and the unstable, multiple trauma patient. Open surgical repair is associated with perioperative mortality of 11%, with 18% of patients requiring prolonged ventilation [1].

The endovascular management of innominate artery aneurysms offers a minimally invasive approach associated with a lower morbidity and mortality in high-risk patients. Despite the attractiveness of an endovascular approach to treat innominate artery aneurysms, the majority of patients have landing zones that are prohibitive to the conventional methods of deploying endoluminal grafts. Coverage of the branch vessels may prove problematic due to the necessity of debranching procedures to maintain arterial flow to the arch vessels. While there are many reasons to consider an endoluminal approach for innominate artery aneurysms, the current experience is limited [2] and open repair remains the standard of care.

The hybrid approach to treating arch aneurysms [3–5] offers a benefit to patients who are at a higher risk for a more demanding operation. The hybrid approach can be performed off cardiopulmonary bypass without any hypothermia and circulatory arrest. Neurological sequelae are few due to a short partial aortic cross-clamp time and if present are more likely due to manipulation of wires in the arch during deployment of endograft. Retrograde arch deployment of endoluminal grafts is often complicated due to difficult arch configurations and specific deployment characteristics of these devices. The antegrade technique of endograft deployment allows precise delivery of the endoluminal graft at the proximal aortic arch, thus avoiding arterial access problems in the groin. Vessel access in the groins can be complicated by vessel tortuosity and the presence of significant, occlusive disease. Threading the wire through the delivery conduit to the femoral artery facilitates the advancement of both the sheath and the endoluminal graft across the aortic arch. It also permits precise deployment of the stent graft within the tube graft on the ascending aorta.

Bergeron *et al.* [4] treated aneurysms and dissections involving the aortic arch in 29 high-risk patients, deploying a variety of commercial stent grafts using preliminary arch vessel transposition in 26 of them. They reported 1 major stroke (3.5%) and 2 deaths (7.7%). The deaths were attributed to procedural complications such as an iliac rupture and perforation of the left ventricle. One patient had a delayed minor stroke. Schumacher *et al.* [5] encountered no neurological complications.

The hybrid procedure [6–12] is a relatively safe procedure that can be successfully performed in patients not suitable for conventional open surgical repair.

## References

1 Kieffer E, Chiche L, Koskas F, Bahnini A. Aneurysms of the innominate artery (surgical treatment of 27 patients). *J Vasc Surg* 2001; **34**: 222–228.

2 Axisa BM, Loftus IM, Fishwick G *et al.* Endovascular repair of an innominate artery false aneurysm following blunt trauma. *J Endovasc Ther* 2000; **7**: 245–250.

3 Kato N, Shimono T, Hirano T *et al.* Aortic arch aneurysms: treatment with extraanatomical bypass and endovascular stent-grafting. *Cardiovasc Intervent Radiol* 2002; **25**: 419–422.

4 Bergeron P, Coulon P, De Chaumaray T *et al.* Great vessels transposition and aortic archexclusion. *J Cardiovasc Surg (Torino)* 2005; **46**: 141–147.

5 Schumacher H, Böckler D, Bardenheuer H *et al.* Endovascular aortic arch reconstruction with supra-aortic transposition for symptomatic contained rupture and dissection: early experience in 8 high-risk patients. *J Endovasc Ther* 2003; **10**: 1066–1074.

6 Carrel TP, Berdat PA, Baumgartner I *et al.* Combined surgical and endovascular approach to treat a complex aortic coarctation without extracorporeal circulation. *Ann Thorac Surg* 2004; **78**: 1462–1465.

7 Svensson LG. Progress in ascending and aortic arch surgery: minimally invasive surgery, blood conservation, and neurological deficit prevention. *Ann Thorac Surg* 2002; **74**: S1786–S1788.

8 Diethrich EB, Ghazoul M, Wheatley GH *et al.* Great vessel transposition for antegrade delivery of the TAG Endoprosthesis in the proximal aortic arch. *J Endovasc Ther* 2005; **12**: 583–587.

9 Greenberg RK, Haddad F, Svensson L *et al.* Hybrid approaches to thoracic aortic aneurysms: the role of endovascular elephant trunk completion. *Circulation* 2005; **112**: 2619–2626.

10 Diethrich EB, Ghazoul M, Wheatley GH, III *et al.* Surgical correction of ascending type A thoracic aortic dissection: simultaneous endoluminal exclusion of the arch and distal aorta. *J Endovasc Ther* 2005; **12**: 660–666.

11 Zhou W, Reardon M, Peden EK, Lin PH, Lumsden AB. Hybrid approach to complex thoracic aortic aneurysms in high risk patients: surgical challenges and clinical outcomes. *J Vasc Surg* 2006; **44**(4): 688–693.

12 Criado FJ, Clark NS, Barnatan MF. Stent graft repair in the aortic arch and descending thoracic aorta: a 4-year experience. *J Vasc Surg* 2002; **36**: 1121–1128.

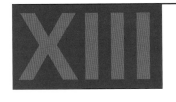

# SECTION XIII

# Future of thoracic aortic endografting

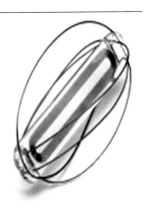

## CASE 43

# Remote wireless pressure sensing for postoperative surveillance of thoracic endoluminal grafts

## Introduction

Thoracic endografting for the treatment of thoracic aortic aneurysms requires lifelong postoperative surveillance using various imaging techniques. Currently, the entirety of exclusion or absence of endoleaks is evaluated by intraoperative angiography and postoperative CT scans. Multiple contrast injections can lead to an increased risk of contrast-induced nephropathy as well as increased radiation to both patient and surgeon. Remote wireless pressure sensor monitoring is a new technology with potential benefit for postoperative surveillance of thoracic endografts without the added risk of radiation exposure or contrast-induced nephropathy.

## Case scenario

A 71-year-old woman with multiple comorbidities including hypertension, severe chronic obstructive pulmonary disease, and renal dysfunction underwent a CT scan of the chest for the assessment of pain that was radiating to her back. She was found to have a 6.5 cm × 5.1 cm saccular aneurysm (Figure 1). She was not a suitable candidate for open surgical repair and was offered a less invasive approach using an endoluminal graft. In order to reduce her exposure to radiation and the risk of contrast-induced nephropathy associated with repeated CT scans, she was chosen to receive an EndoSure wireless pressure sensor (CardioMEMS, Inc., Atlanta, GA) for the surveillance of her thoracic aneurysm. The

sensor would be deployed during the same procedure used to insert and implant the endoluminal graft for her aneurysm (Figure 2).

## Technical details

Under general anesthesia, open retrograde cannulation of the right common femoral artery was performed with an 18-G needle and a 0.035-in. soft-tip angled glide wire was passed into the distal thoracic aorta and exchanged to a 9-F (French) sheath under fluoroscopic visualization. Percutaneous access of the left common femoral artery was similarly performed and a 5-F sheath introduced. Five thousand units of heparin were given to keep the activated clotted time greater than 200 seconds. A 5-F angiographic pigtail catheter was advanced through the left groin sheath into the thoracic aorta. The fluoroscopic C-arm was positioned in a left anterior oblique angle and an oblique thoracic arch aortogram was performed to visualize the arch vessels and the descending thoracic aortic aneurysm (Figure 3). Intravascular ultrasound (IVUS) using an 8.2-F probe (Volcano Therapeutics Inc., Rancho Cordova, CA) was performed. Based on the measurements, a 34 mm × 15 cm Gore TAG graft (W.L. Gore & Associates, Flagstaff, AZ) was chosen. The IVUS catheter was exchanged for an extra-stiff 260-cm Lunderquist wire (Cook Inc., Bloomington, IN). An angiogram was performed to evaluate the aneurysm sac with careful attention paid to the amount of free-flowing blood contained within the

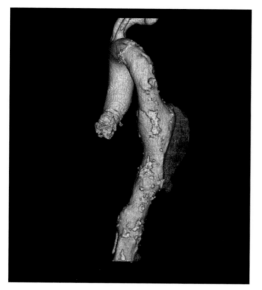

**Figure 1** A 64-slice CT scan of the chest demonstrating a saccular aneurysm measuring 6.5 cm × 5.1 cm.

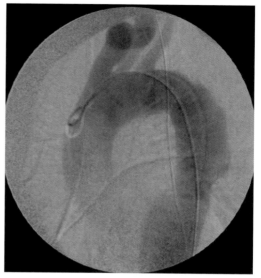

**Figure 3** A predeployment angiogram demonstrating a descending thoracic aneurysm.

sac. To properly deploy the sensor, a pocket free of thrombus would be needed to ensure that the Endo-Sure sensor would not be crushed upon deployment of the endoluminal graft. Crushing of the sensor can lead to erroneous readings. Once eligibility was

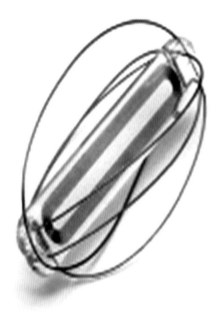

**Figure 2** An EndoSure wireless pressure sensor (CardioMEMS, Inc., Atlanta, GA).

validated, a 30 mm × 15 mm EndoSure wireless pressure sensor (Figure 2) was loaded on a long delivery sheath through the left groin and deployed into the aneurysm sac. The right 9-F sheath was exchanged for a 22-F Gore sheath and a 34 mm × 15 cm TAG stent-graft device was advanced through the Gore sheath and subsequently deployed over an extra-stiff wire. The device was deployed within an area that had previously been identified for suitable landing zones and marked on a "road map" angiogram. A Gore trilobe balloon was used to perform postdeployment balloon angioplasty to the proximal and distal segments of the graft to ensure proper apposition. Pressure readings taken from the sensor before and postexclusion of the aneurysm are shown in Figure 4. An overall reduction in systolic, diastolic, and mean pressures can be seen with the pulse pressure reduced to 0.54 mm Hg immediately after endoluminal graft deployment. A completion angiogram demonstrated exclusion of the aneurysm with no endoleak (Figure 5). All wires and sheaths were removed; the right common femoral artery was closed in a transverse fashion with restoration of flow. A 6-F angioseal closure device was deployed to the left common femoral artery. Prior to leaving the operating room, the patient was extubated and bilateral peripheral pulses were documented. A CT scan of the

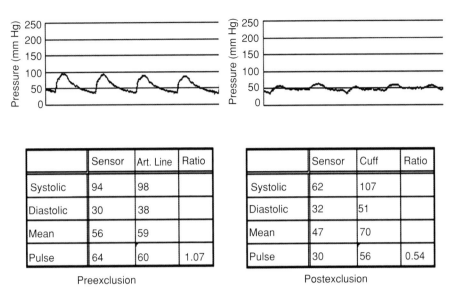

| | Sensor | Art. Line | Ratio |
|---|---|---|---|
| Systolic | 94 | 98 | |
| Diastolic | 30 | 38 | |
| Mean | 56 | 59 | |
| Pulse | 64 | 60 | 1.07 |

Preexclusion

| | Sensor | Cuff | Ratio |
|---|---|---|---|
| Systolic | 62 | 107 | |
| Diastolic | 32 | 51 | |
| Mean | 47 | 70 | |
| Pulse | 30 | 56 | 0.54 |

Postexclusion

**Figure 4** Pre- and postexclusion of pressure tracing readings from the EndoSure wireless pressure sensor (CardioMEMS, Inc., Atlanta, GA).

chest performed the following day showed exclusion of the descending thoracic aneurysm with no endoleak noted (Figure 6). She was discharged home on the second postoperative day in satisfactory condition.

## Discussion

Stent-graft repair of the thoracic aorta is associated with the risk of potential type I, II, and III endoleaks. Endoleak rates of 29% with respect to stent grafting of the thoracic aorta have been

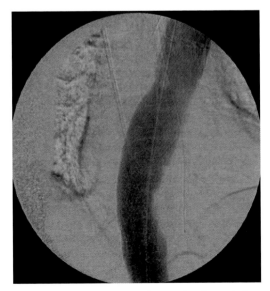

**Figure 5** A postdeployment angiogram showing exclusion of the aneurysm with no demonstrable endoleak.

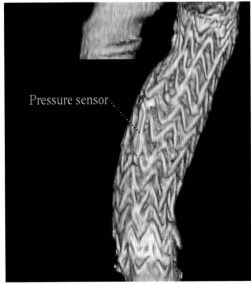

**Figure 6** A 3-D reconstruction documents the position of the wireless pressure sensor within the aneurysm sac.

recently reported by Parmer *et al.* [1]. Extensive coverage of the thoracic aorta with more than one device, a large aneurysm size, the length of aorta covered by stent, and male gender have been shown to be strong predictors of developing an endoleak [1]. Reintervention rates close to 10%, using endovascular techniques, are necessary when such endoleaks are detected [2]. The development of an endoleak can result in a partial repressurization of the aneurysm sac with a potential for rupture despite an incomplete exclusion of the aneurysm by an endoluminal graft. Routine ultrasound technology while useful to monitor abdominal endografts does not translate well to thoracic endografts. Current postoperative surveillance of thoracic endoluminal grafts includes contrast-enhanced CT scans of the chest to monitor aneurysm sac regression, graft migration, and the presence of endoleaks. The CT scans are done periodically with at least four CT scans to be done within the first year of treatment should the manufacturer's suggested follow-up regimen be followed. At the very least, one CT scan should be done annually for the duration of the patient's life. A follow-up schedule like this can put endoluminal graft recipients at risk for radiation exposure and renal dysfunction associated with the use of contrast dye. Disregarding the potential health implications, patients have to endure the cost of the CT scans as well as the investment of their time all of which may compromise patient compliance with a surveillance program. The EndoSure sensor works by having an outside antenna transmit a radiofrequency signal to the implanted sensor. Depending on the pressure inside the aneurysm sac, the sensor will return the signal back to the antenna at a particular frequency. The interpretation of this frequency by computer software can give some insight into the systolic, diastolic, mean, and pulse pressure of the sac. The acute pressure measurement to confirm aneurysm sac exclusion trial (APEX) data demonstrated the efficacy of immediate exclusion of an abdominal aortic aneurysm sac using the pressure sensor with agreement between the sensor measurements and angiography regarding detection of type I and III endoleaks in 92.1% ($n = 70$) with a sensitivity of 94% and a specificity of 80% [3–5]. The data collected in this study led the Food and Drug Administration to approve the device for the implantation in an abdominal aortic aneurysm prior to endoluminal graft exclusion. The first implantation of the EndoSure sensor in a thoracic aneurysm prior to an endoluminal graft was done by Dr Pierre Silveira and Dr Ross Milner in Florianapolis, Brazil [6]. This adjunctive tool can be safely used in a doctor's office with a measurement taken within minutes upon finding the sensor signal. Advantages of this new technology include frequent evaluations with multiple examinations performed on a given patient at any time within the year; systemic pressurization may be detected much earlier within a previously excluded aneurysm and lead to prompt evaluation and treatment. The microelectromechanical technology of the EndoSure sensor is currently being studied for use in the false lumen evaluation of treated type B dissections, blood pressure evaluation, and heart failure monitoring. In conclusion, remote pressure sensing may, in the future, eliminate the need for serial contrast-enhanced CT scans as part of a postoperative surveillance program for thoracic aneurysms.

# References

1 Parmer S, Carpenter JP, Stavropolous W *et al.* Endoleaks after endovascular repair of thoracic aortic aneurysms. *J Vasc Surg* 2006; **44**: 447–452.

2 Sampram EK, Karafa MT, Mascha EJ *et al.* Nature, frequency, and predictors of secondary procedures after endovascular repair of abdominal aortic aneurysm. *J Vasc Surg* 2003; **37**: 930–937.

3 Baum RA, Carpenter JP, Cope C *et al.* Aneurysm sac pressure measurements after endovascular repair of abdominal aortic aneurysms. *J Vasc Surg* 2001; **33**: 32–41.

4 Ohki T, Yadav J, Gargiulo N *et al.* Preliminary results of an implantable wireless aneurysm pressure sensor in a canine model: will surveillance CT scan following endovascular AAA repair become obsolete? *J Endovasc Ther* 2003; **10**(Suppl 1): 32.

5 Ohki T, Ouriel K, Silveira PG *et al.* Initial results of wireless pressure sensing for endovascular aneurysm repair: the APEX trial-acute pressure measurement to confirm aneurysm sac exclusion. *J Vasc Surg* 2007; **45**(2): 236–242.

6 Milner R, Kasirajan K, Chaikof E. Future of endograft surveillance. *Semin Vasc Surg* 2006; **19**: 75–82.

# CASE 44
# Zenith® Dissection™ Case Study

## Introduction

Aortic dissection is a catastrophic cardiovascular disease associated with high morbidity and mortality, affecting approximately 10 per 100,000 of the population per year [1]. Deaths due to aortic dissection exceed those due to ruptured abdominal aortic aneurysm and 35% are not diagnosed before death [2]. Covered stent grafts have recently been advocated to treat the primary entry tear in Type B dissections, and in some centers, have become the treatment of choice. Such treatment has consisted of placing a stent graft across the primary entry tear with the aim of depressurizing the false lumen and inducing proximal false lumen thrombosis. However, due to reentry tears or intimal fenestrations related to branch vessels, false lumen flow often persists in the lower thoracic and abdominal aorta. This flow acts to prevent complete thrombosis of the false lumen. Repair is therefore incomplete and the dissection persists, leaving the potential for aneurysmal change, rupture, or redissection [3–6]. This case study describes a novel treatment of a dissection using a stent graft with bare stents below it for a more holistic repair of the dissected aorta [7].

## Case scenario

A 40-year-old man with a history of poorly controlled hypertension presented to his local hospital with sudden onset of chest and back pain. Two years prior, he had been diagnosed with an uncomplicated Type B aortic dissection. He was then managed conservatively, with antihypertensive therapy using candesartan (an angiotensin II receptor antagonist) and atenolol (a beta-blocker), in conjunction with twice-yearly surveillance CT scanning. During the initial 18 months postdiagnosis, the patient's CT scans demonstrated progressive dilatation of the proximal descending thoracic aorta from 4.5 to 5.5 cm in diameter. Six months later, the patient deteriorated clinically, with the recurrence of severe back and chest pain, suggestive of redissection.

Multislice CT imaging confirmed marked aneurysmal change, with a maximum proximal descending thoracic aortic diameter of 6.5 cm (Figure 1). In addition, dynamic obstruction of the infrarenal aortic true lumen was evident, along with hypoperfusion of the renal arteries and downstream aorta (Figure 2).

Emergent surgical reconstruction of the aorta was considered; however, it was felt that this approach carried an unacceptably high risk of mortality, given the patient's unstable condition with organ malperfusion. Endovascular aortic reconstruction was, therefore, selected with the goal of endograft placement over the primary entry tear aimed at preventing rupture and providing expansion of the true lumen and reperfusion of the renal and infrarenal aortic segments.

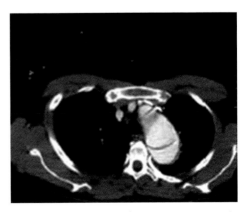

**Figure 1** Axial CT scan image demonstrates aneurysmal changes of the proximal descending thoracic aorta with a diameter of 6.5 cm.

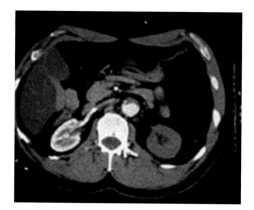

**Figure 2** Axial CT scan of the abdominal aorta demonstrates dynamic obstruction of the infra renal true lumen with hypoperfusion of the renal arteries.

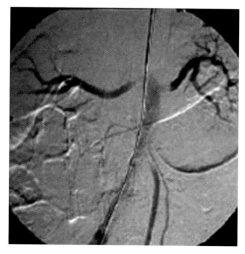

**Figure 4** Angiogram demonstrates severly compromised abdominal and renal perfusion with near static renal flow.

Angiographic evaluation revealed a high-flow primary entry tear just distal to the left subclavian artery, with severely compromised abdominal aortic and renal artery perfusion (Figure 3) Near-static renal perfusion was noted immediately following endograft implantation (Figure 4).

The first stage of the endovascular repair involved implantation of the proximal component of a 34-mm-diameter Zenith® TX2™ TAA Endovascular Graft Proximal Component under transesophageal echocardiography and angiographic guidance. This stent graft covered the origin of the subclavian artery and the primary entry tear,

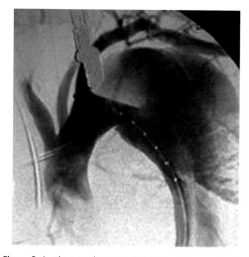

**Figure 3** Angiogram demonstrates a high flow proximal entry tear distal to the left subclavian artery with comppressed true lumen flow.

thereby eliminating inflow into the proximal thoracic false lumen. As part of the same procedure, stenting of the statically obstructed left renal ostium was performed to enable reestablishment of left renal artery inflow. The patient made a satisfactory recovery after the procedure, in terms of both dramatically reduced pain levels and successful reperfusion of the kidneys and lower limbs. Urine output was reestablished and renal function normalized after 4 days.

Follow-up CT scan at 1 week showed thrombosis of the upper thoracic false lumen. However, there was persistent false lumen perfusion distally with reduced true lumen caliber. To address this, bare z-stents (Zenith® Dissection™ Endovascular Stents) were deployed in the aortic true lumen just distal to the stent graft to promote true lumen remodeling and distal fl ow (Figure 5). Follow-up CT scan examination at 1 month demonstrated thrombosis of the thoracic aortic false lumen; however, the abdominal aortic false lumen remained patent because of reentry tears in the abdominal aorta and the left common iliac artery. A third procedure, consisting of stent-graft implantation and coil embolization, successfully obliterated these reentry tears and subsequently induced thrombosis of the abdominal false lumen.

One year later, the patient remained well and asymptomatic. Total false lumen thrombosis was maintained, and significant remodeling of the

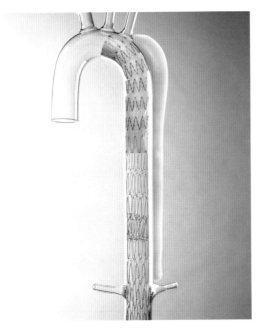

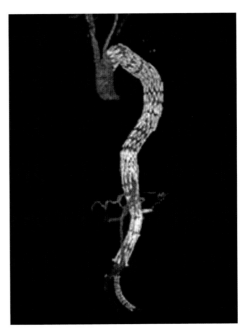

**Figure 5** Glass model of a Cook Zenith dissection endovascular stent graft system.

**Figure 6** 64-slice CT image at 1-year follow-up with complete thrombosis of the false lumen and remodeling of the aortic true lumen.

aortic true lumen had occurred (Figure 6). Currently, the patient remains under close follow-up CT surveillance and is receiving aggressive hypertensive therapy.

The classic endovascular approach to Type B dissection has previously demonstrated advantages over medical treatment [8]. However, it does not address the problem of continued false lumen patency, which in turn promotes remote-phase complications such as progressive aneurysmal change. To address this problem, the more holistic staged endovascular repair of both the thoracic and abdominal aorta can be carried out. This approach permits remodeling to restore normal aortic morphology and is an exciting future direction for endovascular repair of aortic dissection [7].

## References

1 Svensson L. Aortic dissection and aortic aneurysm surgery: clinical observations, experimental investigations, and statistical analyses. Part II. *Curr Prob Surg*, 1992; **29**: 915–1057.

2 Svensson L. *Degenerative Aortic Aneurysms, Cardiovascular and Vascular Disease of The Aorta*. W.B. Saunders Co., Philadelphia, PA, 1997, Chapter 3: 29–41.

3 Lissin LW, Vangelos R. Acute aortic syndrome: a case presentation and review of the literature. Vasc Med, 2002; **7**: 281–287.

4 Umana JP, Miller CD, Mitchell RS. What is the best treatment for patients with acute type B aortic dissection–medical, surgical, or endovascular stent grafting? *Ann Thorac Surg* 2002; **74**: S1840–S1843.

5 Onitsuka S, Akashi H, Tayama K et al. Long term outcome and prognostic predictors of medically treated acute type B aortic dissections. *Ann Thorac Surg* 2004; **78**: 1268–1273.

6 Sueyoshi E, Sakamoto I, Hayashi K, Yamaguchi T, Imada T. Growth rate of aortic diameter in patients with type B aortic dissection during the chronic phase, circulation. 2004; **110** (11, Suppl 1): S11256–S11261.

7 Mossop P. Staged endovascular treatment for type B aortic dissection. *NCP Cardiovasc Med* 2005; **2**(6): 316–321.

8 Dake MD, Kato N, Mitchell RS et al. Endovascular stent-graft placementor the treatment of acute aortic dissection. *N Engl J Med* 1999; **340**: 1546–1552.

# The Road Ahead...

In looking back at the presentations contained within this book, it is important to remember that this technology, in its infancy, was composed of a small group of surgeons customizing commercially available products to fit the needs of their patients. From encapsulating stents with nonpermeable material to stitching grafts together and developing better tools to deliver the device, this book is a testament that endovascular technology, with continuing innovation, will play a larger part in modern medicine. We describe the basic use of endoluminal grafts for the thoracic aorta with future applications for different pathologies. In addressing the spirit of continuing innovation, we also show examples of how surgeons can increase the eligible patient pool for this technology with the use of debranching techniques as well as the potential of hemodynamic sensors to provide real-time information for a surgeon in a convenient manner. Addressing the future of thoracic endovascular technology would be incomplete without mentioning branched or fenestrated endografts and the development of second-generation endoluminal grafts.

Branched or fenestrated grafts represent additional customization of current technology to serve a population for which there is little alternative but the open procedure. Building on the stable endoluminal graft technology foundation and the widespread availability of high-quality imaging and software, surgeons can now order grafts with preplanned fenestrations or covered-stent side branches that will allow the graft to be placed across the aneurysm while preserving arterial flow to the critical vessels. Conceivably, patients with high arch aneurysms or thoracoabdominal aneurysms will be able to benefit from this technology. The most well-known device of this nature is manufactured by Cook Medical. Device characteristics as

demonstrated in Figures 1–4 illustrate the potential of the technology. Patient selection for this type of device is intensive with as many as 85 measurements and assessments needed for the proper sizing of the device. Included in these assessments are ostial diameters, angulation to the aorta, and orientation of the vessel. These customizable aspects of the device make for a device that is not "stock" and would be subject to a build delay. Emergent patients would not be able to benefit from this device but patients who would undergo vessel transposition would be good candidates, provided that their anatomy is within device limits. Technically, the procedure can be complex with multiple cannulations of branch vessels and the need of sufficient intraoperative imaging to allow for accurate placement of the device. Accordingly, this procedure will be reserved only for well-seasoned endovascular specialists. It is also important to note that although this device has seen widespread use in Europe and Australia, but it currently has an investigational status in the United States and available only to a few select sites. The prevailing question for this technology will be how susceptible side branches or fenestrations will be to stenotic or embolic disease.

Having approximately 10 years of clinical information with the first-generation devices, manufacturers are now starting to incorporate feedback from implanting physicians into their next device design. Many of the challenges we highlighted in regard to thoracic endoluminal graft technology will now be addressed. Manufacturers are introducing grafts with both larger and smaller diameters, greater graft lengths, tapered designs, and some changes that will facilitate easier device delivery or apposition to the inner curve of the thoracic arch. Such an example would be a precurved Gore TAG device that is smaller in diameter than the commercial version,

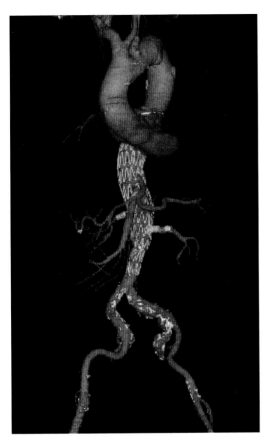

**Figure 1** A 3-D reconstruction of a patient with a thoracoabdominal aneurysm treated with the Cook Zenith Fenestrated AAA Endoluminal Graft. As part of the procedure, each fenestration has a covered stent placed in it. (Courtesy of John Anderson, MD, and Timothy Chuter MD, Cook Medical.)

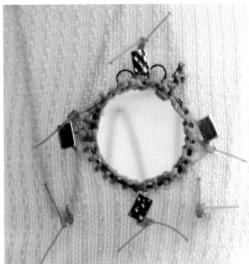

**Figure 2** A close-up picture of the typical fenestration in the Cook fenestrated AAA Endoluminal Graft. Please note the four radiopaque markers surrounding the fenestration for easy visualization and proper placement under fluoroscopy. (Courtesy of John Anderson, MD, and Timothy Chuter, MD, Cook Medical.)

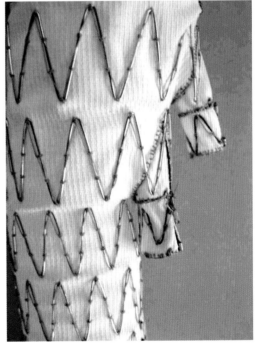

**Figure 3** A close-up view of two side branches intended for the celiac and superior mesenteric arteries on the Cook Branched Thoracoabdominal Endoluminal Graft. (Courtesy of John Anderson, MD, and Timothy Chuter, MD, Cook Medical.)

has no scallops, and has a built-in curve that should give the device an improved handling in the arch (Figure 5). As more information is collected in real-world experiences, manufacturers can better understand the challenges of aortic disease and methods to diminish them.

Medicine is prone to epochal transitions as both technology and knowledge become more refined. From the advent of antibiotics to the introduction of cardiopulmonary bypass, the practice of surgery has reinvented itself. One could argue that the 1950–1960s were a renaissance for cardiothoracic surgery due to the widespread introduction of cardiopulmonary bypass and the pioneering spirit of the surgeons of that age. Looking back at the humble

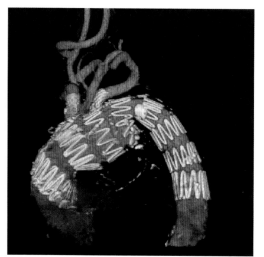

**Figure 4** A 3-D reconstruction of a treated thoracic arch aneurysm using the Cook Zenith TX2 Branched Thoracic Endoluminal Graft. (Courtesy of John Anderson, MD, and Timothy Chuter, MD, Cook Medical.)

origins with its unprecedented growth and potential for the future, we believe that this movement toward endovascular technology, particularly in the chest, represents a revolution. As the American philosopher William James said, "The greatest revolution of our generation is the discovery that human beings, by changing the inner attitudes of their minds, can change the outer aspects of their lives." We hope that this book demonstrated the potential of thoracic endovascular technology and how it may improve both your life and those of the people who surround you.

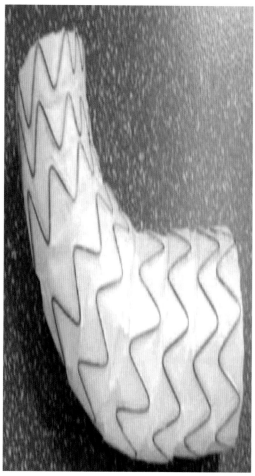

**Figure 5** A prototype of the second-generation TAG device meant specifically for trauma. (Courtesy of Gore Medical.)

# Index